PRINCIPLES OF PROTEOMICS

Edited by
Ian Moore

ArclerPress

Principles of Proteomics

Edited by Ian Moore

Edition 2018

ArclerPress

Published by
Arcler Press LLC
708 3rd Avenue, 6th Floor
New York
NY 10017
United States of America
www.arclerpress.com

ISBN: 978-1-68094-533-1 (Hardback)

Printed in United States of America

Library of Congress Control Number: 2017933105

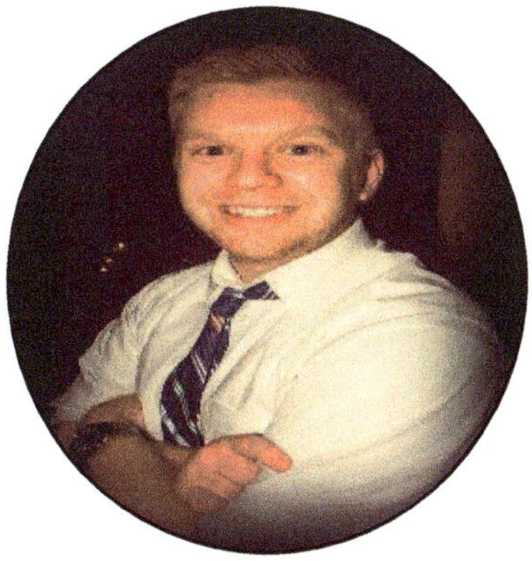

About the Editor

Ian Moore

Ian received his Bachelor of Science from the University of Michigan-Dearborn in 2014. He has interests that include the role of histone modifications in the regulation of gene transcription and the identification of novel protein interactions and their roles in biological processes. He is currently at Wayne State University working as a teaching assistant and completing his graduate thesis.

Table of Contents

5 PROTEIN MICROARRAY AND PROTEIN SEQUENCING

6 PROTEIN HOMEOSTASIS

7 QUANTITATIVE PROTEOMICS

8 POST-TRANSLATIONAL MODIFICATION OF PROTEINS

9 BRADFORD PROTEIN ASSAY

List of Abbreviations

ABPP	Activity-Based Protein Profiling
AMT	Accurate Mass and Time
APCI	Atmospheric Pressure Chemical Ionization
BIRD	Blackbody Infrared Radiative Dissociation
CID	Collision-Induced Dissociation
CTD	Charge Transfer Dissociation
CV	Controlled Vocabularies
CVD	Chemical Vapor Deposition
DART	Direct Analysis in Real Time
DE	Two-Dimensional Gel Electrophoresis
EDD	Electron-Detachment Dissociation
EI	Electron Ionization
ELISA	Enzyme-Linked Immunosorbent Assay
ESI	Electrospray Ionization
FTICR	Fourier Transform Ion Cyclotron Resonance
FTMS	Fourier Transform Mass Spectrometry
GIP	General Import Pore
ICAT	Isotope Coded Affinity Tag
ICP	Inductively Coupled Plasma
ICR	Ion Cyclotron Resonance
IMAC	Immobilized Metal Affinity Chromatography
IRMPD	Infrared Multiphoton Dissociation
LCM	laser Capture Microdissection

MALDI	Matrix-Assisted Laser Desorption/Ionization
MS	Mass spectrometry
NGF	Nerve growth factor
NOE	Nuclear Overhauser Effect
POMC	Pro-Opiomelanocortin
PPI	Protein–Protein Interactions
PTM	Post-Translational Modifi Cation
PVD	Physical Vapor Deposition
RPPA	Reverse Phase Protein Microarray
SCX	Strong Cation Exchange
SDS	Sodium Dodecyl Sulfate
SID	Surface-Induced Dissociation
SILAC	Stable Isotopic Amino Acids In Cell Culture
SIMS	Secondary Ion Mass Spectrometry
SKL	Serine-Lysine-Leucine
SLD	Soft Laser Desorption
SPR	Surface Plasmon Resonance
SRM	Selected Reaction Monitoring
SRP	Signal Recognition Particle
TIMS	Thermal Ionization-Mass Spectrometry
TMT	Tandem Mass Tags
TOF	Time-of-Flight
UPR	Unfolded Protein Response

Preface

Proteomics is the large-scale study of proteomes. A proteome is a set of proteins produced in an organism, system, or biological context. We may refer to, for instance, the proteome of a species (for example, Homo sapiens) or an organ (for example, the liver). The proteome is not constant; it differs from cell to cell and changes over time. However, protein activity (often assessed by the reaction rate of the processes in which the protein is involved) is also modulated by many factors in addition to the expression level of the relevant gene. Several high-throughput technologies have been developed to investigate proteomes in depth. The most commonly applied are mass spectrometry (MS)-based techniques such as Tandem-MS and gel-based techniques such as differential in-gel electrophoresis (DIGE). These high-throughput technologies generate huge amounts of data. Databases are critical for recording and carefully storing this data, allowing the researcher to make connections between their results and existing knowledge. Proteomics is a rapidly growing field of molecular biology that is concerned with the systematic, high-throughput approach to protein expression analysis of a cell or an organism. Typical results of proteomics studies are inventories of the protein content of differentially expressed proteins across multiple conditions. Post-translational modifications, alternative splice products, and proteins intractable to classic separation techniques have presented a challenge towards the realization of the conventional definition of the word. Today, many different areas of study are explored by proteomics. Amongst them are protein-protein interaction studies, protein function, protein modifications, and protein localization studies. The fundamental goal of proteomics is not only to pinpoint all the proteins in a cell, but also to generate a complete three-dimensional map of the cell indicating their exact location. In many ways, proteomics runs parallel to genomics. The starting point for genomics is a gene in order to make inferences about its products (i.e. proteins), whereas proteomics begins with the functionally modified protein and works back to the gene responsible for its production. The techniques for proteome analysis are not as straightforward as those used in transcriptomics. However, the advantage of proteomics is that the real functional molecules of the cell are being studied. Strong gene expression, resulting in an abundant mRNA, does not necessarily mean that the corresponding protein is also abundant or indeed active in the cell. This Text is intended to give the molecular biologist a rudimentary understanding of the technologies behind proteomics and their application to address biological questions.

Content Coverage

Chapters One and *Two* present an introduction of proteome and proteomics, correspondingly. The proteome is the entire set of proteins, produced or modified by an organism or system. Proteins are vital parts of living organisms, with many functions.

Chapters Three and *Four* present a coverage of glycoproteomics and protein structure prediction, respectively. Glycoproteomics is the study of the glycosylation of proteins, a covalent modification which confers altered physico-chemical properties and functional activity on the nascent protein chain, while protein structure prediction is one of the most important goals pursued by bioinformatics and theoretical chemistry; it is highly important in medicine and biotechnology.

Chapter Five is intended to focus on protein microarray and protein sequencing. A protein microarray is a high-throughput method used to track the interactions and activities of proteins, and to determine their function, and determining function on a large scale.

Chapter Six presents an overview of proteostasis that involves a highly complex interconnection of pathways that influence the fate of a protein from synthesis to degradation.

Chapters Seven and *Eight* focus on quantitative proteomics and post-translational modification of proteins, separately. Quantitative proteomics is an analytical chemistry technique for determining the amount of proteins in a sample.

Chapter Nine introduces about the Bradford protein assay which is a spectroscopic analytical procedure used to measure the concentration of protein in a solution.

CHAPTER 1

Introduction of Proteome

Chapter Contents

- **Introduction**
- **Systems**
- **History**
- **Size and Contents**
- **Methods to Study the Proteome**
- **Neuroproteomics**
- **Tandem Mass Spectrometry**

INTRODUCTION

The **proteome** is the entire set of proteins expressed by a genome, cell, tissue, or organism at a certain time. More specifically, it is the set of expressed proteins in a given type of cell or organism, at a given time, under defined conditions. The term is a blend of *proteins* and *genome*. Proteomics is the study of the proteome.

SYSTEMS

The term has been applied to several different types of biological systems. A **cellular proteome** is the collection of proteins found in a particular cell type under a particular set of environmental conditions such as exposure to hormone stimulation. It can also be useful to consider an organism›s **complete proteome**, which can be conceptualized as the complete set of proteins from all of the various cellular proteomes. This is very roughly the protein equivalent of the genome. The term "proteome" has also been used to refer to the collection of proteins in certain sub-cellular biological systems. For example, all of the proteins in a virus can be called a viral proteome.

HISTORY

Marc Wilkins coined the term *proteome* in 1994 in a symposium on «2D Electrophoresis: from protein maps to genomes» held in Siena in Italy. It appeared in print in 1995, with the publication of part of Wilkins›s PhD thesis. Wilkins used the term to describe the entire complement of proteins expressed by a genome, cell, tissue or organism.

SIZE AND CONTENTS

The proteome can be larger than the genome, especially in eukaryotes, as more than one protein can be produced from one gene due to alternative splicing (e.g. human proteome consists 92,179 proteins out of which 71,173 are splicing variants). On the other hand, not all genes are translated to proteins, and many known genes encode only RNA which is the final functional product. Moreover, complete proteome size vary depending the kingdom of life. For instance, eukaryotes, bacteria, Archaea and viruses have on average 15145, 3200, 2358 and 42 proteins respectively encoded in their genomes.

Dark Proteome

Perdigão and co-workers surveyed the "dark" proteome – that is, regions of proteins never observed by experimental structure determination and inaccessible to homology modeling. For 546,000 Swiss-Prot proteins, they found that 44–54% of the proteome in eukaryotes and viruses was "dark", compared with only ~14% in archaea and bacteria. Surprisingly, most of the dark proteome could not be accounted for by conventional explanations, such as intrinsic disorder or transmembrane regions. Nearly half of the dark proteome comprised dark proteins, in which the entire sequence lacked similarity to any known structure. Dark proteins fulfill a wide variety of functions, but a subset showed distinct and largely unexpected features, such as association with secretion, specific tissues, the endoplasmic reticulum, disulfide bonding, and proteolytic cleavage.

METHODS TO STUDY THE PROTEOME

Numerous methods are available to study proteins, sets of proteins, or the whole proteome. In fact, proteins are often studied indirectly, e.g. using computational methods and analyses of genomes. Only a few examples are given below.

Separation Techniques and Electrophoresis

Proteomics, the study of the proteome, has largely been practiced through the separation of proteins by two dimensional gel electrophoresis. In the first dimension, the proteins are separated by isoelectric focusing, which resolves proteins on the basis of charge. In the second dimension, proteins are separated by molecular weight using SDS-PAGE. The gel is dyed with Coomassie Brilliant Blue or silver to visualize the proteins. Spots on the gel are proteins that have migrated to specific locations.

Mass Spectrometry

Mass spectrometry has augmented proteomics. Peptide mass fingerprinting identifies a protein by cleaving it into short peptides and then deduces the protein's identity by matching the observed peptide masses against a sequence database. Tandem mass spectrometry, on the other hand, can get sequence information from individual peptides by isolating them, colliding them with a non-reactive gas, and then cataloguing the fragment ions produced.

In May 2014, a draft map of the human proteome was published in *Nature*. This map was generated using high-resolution Fourier-transform mass spectrometry. This study profiled 30 histologically normal human samples resulting in the identification of proteins coded by 17,294 genes. This accounts for around 84% of the total annotated protein-coding genes.

Protein Complementation Assays and Interaction Screens

Protein fragment complementation assays are often used to detect protein–protein interactions. The yeast two-hybrid assay is the most popular of them but there are numerous variations, both used *in vitro* and *in vivo*.

NEUROPROTEOMICS

Neuroproteomics is the study of the protein complexes and species that make up the nervous system. These proteins interact to make the neurons connect in such a way to create the intricacies that nervous system is known for. Neuroproteomics is a complex field that has a long way to go in terms of profiling the entire neuronal proteome. It is a relatively recent field that has many applications in therapy and science. So far, only small subsets of the neuronal proteome have been mapped, and then only when applied to the proteins involved in the synapse.

History

Origins

The word *proteomics* was first used in 1994 by Marc Wilkins as the study of "the protein equivalent of a genome". It is defined as all of the proteins expressed in a biological system under specific physiologic conditions at a certain point in time. It can change with any biochemical alteration, and so it can only be defined under certain conditions. Neuroproteomics is a subset of this field dealing with the complexities and multi-system origin of neurological disease. Neurological function is based on the interactions of many proteins of different origin, and so requires a systematic study of subsystems within its proteomic structure.

Modern Times

Neuroproteomics has the difficult task of defining on a molecular level the pathways of consciousness, senses, and self. Neurological disorders are unique in that they do not always exhibit outward symptoms. Defining the disorders becomes difficult and so neuroproteomics is a step in the right direction of identifying bio-markers that can be used to detect diseases. Not only does the field have to map out the different proteins possible from the genome, but there are many modifications that happen after transcription that affect function as well. Because neurons are such dynamic structures, changing with every action potential that travels through them, neuroproteomics offers the most potential for mapping out the molecular template of their function. Genomics offers a static roadmap of the cell, while proteomics can offer a glimpse into structures smaller than the cell because of its specific nature to each moment in time.

Mechanisms of Use

Protein Separation

In order for neuroproteomics to function correctly, proteins must be separated in terms of the proteome from which they came. For example, one set might be under normal conditions, while another might be under diseased conditions. Proteins are commonly separated using two-dimensional polyacrylamide gel electrophoresis (2D PAGE). For this technique, proteins are run across an immobile gel with a pH gradient until they stop at the point where their net charge is neutral. After separating by charge in one direction, sodium dodecyl sulfate is run in the other direction to separate the proteins by size. A two-dimensional map is created using this technique that can be used to match additional proteins later. One can usually match the function of a protein by identifying in an 2D PAGE in simple proteomics because many intracellular somatic pathways are known. In neuroproteomics, however, many proteins combine to give an end result that may be neurological disease or breakdown. It is necessary then to study each protein individually and find a correlation between the different proteins to determine the cause of a neurological disease. New techniques are being developed that can identify proteins once they are separated out using 2D PAGE.

Protein Identification

Protein separate techniques, such as 2D PAGE, are limitd in that they cannot handle very high or low molecular weight protein species. Alternative methods have been developed to deal with such cases. These include liquid chromatography mass spectrometry along with sodium dodecyl sulfate polyacrylamide gel electrophoresis, or liquid chromatography mass spectrometry run in multiple dimensions. Compared to simple 2D page, liquid chromatography mass spectrometry can handle a larger range of protein species size, but it is limited in the amount of protein sample it handle at once. Liquid chromatography mass spectrometry is also limited in its lack of a reference map from which to work with. Complex algorithms are usually used to analyze the fringe results that occur after a procedure is run. The unknown portions of the protein species are usually not analyzed in favor of familiar proteomes, however. This fact reveals a fault with current technology; new techniques are needed to increase both the specificity and scope of proteome mapping.

Applications

Drug Addiction

It is commonly known that drug addiction involves combining the terms permanent and plasticity seem counter to each other. Neuroproteomics is being applied to study the effect of drug addiction across the synapse. Research is being conducted by isolating distinct regions of the brain in which synaptic transmission takes place and defining the proteome for that particular region. Different stages of drug abuse must be studied, however, in order to map out the progression of protein changes along the course of the drug addiction. These stages include enticement, ingesting, withdrawal, addiction, and removal. It begins with the change in the genome through transcription that occurs due to the abuse of drugs. It continues to identify the most likely proteins to be affected by the drugs and focusing in on that area. For drug addiction, the synapse is the most likely target as it involves communication between neurons. Lack of sensory communication in neurons is often an outward sign of drug abuse, and so neuroproteomics is being applied to find out what proteins are being affected to prevent the transport of neurotransmitters. In particular, the vesicle releasing process is being studied to identify the proteins involved in the synapse during drug abuse. Proteins such as synaptotagmin and synaptobrevin interact to fuse the vesicle into the membrane. Phosphorylation also has its own set of proteins involved that work together to allow the synapse to function properly. Drugs such as morphine change properties such as cell adhesion, neurotransmitter volume, and synaptic traffic. After significant morphine application, tyrosine kinases received less phosphorylation and thus send fewer signals inside the cell. These receptor proteins are unable to initiate the intracellular signaling processes that enable the neuron to live, and necrosis or apoptosis may be the result. With more and more neurons affected along this chain of cell death, permanent loss of sensory or motor function may be the result. By identifying the proteins that are changed with drug abuse, neuroproteomics may give clinicians even earlier biomarkers to test for to prevent permanent neurological damage.

Recently, a novel terminology (Psychoproteomics) has been coined by the University of Florida researchers from Dr. Mark S Gold Lab. Kobeissy et al. defined Psychoproteomics as integral proteomics approach dedicated to studying proteomic changes in the field of psychiatric disorders, particularly substance-and drug-abuse neurotoxicity.

Brain Injury

Traumatic brain injury is defined as a “direct physical impact or trauma to the head followed by a dynamic series of injury and repair events”. Recently, neuroproteomics have been applied to studying the disability that over 5.4 million Americans live with. In addition to physically injuring the brain tissue, traumatic brain injury induces the release of glutamate that interacts with ionotropic glutamate receptors (iGluRs). These glutamate receptors acidify the surrounding intracranial fluid, causing further injury on the molecular level to nearby neurons. The death of the surrounding neurons is induced through normal apoptosis mechanisms, and it is this cycle that is being studied with neuroproteomics. Three different cysteine protease derivatives are involved in the apoptotic pathway induced by the acidic environment triggered by glutamate. These cysteine proteases include calpain, caspase, and cathepsin. These three proteins are examples of detectable signs of traumatic brain injury that are much more specific than temperature, oxygen level, or intracranial pressure. Proteomics thus also offers a tracking mechanism by which researchers can monitor the progression of traumatic brain injury, or a chronic disease such as Alzheimer's or Parkinson's. Especially in Parkinson's, in which neurotransmitters play a large role, recent proteomic research has involved the study of synaptotagmin. Synaptotagmin is involved in the calcium-induced budding of vesicle containing neurotransmitters from the presynaptic membrane. By studying the intracellular mechanisms involved in neural apoptosis after traumatic brain injury, researchers can create a map that genetic changes can follow later on.

Nerve Growth

One group of researchers applied the field of neuroproteomics to examine how different proteins affect the initial growth of neuritis. The experiment compared the protein activity of control neurons with the activity of neurons treated with nerve growth factor (NGF) and JNJ460, an "immunophilin ligand." JNJ460 is an offspring of another drug that is used to prevent immune attack when organs are transplanted. It is not an immunosuppressant, however, but rather it acts as a shield against microglia. NGF promotes neuron viability and differentiation by binding to TrkA, a tyrosine receptor kinase. This receptor is important in initiating intracellular metabolic pathways, including Ras, Rak, and MAP kinase.

Protein differentiation was measured in each cell sample with and without treatment by NGF and JNJ460. A peptide mixture was made by washing off unbound portions of the amino acid sequence in a reverse column. The resulting mixture was then suspended a peptide mixture in a bath of cation exchange fluid. The proteins were identified by splicing them with trypsin and then searching through the results of passing the product through a mass spectrometer. This applies a form of liquid chromatography mass spectrometry to identify proteins in the mixture

JNJ460 treatment resulted in an increase in "signal transduction" proteins, while NGF resulted in an increase in proteins associated with the ribosome and synthesis of other proteins. JNJ460 also resulted in more structural proteins associated with intercellular growth, such as actin, myosin, and troponin. With NGF treatment, cells increased protein synthesis and creation of ribosomes. This method allows the analysis of all of the protein patterns overall, rather than a single change in an amino acid. Western blots confirmed the results, according to the researchers, though the changes in proteins were not as obvious in their protocol.

The main significance to these findings are that JNJ460 are NGF are distinct processes that both control the protein output of the cell. JNJ460 resulted in increased neuronal size and stability while NGF resulted in increased membrane proteins. When combined together, they significantly increase a neuron's chance of growth. While JNJ460 may "prime" some parts of the cell for NGF treatment, they do not work together. JNJ460 is thought to interact with Schwann cells in regenerating actin and myosin, which are key players in axonal growth. NGF helps the neuron grow as a whole. These two proteins do not play a part in communication with other neurons, however. They merely increase the size of the membrane down which a signal can be sent. Other neurotrophic factor proteomes are needed to guide neurons to each other to create synapses.

Limitations

As there is a large amount of raw neuronal proteins available to create proteomic maps, it is essential that small areas of neurons are selected for to maintain specificity. When taking samples, there are a few places that interest neurologists most. The most important place to start for neurologists is the plasma membrane. This is where most of the communication between neurons takes place. The proteins being mapped here include ion channels, neurotransmitter receptors, and molecule transporters. Along the plasma membrane, the proteins involved in creating cholesterol-rich lipid rafts are being studied because they have been shown to be crucial for glutamate uptake during the initial stages of neuron formation. As mentioned before, vesicle proteins are also being studied closely because they are involved in disease. Collecting samples to study, however, requires special consideration to ensure that the reproducibility of the samples is not compromised. When taking a global sample of one area of the brain for example, proteins that are ubiquitous and relatively unimportant show up very clear in the SDS PAGE. Other unexplored, more specific proteins barely show up and are therefore ignored. It is usually necessary to divide up the plasma membrane proteome, for example, into subproteomes characterized by specific function. This allows these more specific classes of peptides to show up more clearly. In a way, dividing into subproteomes is simply applying a magnifying lens to a specific section of a global proteome's SDS PAGE map. This method seems to be most effective when applied to each cellular organelle separately. Mitochondrial proteins, for example, which are more effective at transporting electrons across its membrane, can be specifically targeted effectively in order to match their electron-transporting ability to their amino acid sequence.

TANDEM MASS SPECTROMETRY

Tandem mass spectrometry, also known as **MS/MS** or **MS^2**, involves multiple steps of mass spectrometry selection, with some form of fragmentation occurring in between the stages. In a tandem mass spectrometer, ions are formed in the ion source and separated by mass-to-charge ratio in the first stage of mass spectrometry (MS1). Ions of a particular mass-to-charge ratio (precursor ions) are selected and fragment ions (product ions) are created by

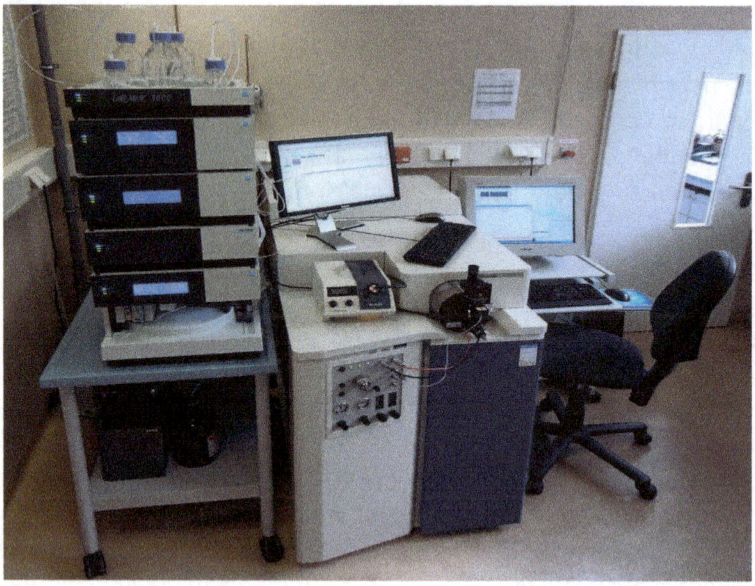

A quadrupole time-of-flight hybrid tandem mass spectrometer.

Instrumentation

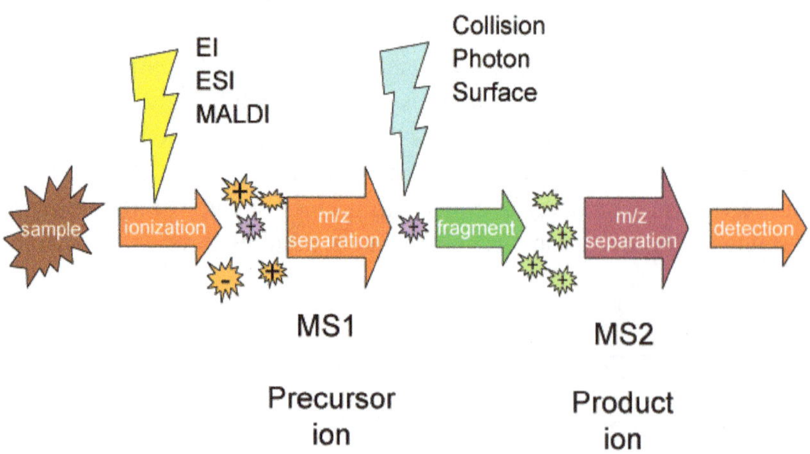

Schematic of tandem mass spectrometry

For tandem mass spectrometry in space, the different elements are often noted in shorthand. Multiple stages of mass analysis separation can be accomplished with individual mass spectrometer elements separated in space or using a single mass spectrometer with the MS steps separated in time.

Tandem in space

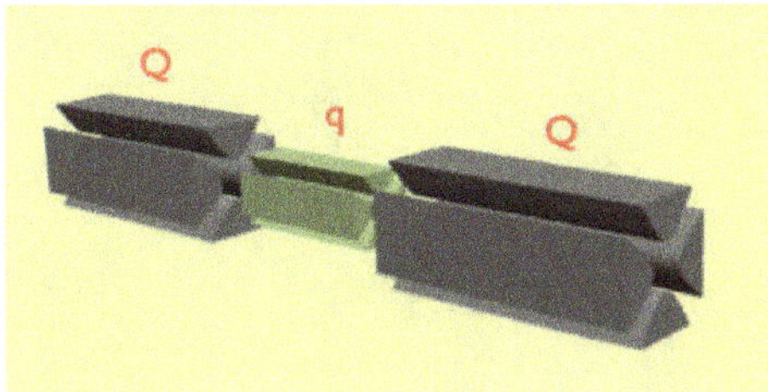

Triple quadrupole diagram; and example of tandem mass spectrometry in space.

In tandem mass spectrometry *in space*, the separation elements are physically separated and distinct, although there is a physical connection between the elements to maintain high vacuum. These elements can be sectors, transmission quadrupole, or time-of-flight. When using multiple quadrupoles, they can act as both mass analyzers and collision chambers.

Q – Quadrupole mass analyzer

q – Radio frequency collision quadrupole

TOF – Time-of-flight mass analyzer

B – Magnetic sector

E – Electric sector

The notation can be combined to indicate various hybrid instrument, for example

QqQ – Triple quadrupole mass spectrometer

QTOF – Quadrupole time-of-flight mass spectrometer (also QqTOF)

BEBE – Four-sector (reverse geometry) mass spectrometer

Tandem in Time

By doing tandem mass spectrometry *in time*, the separation is accomplished with ions trapped in the same place, with multiple separation steps taking place over time. A quadrupole ion trap or Fourier transform ion cyclotron resonance (FTICR) instrument can be used for such an analysis. Trapping instruments can perform multiple steps of analysis, which is sometimes referred to as MS^n (MS to the n). Often the number of steps, n, is not indicated, but occasionally the value is specified; for example MS^3indicates three stages of separation. Tandem in time MS instruments do not use the modes described next, but typically collect all of the information from a precursor ion scan and a parent ion scan of the entire spectrum. Each instrumental configuration utilizes a unique mode of mass identification.

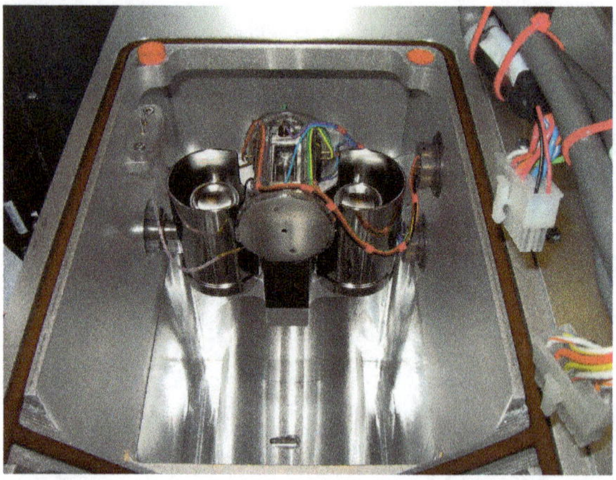

An ion trap mass spectrometer is an example of a tandem mass spectrometry in time instrument.

Tandem in space MS/MS Modes

When tandem MS is performed with an in space design, the instrument must operate in one of a variety of modes. There are a number of different tandem MS/MS experimental setups and each mode has its own applications and provides different information. Tandem MS in space uses the coupling of two instrument components which measure the same mass spectrum range but with a controlled fractionation between them in space, while tandem MS in time involves the use of an ion trap.

There are four main scan experiments possible using MS/MS: precursor ion scan, product ion scan, neutral loss scan, and selected reaction monitoring.

For a precursor ion scan, the product ion is selected in the second mass analyzer, and the precursor masses are scanned in the first mass analyzer. Note that precursor ion is synonymous with parent ion and product ion with daughter ion; however the use of these anthropomorphic terms is discouraged.

In a product ion scan, a precursor ion is selected in the first stage, allowed to fragment and then all resultant masses are scanned in the second mass analyzer and detected in the detector that is positioned after the second mass analyzer. This experiment is commonly performed to identify transitions used for quantification by tandem MS.

In a neutral loss scan, the first mass analyzer scans all the masses. The second mass analyzer also scans, but at a set offset from the first mass analyzer. This offset corresponds to a neutral loss that is commonly observed for the class of compounds. In a constant-neutral-loss scan, all precursors that undergo the loss of a specified common neutral are monitored. To obtain this information, both mass analyzers are scanned simultaneously, but with a mass offset that correlates with the mass of the specified neutral. Similar to the precursor-ion scan, this technique is also useful in the selective identification of closely related class of compounds in a mixture.

In selected reaction monitoring, both mass analyzers are set to a selected mass. This mode is analogous to selected ion monitoring for MS experiments.

Fragmentation

Fragmentation of gas-phase ions is essential to tandem mass spectrometry and occurs between different stages of mass analysis. There are many methods used to fragment the ions and these can result in different types of fragmentation and thus different information about the structure and composition of the molecule.

In-source Fragmentation

Often, the ionization process is sufficiently violent to leave the resulting ions with sufficient internal energy to fragment within the mass spectrometer. If the product ions persist in their non-equilibrium state for a moderate amount of time before auto-dissociation this process is called metastable fragmentation. Nozzle-skimmer fragmentation refers to the purposeful induction of in-source fragmentation by increasing the nozzle-skimmer potential on usually electrospray based instruments. Although in-source fragmentation allows for fragmentation analysis, it is not technically tandem mass spectrometry unless metastable ions are mass analyzed or selected before auto-dissociation and a second stage of analysis is performed on the resulting fragments. In-source fragmentation is often used in addition to tandem mass spectrometry (with post-source fragmentation) to allow for two steps of fragmentation in a pseudo MS^3-type of experiment.

Collision-Induced Dissociation

Post-source fragmentation is most often what is being used in a tandem mass spectrometry experiment. Energy can also be added to the ions, which are usually already vibrationally excited, through post-source collisions with neutral atoms or molecules, the absorption of radiation, or the transfer or capture of an electron by a multiply charged ion. Collision-induced dissociation (CID), also called collisionally activated dissociation (CAD), involves the collision of an ion with a neutral atom or molecule in the gas phase and subsequent dissociation of the ion. For example, consider

$$\mathrm{AB^+ + M \longrightarrow A + B^+ + M}$$

where the ion AB^+ collides with the neutral species M and subsequently breaks apart. The details of this process are described by collision theory.

Higher-energy collisional dissociation (HCD) is a CID technique specific to orbitrap mass spectrometers in which fragmentation takes place external to the trap.

Electron capture and Transfer Methods

The energy released when an electron is transferred to or captured by a multiply charged ion can induce fragmentation.

Electron Capture Dissociation

If an electron is added to a multiply charged positive ion, the Coulomb energy is liberated. Adding a free electron is called electron capture dissociation (ECD), and is represented by

$$[\mathrm{M}+n\mathrm{H}]^{n+} + \mathrm{e}^- \longrightarrow \left[[\mathrm{M}+(n-1)\mathrm{H}]^{(n-1)+}\right]^* \longrightarrow \textbf{fragments}$$

for a multiply protonated molecule M.

Electron Transfer Dissociation

Adding an electron through an ion-ion reaction is called electron transfer dissociation (ETD).Similar to electron-capture dissociation, ETD induces fragmentation of cations (e.g. peptides or proteins) by transferring electrons to them. It was invented by Donald F. Hunt, Joshua Coon, John E. P. Syka and Jarrod Marto at the University of Virginia.

ETD does not use free electrons but employs radical anions (e.g. anthracene or azobenzene) for this purpose:

$$[\mathrm{M}+n\mathrm{H}]^{n+} + \mathrm{A}^- \longrightarrow \left[[\mathrm{M}+(n-1)\mathrm{H}]^{(n-1)+}\right]^* + \mathrm{A} \longrightarrow \textbf{fragments}$$

where A is the anion.

ETD cleaves randomly along the peptide backbone (c and z ions) while side chains and modifications such as phosphorylation are left intact. The technique only works well for higher charge state ions ($z>2$), however relative to collision-induced dissociation (CID), ETD is advantageous for the fragmentation of longer peptides or even entire proteins. This makes the technique important for top-down proteomics. Much like ECD, ETD is effective for peptides with modifications such as phosphorylation.

Electron-transfer and higher-energy collision dissociation (EThcD) is a combination ETD and HCD where the peptide precursor is initially subjected to an ion/ion reaction with fluoranthene anions in a linear ion trap, which generates c- and z-ions. In the second step HCD all-ion fragmentation is applied to all ETD derived ions to generate b- and y- ions prior to final analysis in the orbitrap analyzer. This method employs dual fragmentation to generate ion- and thus data-rich MS/MS spectra for peptide sequencing and PTM localization.

Negative Electron Transfer Dissociation

Fragmentation can also occur with a deprotonated species, in which an electron is transferred from the specie to an cationic reagent in a negative electron transfer dissociation (NETD):

$$[\mathrm{M}-n\mathrm{H}]^{n-} + \mathrm{A}^+ \longrightarrow \left[[\mathrm{M}-n\mathrm{H}]^{(n+1)-}\right]^* + \mathrm{A} \longrightarrow \textbf{fragments}$$

Following this transfer event, the electron deficient anion undergoes internal rearrangement and fragments. NETD is the ion/ion analogue of electron-detachment dissociation (EDD).

NETD is compatible with fragmenting peptide and proteins along the backbone at the C_α-C bond. The resulting fragments are usually a•- and x-type product ions.

Electron-Detachment Dissociation

Electron-detachment dissociation (EDD) is a method for fragmenting anionic species in mass spectrometry. It serves as a negative counter mode to electron capture dissociation. Negatively charged ions are activated by irradiation with electrons of moderate kinetic energy. The result is ejection of electrons from the parent ionic molecule, which causes dissociation via recombination.

Charge Transfer Dissociation

Reaction between positively charged peptides and cationic reagents, also known as charge transfer dissociation (CTD), has recently been demonstrated as an alternative high-energy fragmentation pathway for low-charge state (1+ or 2+) peptides. The proposed mechanism of CTD using helium cations as the reagent is:

$$[\mathbf{M}+\mathbf{H}]^{1+}+\mathbf{He}^{+}\longrightarrow\left[[\mathbf{M}+\mathbf{H}]^{2+}\right]^{*}+\mathbf{He}^{0}\longrightarrow\mathbf{fragments}$$

Initial reports are that CTD causes backbone C_α-C bond cleavage of peptides and provides a•- and x-type product ions.

Photodissociation

The energy required for dissociation can be added by photon absorption, resulting in ion photodissociation and represented by

$$\mathrm{AB}^{+}+h\nu\longrightarrow\mathrm{A}+\mathrm{B}^{+}$$

where $h\nu$ represents the photon absorbed by the ion. Ultraviolet lasers can be used, but can lead to excessive fragmentation of biomolecules.

Infrared Multiphoton Dissociation

Infrared photons will heat the ions and cause dissociation if enough of them are absorbed. This process is called infrared multiphoton dissociation (IRMPD) and is often accomplished with a carbon dioxide laser and an ion trapping mass spectrometer such as a FTMS.

Blackbody infrared Radiative Dissociation

Blackbody radiation can be used for photodissociation in a technique known as blackbody infrared radiative dissociation (BIRD). In the BIRD method, the entire mass spectrometer vacuum chamber is heated to create infrared radiation. BIRD uses the light from black body radiation to thermally (vibrationally) excite the ions until a bond breaks. This is similar to infrared multiphoton dissociation with the exception of the source of radiation.

This technique is most often used with Fourier transform ion cyclotron resonance mass spectrometers.

Surface Induced Dissociation

With surface-induced dissociation (SID), the fragmentation is a result of the collision of an ion with a surface under high vacuum.

Quantitative Proteomics

Quantitative proteomics is used to determine the relative or absolute amount of proteins in a sample. Several quantitative proteomics methods are based on tandem mass spectrometry. MS/MS has become a benchmark procedure for the structural elucidation of complex biomolecules.

Isobaric tag for Relative and Absolute Quantitation

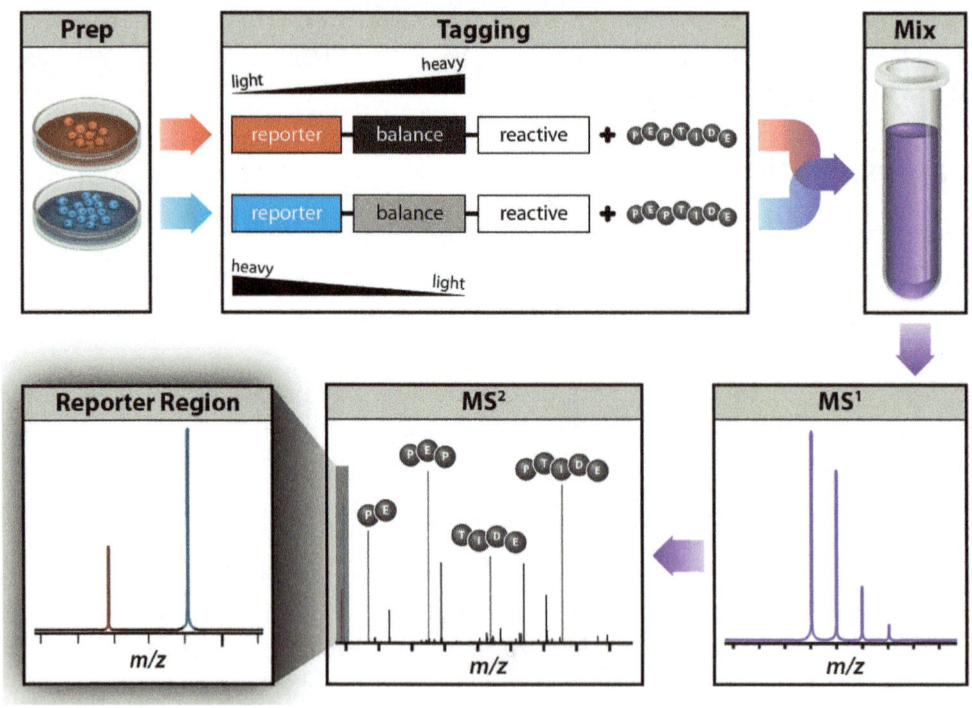

Isobaric labeling for tandem mass spectrometry: proteins are extracted from cells, digested, and labeled with tags of the same mass. When fragmented during MS/MS, the reporter ions show the relative amount of the peptides in the samples.

An isobaric tag for relative and absolute quantitation (iTRAQ) is a reagent for tandem mass spectrometry that is used to determine the amount of proteins from different sources in a single experiment. It uses stable isotope labeled molecules that can form a covalent bond with the N-terminus and side chain amines of proteins. The iTRAQ reagents are used to label peptides from different samples that are pooled and analyzed by liquid chromatography and tandem mass spectrometry. The fragmentation of the attached tag generates a low molecular mass reporter ion that can be used to relatively quantify the peptides and the proteins from which they originated.

Tandem Mass Tag

A tandem mass tag (TMT) is an isobaric mass tag chemical label used for protein quantification and identification. The tags contain four regions: mass reporter, cleavable linker, mass normalization, and protein reactive group.

Applications

Peptides

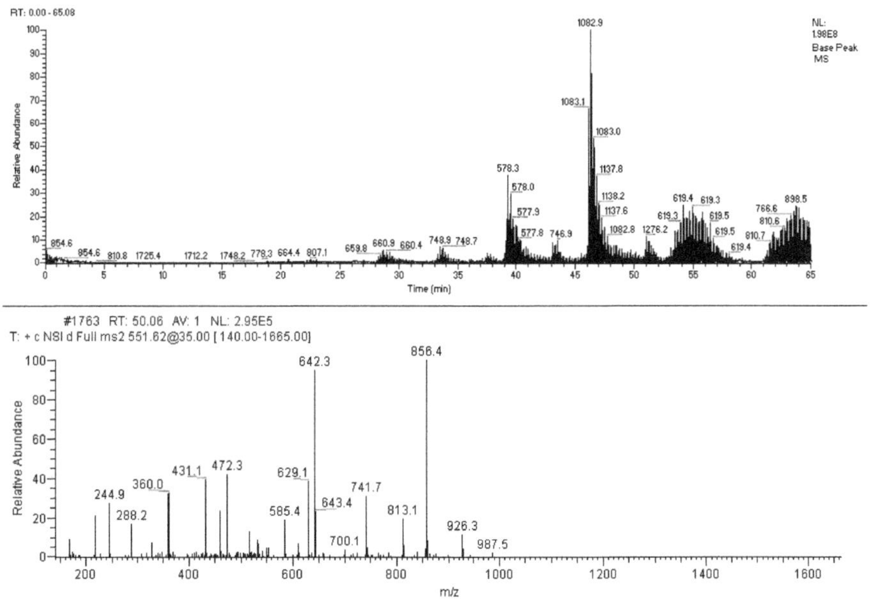

Chromatography trace (top) and tandem mass spectrum (bottom) of a peptide.

Tandem mass spectrometry can be used for protein sequencing. When intact proteins are introduced to a mass analyzer, this is called "top-down proteomics" and when proteins are digested into smaller peptides and subsequently introduced into the mass spectrometer, this is called "bottom-up proteomics». Shotgun proteomics is a variant of bottom up proteomics in which proteins in a mixture are digested prior to separation and tandem mass spectrometry.

Tandem mass spectrometry can produce a peptide sequence tag that can be used to identify a peptide in a protein database. A notation has been developed for indicating peptide fragments that arise from a tandem mass spectrum. Peptide fragment ions are indicated by a, b, or c if the charge is retained on the N-terminus and by x, y or z if the charge is maintained on the C-terminus. The subscript indicates the number of amino acid residues in the fragment. Superscripts are sometimes used to indicate neutral losses in addition to the backbone fragmentation, * for loss of ammonia and ° for loss of water. Although peptide backbone cleavage is the most useful for sequencing and peptide identification other fragment ions may be observed under high energy dissociation conditions. These include the side chain loss ions d, v, w and ammonium ionsand additional sequence-specific fragment ions associated with particular amino acid residues.

Oligosaccharides

Oligosaccharides may be sequenced using tandem mass spectrometry in a similar manner to peptide sequencing. Fragmentation generally occurs on either side of the glycosidic bond (b, c, y and z ions) but also under more energetic conditions through the sugar ring structure in a cross-ring cleavage (x ions). Again trailing subscripts are used to indicate position of the cleavage along the chain. For cross ring cleavage ions the nature of the cross ring cleavage is indicated by preceding superscripts.

Oligonucleotides

Tandem mass spectrometry has been applied to DNA and RNA sequencing. A notation for gas-phase fragmentation of oligonucleotide ions has been proposed.

Newborn Screening

Newborn screening is the process of testing newborn babies for treatable genetic, endocrinologic, metabolic and hematologic diseases. The development of tandem mass spectrometry screening in the early 1990s led to a large expansion of potentially detectable congenital metabolic diseases that affect blood levels of organic acids.

REFERENCES

1. Alzate O. "Neuroproteomics." Frontiers in Neuroscience Series (October 2010) C.R.C. Press. ISBN 978-1-4200-7625-7
2. Abul-Husn, Noura S., Lakshmi A. Devi. "Neuroproteomics of the Synapse and Drug Addiction." The Journal of Pharmacology and Experimental Therapeutics 138 (2006): 461-468.
3. Becker, Michael, Jens Schindler, Hans G. Nothwang. "Neuroproteomics - the Tasks Lying Ahead." Electrophoresis 27 (2006): 2819-2829.
4. Butcher, James. "Neuroproteomics Comes of Age." The Lancet Neurology 6 (2007): 851-852.

5. Kim, Sandra I., Hans Voshol, Jan van Oostrum, Terri G. Hastings, Michael Casico, Marc J. Glucksmann. "Neuroproteomics: Expression Profiling of the Brain's Proteomes in Health and Disease." Neurochemical Research 29 (2004): 1317-1331

6. Kobeissy, Firas H., Andrew K. Ottens, Zhiqun Zhang, Ming Cheng Liu, Nancy D. Denslow, Jitendra R. Dave, Frank C. Tortella, Ronald L. Hayes, Kevin K. Wang. "Novel Differential Neuroproteomics Analysis of Traumatic Brain Injury in Rats." Molecular & Cellular Proteomics 5 (2006): 1887-1898.

7. Liu, Tong, Veera D'mello, Longwen Deng, Jun Hu, Michael Ricardo, Sanqiang Pan, Xiaodong Lu, Scott Wadsworth, John Siekierka, Raymond Birge, Hong Li. "A Multiplexed Proteomics Approach to Differentiate Neurite Outgrowth Patterns." Journal of Neuroscience Methods 158 (2006): 22-29.

8. Ottens, Andrew K., Firas H. Kobeissy, Erin C. Golden, Zhiqun Zhang, William E. Haskins, Su-Shing Chen, Ronald L. Hayes, Kevin K. Wang, Nancy D. Denslow. "Neuroproteomics in Neurotrauma." Mass Spectrometry Review 25 (2006): 380-406.

9. Ottens, Andrew K. "The methodology of neuroproteomics." Methods Mol Biol. (2009) 566:1-21.

10. Southey, Bruce R., Andinet Amare, Tyler A. Zimmerman, Sandra L. Rodriguez, Jonathan V. Sweedler. "NeuroPred: a Tool to Predict Cleavage Sites in Neuropeptide Precursors and Provide the Masses of the Resulting Peptides." Nucleic Acids Research 34 (2006): 267-272.

11. Tribl, F, K Marcus, G Bringmann, H.E. Meyer, M Gerlach, P Riederer. "Proteomics of the Human Brain: Sub-Proteomes Might Hold the Key to Handle Brain Complexity." Journal of Neural Transmission 113 (2006): 1041-1054.

12. Williams, Kenneth, Terence Wu, Christopher Colangelo, Angus C. Nairn. "Recent Advances in Neuroproteomics and Potential Application to Studies of Drug Addiction." Neuropharmacology 47 (2004): 148-166.

13. Kobeissy, Firas H., Sadasivan S, Liu J, Mark S Gold, Kevin K. Wang. "Psychiatric research: psychoproteomics, degradomics and systems biology." Expert Rev Proteomics 5 (2008): 293-314.

14. IUPAC, Compendium of Chemical Terminology, 2nd ed. (the "Gold Book") (1997). Online corrected version: (2006–) "tandem mass spectrometer".

15. IUPAC, Compendium of Chemical Terminology, 2nd ed. (the "Gold Book") (1997). Online corrected version: (2006–) "precursor ion".

16. IUPAC, Compendium of Chemical Terminology, 2nd ed. (the "Gold Book") (1997). Online corrected version: (2006–) "parent ion".

17. IUPAC, Compendium of Chemical Terminology, 2nd ed. (the "Gold Book") (1997). Online corrected version: (2006–) "product ion".

18. IUPAC, Compendium of Chemical Terminology, 2nd ed. (the "Gold Book") (1997). Online corrected version: (2006–) "daughter ion".

19. Bursey, Maurice M. (1991). "Comment to readers: Style and the lack of it". Mass Spectrometry Reviews. 10: 1–2. doi:10.1002/mas.1280100102.
20. Adams, J. (1992). "To the editor". Journal of the American Society for Mass Spectrometry. 3 (4): 473. doi:10.1016/1044-0305(92)87078-D.
21. Louris JN, Wright LG, Cooks RG, Schoen AE (1985). "New scan modes accessed with a hybrid mass spectrometer". Analytical Chemistry. 57 (14): 2918–2924. doi:10.1021/ac00291a039.
22. deHoffman, Edmond; Stroobant, Vincent (2003). Mass Spectrometry: Principles and Applications. Toronto: Wiley. p. 133. ISBN 0-471-48566-7.
23. IUPAC gold book definition of metastable ion (in mass spectrometry)
24. IUPAC gold book definition of transient (chemical) species
25. Körner R, Wilm M, Morand K, Schubert M, Mann M (February 1996). "Nano electrospray combined with a quadrupole ion trap for the analysis of peptides and protein digests". Journal of the American Society for Mass Spectrometry. 7 (2): 150–6. doi:10.1016/1044-0305(95)00626-5. PMID 24203235.
26. Wells JM, McLuckey SA (2005). "Collision-induced dissociation (CID) of peptides and proteins". Methods in Enzymology. 402: 148–85. doi:10.1016/S0076-6879(05)02005-7. PMID 16401509.
27. Sleno L, Volmer DA (October 2004). "Ion activation methods for tandem mass spectrometry". Journal of Mass Spectrometry. 39 (10): 1091–112. doi:10.1002/jms.703. PMID 15481084.
28. Olsen JV, Macek B, Lange O, Makarov A, Horning S, Mann M (September 2007). "Higher-energy C-trap dissociation for peptide modification analysis". Nature Methods. 4 (9): 709–12. doi:10.1038/nmeth1060. PMID 17721543.
29. Cooper HJ, Håkansson K, Marshall AG (2005). "The role of electron capture dissociation in biomolecular analysis". Mass Spectrometry Reviews. 24 (2): 201–22. doi:10.1002/mas.20014. PMID 15389856.
30. Syka JE, Coon JJ, Schroeder MJ, Shabanowitz J, Hunt DF (June 2004). "Peptide and protein sequence analysis by electron transfer dissociation mass spectrometry". Proceedings of the National Academy of Sciences of the United States of America. 101 (26): 9528–33. Bibcode:2004PNAS..101.9528S. doi:10.1073/pnas.0402700101. PMC 470779 . PMID 15210983.
31. Mikesh LM, Ueberheide B, Chi A, Coon JJ, Syka JE, Shabanowitz J, Hunt DF (December 2006). "The utility of ETD mass spectrometry in proteomic analysis". Biochimica et Biophysica Acta. 1764 (12): 1811–22. doi:10.1016/j.bbapap.2006.10.003. PMC 1853258 . PMID 17118725.
32. US patent 7534622, Donald F. Hunt, Joshua J. Coon, John E.P. Syka, Jarrod A. Marto, "Electron transfer dissociation for biopolymer sequence mass spectrometric analysis", issued 2009-05-19
33. McLuckey SA, Stephenson JL (1998). "Ion/ion chemistry of high-mass multiply charged ions". Mass Spectrometry Reviews. 17 (6): 369–407. doi:10.1002/(SICI)1098-2787(1998)17:6<369::AID-MAS1>3.0.CO;2-J. PMID 10360331.

34. Chi A, Huttenhower C, Geer LY, Coon JJ, Syka JE, Bai DL, Shabanowitz J, Burke DJ, Troyanskaya OG, Hunt DF (February 2007). "Analysis of phosphorylation sites on proteins from Saccharomyces cerevisiae by electron transfer dissociation (ETD) mass spectrometry". Proceedings of the National Academy of Sciences of the United States of America. 104 (7): 2193–8. Bibcode:2007PNAS..104.2193C. doi:10.1073/pnas.0607084104. PMC 1892997 . PMID 17287358.

35. Frese CK, Altelaar AF, van den Toorn H, Nolting D, Griep-Raming J, Heck AJ, Mohammed S (November 2012). "Toward full peptide sequence coverage by dual fragmentation combining electron-transfer and higher-energy collision dissociation tandem mass spectrometry". Analytical Chemistry. 84 (22): 9668–73. doi:10.1021/ac3025366. PMID 23106539.

36. Frese CK, Zhou H, Taus T, Altelaar AF, Mechtler K, Heck AJ, Mohammed S (March 2013). "Unambiguous phosphosite localization using electron-transfer/higher-energy collision dissociation (EThcD)". Journal of Proteome Research. 12 (3): 1520–5. doi:10.1021/pr301130k. PMC 3588588 . PMID 23347405.

37. Coon JJ, Shabanowitz J, Hunt DF, Syka JE (June 2005). "Electron transfer dissociation of peptide anions". Journal of the American Society for Mass Spectrometry. 16 (6): 880–2. doi:10.1016/j.jasms.2005.01.015. PMID 15907703.

38. Budnik BA, Haselmann KF, Zubarev RA (2001). "Electron detachment dissociation of peptide di-anions: an electron–hole recombination phenomenon". Chemical Physics Letters. 342 (3-4): 299–302. Bibcode:2001CPL...342..299B. doi:10.1016/S0009-2614(01)00501-2.

39. Chingin K, Makarov A, Denisov E, Rebrov O, Zubarev RA (January 2014). "Fragmentation of positively-charged biological ions activated with a beam of high-energy cations". Analytical Chemistry. 86 (1): 372–9. doi:10.1021/ac403193k.

40. Hoffmann WD, Jackson GP (November 2014). "Charge transfer dissociation (CTD) mass spectrometry of peptide cations using kiloelectronvolt helium cations". Journal of the American Society for Mass Spectrometry. 25 (11): 1939–43. Bibcode:2014JASMS.tmp..208H. doi:10.1007/s13361-014-0989-6.

41. Morgan JW, Hettick JM, Russell DH (2005). "Peptide sequencing by MALDI 193-nm photodissociation TOF MS". Methods in Enzymology. 402: 186–209. doi:10.1016/S0076-6879(05)02006-9. PMID 16401510.

42. Little DP, Speir JP, Senko MW, O'Connor PB, McLafferty FW (September 1994). "Infrared multiphoton dissociation of large multiply charged ions for biomolecule sequencing". Analytical Chemistry. 66 (18): 2809–15. doi:10.1021/ac00090a004. PMID 7526742.

43. Schnier PD, Price WD, Jockusch RA, Williams ER (July 1996). "Blackbody infrared radiative dissociation of bradykinin and its analogues: energetics, dynamics, and evidence for salt-bridge structures in the gas phase". Journal of the American Chemical Society. 118 (30): 7178–89. doi:10.1021/ja9609157. PMC 1393282 . PMID 16525512.

44. Dunbar RC (2004). "BIRD (blackbody infrared radiative dissociation): evolution,

principles, and applications". Mass Spectrometry Reviews. 23 (2): 127–58. doi:10.1002/mas.10074. PMID 14732935.

45. Grill V, Shen J, Evans C, Cooks RG (2001). "Collisions of ions with surfaces at chemically relevant energies: Instrumentation and phenomena". Review of Scientific Instruments. 72 (8): 3149. Bibcode:2001RScI...72.3149G. doi:10.1063/1.1382641.
46. Mabud, M. (1985). "Surface-induced dissociation of molecular ions". International Journal of Mass Spectrometry and Ion Processes. 67 (3): 285–294. Bibcode:1985IJMSI..67..285M. doi:10.1016/0168-1176(85)83024-X.
47. Ong SE, Mann M (October 2005). "Mass spectrometry-based proteomics turns quantitative". Nature Chemical Biology. 1 (5): 252–62. doi:10.1038/nchembio736. PMID 16408053.
48. Bantscheff M, Schirle M, Sweetman G, Rick J, Kuster B (October 2007). "Quantitative mass spectrometry in proteomics: a critical review". Analytical and Bioanalytical Chemistry. 389 (4): 1017–31. doi:10.1007/s00216-007-1486-6. PMID 17668192.
49. Nikolov M, Schmidt C, Urlaub H (2012). "Quantitative mass spectrometry-based proteomics: an overview". Methods in Molecular Biology. 893: 85–100. doi:10.1007/978-1-61779-885-6_7. PMID 22665296.
50. Maher S, Jjunju FP, Taylor S (2015). "100 years of mass spectrometry: Perspectives and future trends". Rev. Mod. Phys. 87 (1): 113–135. Bibcode:2015RvMP...87..113M. doi:10.1103/RevModPhys.87.113.
51. Ross PL, Huang YN, Marchese JN, Williamson B, Parker K, Hattan S, Khainovski N, Pillai S, Dey S, Daniels S, Purkayastha S, Juhasz P, Martin S, Bartlet-Jones M, He F, Jacobson A, Pappin DJ (December 2004). "Multiplexed protein quantitation in Saccharomyces cerevisiae using amine-reactive isobaric tagging reagents". Molecular & Cellular Proteomics. 3 (12): 1154–69. doi:10.1074/mcp.M400129-MCP200. PMID 15385600.
52. Zieske LR (2006). "A perspective on the use of iTRAQ reagent technology for protein complex and profiling studies". Journal of Experimental Botany. 57 (7): 1501–8. doi:10.1093/jxb/erj168. PMID 16574745.
53. Gafken PR, Lampe PD (2006). "Methodologies for characterizing phosphoproteins by mass spectrometry". Cell Communication & Adhesion. 13 (5-6): 249–62. doi:10.1080/15419060601077917. PMC 2185548 . PMID 17162667.
54. Thompson A, Schäfer J, Kuhn K, Kienle S, Schwarz J, Schmidt G, Neumann T, Johnstone R, Mohammed AK, Hamon C (April 2003). "Tandem mass tags: a novel quantification strategy for comparative analysis of complex protein mixtures by MS/MS". Analytical Chemistry. 75 (8): 1895–904. doi:10.1021/ac0262560. PMID 12713048.
55. Angel TE, Aryal UK, Hengel SM, Baker ES, Kelly RT, Robinson EW, Smith RD (May 2012). "Mass spectrometry-based proteomics: existing capabilities and future directions". Chemical Society Reviews. 41 (10): 3912–28. doi:10.1039/c2cs15331a. PMC 3375054 . PMID 22498958.

56. Hardouin J (2007). "Protein sequence information by matrix-assisted laser desorption/ionization in-source decay mass spectrometry". Mass Spectrometry Reviews. 26 (5): 672–82. doi:10.1002/mas.20142. PMID 17492750.

57. Shadforth I, Crowther D, Bessant C (November 2005). "Protein and peptide identification algorithms using MS for use in high-throughput, automated pipelines". Proteomics. 5 (16): 4082–95. doi:10.1002/pmic.200402091. PMID 16196103.

58. Mørtz E, O'Connor PB, Roepstorff P, Kelleher NL, Wood TD, McLafferty FW, Mann M (August 1996). "Sequence tag identification of intact proteins by matching tanden mass spectral data against sequence data bases". Proceedings of the National Academy of Sciences of the United States of America. 93 (16): 8264–7. Bibcode:1996PNAS...93.8264M. doi:10.1073/pnas.93.16.8264. PMC 38658 . PMID 8710858.

59. Roepstorff P, Fohlman J (November 1984). "Proposal for a common nomenclature for sequence ions in mass spectra of peptides". Biomedical Mass Spectrometry. 11 (11): 601. doi:10.1002/bms.1200111109. PMID 6525415.

60. Johnson RS, Martin SA, Biemann K (December 1988). "Collision-induced fragmentation of (M + H)+ ions of peptides. Side chain specific sequence ions". International Journal of Mass Spectrometry and Ion Processes. 86: 137–154. doi:10.1016/0168-1176(88)80060-0.

61. Falick AM, Hines WM, Medzihradszky KF, Baldwin MA, Gibson BW (November 1993). "Low-mass ions produced from peptides by high-energy collision-induced dissociation in tandem mass spectrometry". Journal of the American Society for Mass Spectrometry. 4 (11): 882–93. doi:10.1016/1044-0305(93)87006-X. PMID 24227532.

62. Downard KM, Biemann K (January 1995). "Methionine specific sequence ions formed by the dissociation of protonated peptides at high collision energies". Journal of Mass Spectrometry. 30 (1): 25–32. doi:10.1002/jms.1190300106.

63. Zaia J (2004). "Mass spectrometry of oligosaccharides". Mass Spectrometry Reviews. 23 (3): 161–227. doi:10.1002/mas.10073. PMID 14966796.

64. Bruno Domon; Catherine E Costello (1988). "A systematic nomenclature for carbohydrate fragmentations in FAB-MS/MS spectra of glycoconjugates". Glycoconj. J. 5 (4): 397–409. doi:10.1007/BF01049915.

65. Spina E, Cozzolino R, Ryan E, Garozzo D (August 2000). "Sequencing of oligosaccharides by collision-induced dissociation matrix-assisted laser desorption/ionization mass spectrometry". Journal of Mass Spectrometry. 35 (8): 1042–8. doi:10.1002/1096-9888(200008)35:8<1042::AID-JMS33>3.0.CO;2-Y. PMID 10973004.

66. Banoub JH, Newton RP, Esmans E, Ewing DF, Mackenzie G (May 2005). "Recent developments in mass spectrometry for the characterization of nucleosides, nucleotides, oligonucleotides, and nucleic acids". Chemical Reviews. 105 (5): 1869–915. doi:10.1021/cr030040w. PMID 15884792.

67. Thomas B, Akoulitchev AV (March 2006). "Mass spectrometry of RNA". Trends

in Biochemical Sciences. 31 (3): 173–81. doi:10.1016/j.tibs.2006.01.004. PMID 16483781.

68. Wu J, McLuckey SA (2004). "Gas-phase fragmentation of oligonucleotide ions". International Journal of Mass Spectrometry. 237 (2–3): 197–241. Bibcode:2004IJMSp.237..197W. doi:10.1016/j.ijms.2004.06.014.
69. Tarini BA (August 2007). "The current revolution in newborn screening: new technology, old controversies". Archives of Pediatrics & Adolescent Medicine. 161 (8): 767–72. doi:10.1001/archpedi.161.8.767. PMID 17679658.
70. Kayton A (2007). "Newborn screening: a literature review". Neonatal Network. 26 (2): 85–95. doi:10.1891/0730-0832.26.2.85. PMID 17402600.
71. Chace DH, Kalas TA, Naylor EW (November 2003). "Use of tandem mass spectrometry for multianalyte screening of dried blood specimens from newborns". Clinical Chemistry. 49 (11): 1797–817. doi:10.1373/clinchem.2003.022178. PMID 14578311.

CHAPTER 2

Proteomics: The Study of Proteomes

Chapter Contents

- **Introduction**
- **Complexity of the Problem**
- **Limitations of Genomics and Proteomics Studies**
- **Methods of Studying Proteins**
- **Practical Applications of Proteomics**
- **Emerging Trends in Proteomics**
- **Activity-Based Proteomics**
- **Bottom-Up Proteomics**
- **Top-Down Proteomics**
- **Shotgun Proteomics**
- **Proteomics Identifications Database**

The focus of proteomics is a biological group called the proteome. The proteome is dynamic, defined as the set of proteins expressed in a specific cell, given a particular set of conditions. Within a given human proteome, the number of proteins can be as large as 2 million.

INTRODUCTION

Proteomics is the large-scale study of proteins. Proteins are vital parts of living organisms, with many functions. The term *proteomics* was coined in 1997 in analogy with genomics, the study of the genome. The word *proteome* is a portmanteau of *prote*in and gen*ome*, and was coined by Marc Wilkins in 1994 while working on the concept as a PhD student.

The proteome is the entire set of proteins, produced or modified by an organism or system. This varies with time and distinct requirements, or stresses, that a cell or organism undergoes. Proteomics is an interdisciplinary domain that has benefited greatly from the genetic information of the Human Genome Project; it is also emerging scientific research and exploration of proteomes from the overall level of intracellular protein composition, structure, and its own unique activity patterns. It is an important component of functional genomics.

While *proteomics* generally refers to the large-scale experimental analysis of proteins, it is often specifically used for protein purification and mass spectrometry.

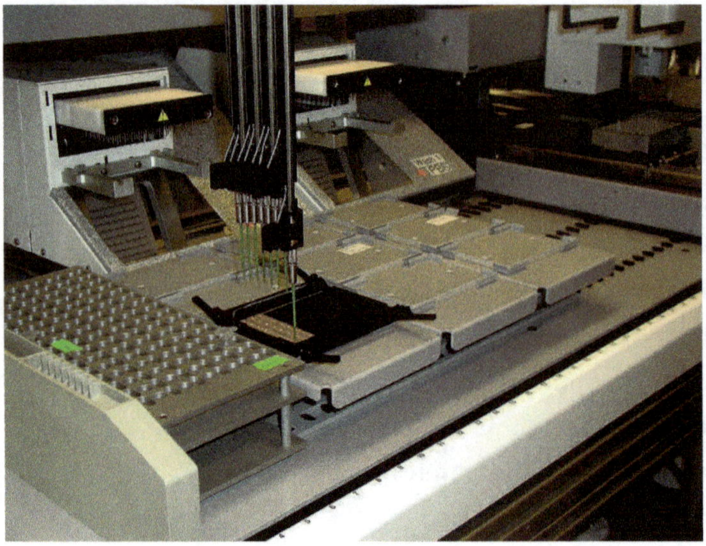

Robotic preparation of MALDI mass spectrometry samples on a sample carrier.

COMPLEXITY OF THE PROBLEM

After genomics and transcriptomics, proteomics is the next step in the study of biological systems. It is more complicated than genomics because an organism's genome is more or less constant, whereas the proteome differs from cell to cell and from time to time. Distinct genes are expressed in different cell types, which means that even the basic set of proteins that are produced in a cell needs to be identified.

In the past this phenomenon was done by RNA analysis, but it was found not to correlate with protein content. It is now known that mRNA is not always translated into protein, and the amount of protein produced for a given amount of mRNA depends on the gene it is transcribed from and on the current physiological state of the cell. Proteomics confirms the presence of the protein and provides a direct measure of the quantity present.

Post-Translational Modifications

Not only does the translation from mRNA cause differences, but many proteins are also subjected to a wide variety of chemical modifications after translation. Many of these post-translational modifications are critical to the protein's function.

Phosphorylation

One such modification is phosphorylation, which happens to many enzymes and structural proteins in the process of cell signaling. The addition of a phosphate to particular amino acids—most commonly serine and threonine mediated by serine/threonine kinases, or more rarely tyrosine mediated by tyrosine kinases—causes a protein to become a target for binding or interacting with a distinct set of other proteins that recognize the phosphorylated domain.

Because protein phosphorylation is one of the most-studied protein modifications, many "proteomic" efforts are geared to determining the set of phosphorylated proteins in a particular cell or tissue-type under particular circumstances. This alerts the scientist to the signaling pathways that may be active in that instance.

Ubiquitination

Ubiquitin is a small protein that can be affixed to certain protein substrates by enzymes called E3 ubiquitin ligases. Determining which proteins are poly-ubiquitinated helps understand how protein pathways are regulated. This is, therefore, an additional legitimate "proteomic" study. Similarly, once a researcher determines which substrates are ubiquitinated by each ligase, determining the set of ligases expressed in a particular cell type is helpful.

Additional Modifications

In addition to phosphorylation and ubiquitination, proteins can be subjected to (among others) methylation, acetylation, glycosylation, oxidation and nitrosylation. Some proteins undergo all these modifications, often in time-dependent combinations. This illustrates the potential complexity of studying protein structure and function.

Distinct Proteins are made under Distinct Settings

A cell may make different sets of proteins at different times or under different conditions, for example during development, cellular differentiation, cell cycle, or carcinogenesis. Further increasing proteome complexity, as mentioned, most proteins can undergo a wide range of post-translational modifications.

Therefore, a "proteomics" study can quickly become complex, even if the topic of study is restricted. In more ambitious settings, such as when a biomarker for a specific cancer subtype is sought, the proteomics scientist might elect to study multiple blood serum samples from multiple cancer patients to minimize confounding factors and account for experimental noise. Thus, complicated experimental designs are sometimes necessary to account for the dynamic complexity of the proteome.

LIMITATIONS OF GENOMICS AND PROTEOMICS STUDIES

Proteomics gives a different level of understanding than genomics for many reasons:

- the level of transcription of a gene gives only a rough estimate of its *level of translation* into a protein. An mRNA produced in abundance may be degraded rapidly or translated inefficiently, resulting in a small amount of protein.
- as mentioned above many proteins experience *post-translational modifications* that profoundly affect their activities; for example some proteins are not active until they become phosphorylated. Methods such as phosphoproteomics and glycoproteomics are used to study post-translational modifications.
- many transcripts give rise to more than one protein, through alternative splicing or alternative post-translational modifications.
- many proteins form complexes with other proteins or RNA molecules, and only function in the presence of these other molecules.
- protein degradation rate plays an important role in protein content.

Reproducibility. One major factor affecting reproducibility in proteomics experiments is the simultaneous elution of many more peptides than can be measured by mass spectrometers. This causes stochastic differences between experiments due to data-dependant acquisition of tryptic peptides. Although early large-scale shotgun proteomics analyses showed considerable variability between laboratories, presumably due in part to technical and experimental differences between labs, reproducibility has been improved in more recent mass spectrometry analysis, particularly on the protein level and using Orbitrap mass spectrometers. Notably, targeted proteomics shows increased reproducibility and repeatability compared with shotgun methods, although at the expense of data density and effectiveness.

METHODS OF STUDYING PROTEINS

In proteomics, there are multiple methods to study proteins. Generally, proteins can either be detected using antibodies (immunoassays) or using mass spectrometry. If a complex biological sample is analyzed, then biochemical separation has to be used before the detection step as there are too many analytes in the sample to perform accurate detection and quantification.

Protein Detection with Antibodies (Immunoassays)

Antibodies to particular proteins or to their modified forms have been used in biochemistry and cell biology studies. These are among the most common tools used by molecular biologists today. There are several specific techniques and protocols that use antibodies for protein detection. The enzyme-linked immunosorbent assay (ELISA) has been used for decades to detect and quantitatively measure proteins in samples. The Western blot can be used for detection and quantification of individual proteins, where in an initial step a complex protein mixture is separated using SDS-PAGE and then the protein of interest is identified using an antibody.

Modified proteins can be studied by developing an antibody specific to that modification. For example, there are antibodies that only recognize certain proteins when they are tyrosine-phosphorylated, known as phospho-specific antibodies. Also, there are antibodies specific to other modifications. These can be used to determine the set of proteins that have undergone the modification of interest.

Antibody-Free Protein Detection

While protein detection with antibodies are still very common in molecular biology, also other methods have been developed that do not rely on an antibody. These methods offer various advantages, for instance they are often able to determine the sequence of a protein or peptide, they may have higher throughput than antibody-based and they sometimes can identify and quantify proteins for which no antibody exists.

Detection Methods

One of the earliest method for protein analysis has been Edman degradation (introduced in 1967) where a single peptide is subjected to multiple steps of chemical degradation to resolve its sequence. These methods have mostly been supplanted by technologies that offer higher throughput.

More recent methods use mass spectrometry-based techniques, a development that was made possible by the discovery of "soft ionization" methods such as matrix-assisted laser desorption/ionization (MALDI) and electrospray ionization (ESI) developed in the 1980s. These methods gave rise to the top-down and the bottom-up proteomics workflows where often additional separation is performed before analysis (see below).

Separation Methods

For the analysis of complex biological samples, a reduction of sample complexity is required. This can be performed off-line by one-dimensional or two dimensional separation. More recently, on-line methods have been developed where individual peptides (in bottom-up proteomics approaches) are separated using Reversed-phase chromatography and then directly ionized using ESI; the direct coupling of separation and analysis explains the term "on-line" analysis.

Hybrid Technologies

There are several hybrid technologies that use antibody-based purification of individual analytes and then perform mass spectrometric analysis for identification and quantification. Examples of these methods are the MSIA (mass spectrometric immunoassay) developed by Randall Nelson in 1995 and the SISCAPA (Stable Isotope Standard Capture with Anti-Peptide Antibodies) method, introduced by Leigh Anderson in 2004.

Current Research Methodologies

Fluorescence two-dimensional differential gel electrophoresis (2-D DIGE) can be used to quantify variation in the 2-D DIGE process and establish statistically valid thresholds for assigning quantitative changes between samples.

Comparative proteomic analysis can reveal the role of proteins in complex biological systems, including reproduction. For example, treatment with the insecticide triazophos causes an increase in the content of brown planthopper (*Nilaparvata lugens* (Stål)) male accessory gland proteins (Acps) that can be transferred to females via mating, causing an increase in fecundity (i.e. birth rate) of females. To identify changes in the types of accessory gland proteins (Acps) and reproductive proteins that mated female planthoppers received from male planthoppers, researchers conducted a comparative proteomic analysis of mated *N. lugens* females. The results indicated that these proteins participate in the reproductive process of *N. lugens* adult females and males.

Proteome analysis of *Arabidopsis peroxisomes* has been established as the major unbiased approach for identifying new peroxisomal proteins on a large scale.

There are many approaches to characterizing the human proteome, which is estimated to contain between 20,000 and 25,000 non-redundant proteins. The number of unique protein species will likely increase by between 50,000 and 500,000 due to RNA splicing and proteolysis events, and when post-translational modification are also considered, the total number of unique human proteins is estimated to range in the low millions.

In addition, the first promising attempts to decipher the proteome of animal tumors have recently been reported. This method used as a functional method in *Macrobrachium rosenbergii* protein profiling.

High-Throughput Proteomic Technologies

Proteomics has steadily gained momentum over the past decade with the evolution of several approaches. Few of these are new and others build on traditional methods. Mass spectrometry-based methods and micro arrays are the most common technologies for large-scale study of proteins.

Mass Spectrometry and Protein Profiling

There are two mass spectrometry-based methods currently used for protein profiling. The more established and widespread method uses high resolution, two-dimensional electrophoresis to separate proteins from different samples in parallel, followed by selection and staining of differentially expressed proteins to be identified by mass spectrometry. Despite the advances in 2DE and its maturity, it has its limits as well. The central concern is the inability to resolve all the proteins within a sample, given their dramatic range in expression level and differing properties.

The second quantitative approach uses stable isotope tags to differentially label proteins from two different complex mixtures. Here, the proteins within a complex mixture are labeled first isotopically, and then digested to yield labeled peptides. The labeled mixtures are then combined, the peptides separated by multidimensional liquid chromatography and analyzed by tandem mass spectrometry. Isotope coded affinity tag (ICAT) reagents are the widely used isotope tags. In this method, the cysteine residues of proteins get covalently attached to the ICAT reagent, thereby reducing the complexity of the mixtures omitting the non-cysteine residues.

Quantitative proteomics using stable isotopic tagging is an increasingly useful tool in modern development. Firstly, chemical reactions have been used to introduce tags into specific sites or proteins for the purpose of probing specific protein functionalities. The isolation of phosphorylated peptides has been achieved using isotopic labeling and selective chemistries to capture the fraction of protein among the complex mixture. Secondly, the ICAT technology was used to differentiate between partially purified or purified macromolecular complexes such as large RNA polymerase II pre-initiation complex and the proteins complexed with yeast transcription factor. Thirdly, ICAT labeling was recently combined with chromatin isolation to identify and quantify chromatin-associated proteins. Finally ICAT reagents are useful for proteomic profiling of cellular organelles and specific cellular fractions.

Another quantitative approach is the Accurate Mass and Time (AMT) tag approach developed by Richard D. Smith and coworkers at Pacific Northwest National Laboratory. In this approach, increased throughput and sensitivity is achieved by avoiding the need for tandem mass spectrometry, and making use of precisely determined separation time information and highly accurate mass determinations for peptide and protein identifications.

Protein Chips

Balancing the use of mass spectrometers in proteomics and in medicine is the use of protein micro arrays. The aim behind protein micro arrays is to print thousands of protein detecting features for the interrogation of biological samples. Antibody arrays are an example in which a host of different antibodies are arrayed to detect their respective antigens from a sample of human blood. Another approach is the arraying of multiple protein types for the study of properties like protein-DNA, protein-protein and protein-ligand interactions. Ideally, the functional proteomic arrays would contain the entire complement of the proteins of a given organism. The first version of such arrays consisted of 5000 purified proteins from yeast deposited onto glass microscopic slides. Despite the success of first chip, it was a greater challenge for protein arrays to be implemented. Proteins are inherently much more difficult to work with than DNA. They have a broad dynamic range, are less stable than DNA and their structure is difficult to preserve on glass slides, though they are essential for most assays. The global ICAT technology has striking advantages over protein chip technologies.

Reverse-Phased Protein Microarrays

This is a promising and newer microarray application for the diagnosis, study and treatment of complex diseases such as cancer. The technology merges laser capture microdissection

(LCM) with micro array technology, to produce reverse phase protein microarrays. In this type of microarrays, the whole collection of protein themselves are immobilized with the intent of capturing various stages of disease within an individual patient. When used with LCM, reverse phase arrays can monitor the fluctuating state of proteome among different cell population within a small area of human tissue. This is useful for profiling the status of cellular signaling molecules, among a cross section of tissue that includes both normal and cancerous cells. This approach is useful in monitoring the status of key factors in normal prostate epithelium and invasive prostate cancer tissues. LCM then dissects these tissue and protein lysates were arrayed onto nitrocellulose slides, which were probed with specific antibodies. This method can track all kinds of molecular events and can compare diseased and healthy tissues within the same patient enabling the development of treatment strategies and diagnosis. The ability to acquire proteomics snapshots of neighboring cell populations, using reverse phase microarrays in conjunction with LCM has a number of applications beyond the study of tumors. The approach can provide insights into normal physiology and pathology of all the tissues and is invaluable for characterizing developmental processes and anomalies.

PRACTICAL APPLICATIONS OF PROTEOMICS

One major development to come from the study of human genes and proteins has been the identification of potential new drugs for the treatment of disease. This relies on genome and proteome information to identify proteins associated with a disease, which computer software can then use as targets for new drugs. For example, if a certain protein is implicated in a disease, its 3D structure provides the information to design drugs to interfere with the action of the protein. A molecule that fits the active site of an enzyme, but cannot be released by the enzyme, inactivates the enzyme. This is the basis of new drug-discovery tools, which aim to find new drugs to inactivate proteins involved in disease. As genetic differences among individuals are found, researchers expect to use these techniques to develop personalized drugs that are more effective for the individual.

Proteomics is also used to reveal complex plant-insect interactions that help identify candidate genes involved in the defensive response of plants to herbivory.

Interaction Proteomics and Protein Networks

Interaction proteomics is the analysis of protein interactions from scales of binary interactions to proteome- or network-wide. Most proteins function via protein-protein interactions, and one goal of interaction proteomics is to identify binary protein interactions, protein complexes, and interactomes.

Several methods are available to probe protein–protein interactions. While the most traditional method is yeast two-hybrid analysis, a powerful emerging method is affinity purification followed by protein mass spectrometry using tagged protein baits. Other methods include surface plasmon resonance (SPR), protein microarrays, dual polarisation interferometry, microscale thermophoresis and experimental methods such as phage display and *in silico* computational methods.

Knowledge of protein-protein interactions is especially useful in regard to biological networks and systems biology, for example in cell signaling cascades and gene regulatory networks (GRNs, where knowledge of protein-DNA interactions is also informative). Proteome-wide analysis of protein interactions, and integration of these interaction patterns into larger biological networks, is crucial towards understanding systems-level biology.

Expression Proteomics

Expression proteomics includes the analysis of protein expression at larger scale. It helps identify main proteins in a particular sample, and those proteins differentially expressed in related samples—such as diseased vs. healthy tissue. If a protein is found only in a diseased sample then it can be a useful drug target or diagnostic marker. Proteins with same or similar expression profiles may also be functionally related. There are technologies such as 2D-PAGE and mass spectrometry that are used in expression proteomics.

Biomarkers

The National Institutes of Health has defined a biomarker as "a characteristic that is objectively measured and evaluated as an indicator of normal biological processes, pathogenic processes, or pharmacologic responses to a therapeutic intervention."

Understanding the proteome, the structure and function of each protein and the complexities of protein–protein interactions is critical for developing the most effective diagnostic techniques and disease treatments in the future. For example, proteomics is highly useful in identification of candidate biomarkers (proteins in body fluids that are of value for diagnosis), identification of the bacterial antigens that are targeted by the immune response, and identification of possible immunohistochemistry markers of infectious or neoplastic diseases.

An interesting use of proteomics is using specific protein biomarkers to diagnose disease. A number of techniques allow to test for proteins produced during a particular disease, which helps to diagnose the disease quickly. Techniques include western blot, immunohistochemical staining, enzyme linked immunosorbent assay (ELISA) or mass spectrometry. Secretomics, a subfield of proteomics that studies secreted proteins and secretion pathways using proteomic approaches, has recently emerged as an important tool for the discovery of biomarkers of disease.

Proteogenomics

In proteogenomics, proteomic technologies such as mass spectrometry are used for improving gene annotations. Parallel analysis of the genome and the proteome facilitates discovery of post-translational modifications and proteolytic events, especially when comparing multiple species (comparative proteogenomics).

Structural Proteomics

Structural proteomics includes the analysis of protein structures at large-scale. It compares protein structures and helps identify functions of newly discovered genes. The structural analysis also helps to understand that where drugs bind to proteins and also show where proteins interact with each other. This understanding is achieved using different technologies such as X-ray crystallography and NMR spectroscopy.

Bioinformatics for Proteomics (Proteome Informatics)

Much proteomics data is collected with the help of high throughput technologies such as mass spectrometry and microarray. It would often take weeks or months to analyze the data and perform comparisons by hand. For this reason, biologists and chemists are collaborating with computer scientists and mathematicians to create programs and pipeline to computationally analyze the protein data. Using bioinformatics techniques, researchers are capable of faster analysis and data storage. A good place to find lists of current programs and databases is on the ExPASy bioinformatics resource portal <http://www.expasy.org/proteomics>. The applications of bioinformatics-based proteomics includes medicine, disease diagnosis, biomarker identification, and many more.

Protein Identification

Mass spectrometry and microarray produce peptide fragmentation information but do not give identification of specific proteins present in the original sample. Due to the lack of specific protein identification, past researchers were forced to decipher the peptide fragments themselves. However, there are currently programs available for protein identification. These programs take the peptide sequences output from mass spectrometry and microarray and return information about matching or similar proteins. This is done through algorithms implemented by the program which perform alignments with proteins from known databases such as UniProt and PROSITE to predict what proteins are in the sample with a degree of certainty.

Protein Structure

The biomolecular structure forms the 3D configuration of the protein. Understanding the protein's structure aids in identification of the protein's interactions and function. It used to be that the 3D structure of proteins could only be determined using X-ray crystallography and NMR spectroscopy. Now, through bioinformatics, there are computer programs that can predict and model the structure of proteins. These programs use the chemical properties of amino acids and structural properties of known proteins to predict the 3D model of sample proteins. This also allows scientists to take a look at protein interactions on a larger scale. In addition, biomedical engineers are developing methods to factor in the flexibility of protein structures to make comparisons and predictions.

Post-Translational Modifications

Unfortunately, most programs available for protein analysis are not written for proteins that have undergone post-translational modifications. Some programs will accept post-translational modifications to aid in protein identification but then ignore the modification during further protein analysis. It is important to account for these modifications since they can affect the protein's structure. In turn, computational analysis of post-translational modifications has gained the attention of the scientific community. The current post-translational modification programs are only predictive. Chemists, biologists and computer scientists are working together to create and introduce new pipelines that allow for analysis of post-translational modifications that have been experimentally identified for their effect on the protein's structure and function.

Computational Methods in Studying Protein Biomarkers

One example of the use of bioinformatics and the use of computational methods is the study of protein biomarkers. Computational predictive models have shown that extensive and diverse feto-maternal protein trafficking occurs during pregnancy and can be readily detected non-invasively in maternal whole blood. This computational approach circumvented a major limitation, the abundance of maternal proteins interfering with the detection of fetal proteins, to fetal proteomic analysis of maternal blood. Computational models can use fetal gene transcripts previously identified in maternal whole blood to create a comprehensive proteomic network of the term neonate. Such work shows that the fetal proteins detected in pregnant woman's blood originate from a diverse group of tissues and organs from the developing fetus. The proteomic networks contain many biomarkers that are proxies for development and illustrate the potential clinical application of this technology as a way to monitor normal and abnormal fetal development.

An information theoretic framework has also been introduced for biomarker discovery, integrating biofluid and tissue information. This new approach takes advantage of functional synergy between certain biofluids and tissues with the potential for clinically significant findings not possible if tissues and biofluids were considered individually. By conceptualizing tissue-biofluid as information channels, significant biofluid proxies can be identified and then used for guided development of clinical diagnostics. Candidate biomarkers are then predicted based on information transfer criteria across the tissue-biofluid channels. Significant biofluid-tissue relationships can be used to prioritize clinical validation of biomarkers.

EMERGING TRENDS IN PROTEOMICS

A number of emerging concepts have the potential to improve current features of proteomics. Obtaining absolute quantification of proteins and monitoring post-translational modifications are the two tasks that impact the understanding of protein function in healthy and diseased cells. For many cellular events, the protein concentrations do not change; rather, their function is modulated by post-transitional modifications (PTM). Methods of monitoring PTM are an underdeveloped area in proteomics. Selecting a particular subset of protein for analysis substantially reduces protein complexity, making it advantageous for diagnostic purposes where blood is the starting material. Another important aspect of proteomics, yet not addressed, is that proteomics methods should focus on studying proteins in the context of the environment. The increasing use of chemical cross linkers, introduced into living cells to fix protein-protein, protein-DNA and other interactions, may ameliorate this problem partially. The challenge is to identify suitable methods of preserving relevant interactions. Another goal for studying protein is to develop more sophisticated methods to image proteins and other molecules in living cells and real time.

Proteomics for Systems Biology

Advances in quantitative proteomics would clearly enable more in-depth analysis of cellular systems. Biological systems are subject to a variety of perturbations (cell cycle, cellular differentiation, carcinogenesis, environment (biophysical), etc.). Transcriptional and translational responses to these perturbations results in functional changes to the proteome implicated in response to the stimulus. Therefore, describing and quantifying proteome-wide changes in protein abundance is crucial towards understanding biological phenomenon more holistically, on the level of the entire system. In this way, proteomics can be seen as complementary to genomics, transcriptomics, epigenomics, metabolomics, and other -omics approaches in integrative analyses attempting to define biological phenotypes more comprehensively. As an example, *The Cancer Proteome Atlas* provides quantitative protein expression data for ~200 proteins in over 4,000 tumor samples with matched transcriptomic and genomic data from The Cancer Genome Atlas. Similar datasets in other cell types, tissue types, and species, particularly using deep shotgun mass spectrometry, will be an immensely important resource for research in fields like cancer biology, developmental and stem cell biology, medicine, and evolutionary biology.

Human Plasma Proteome

Characterizing the human plasma proteome has become a major goal in the proteomics arena. The plasma proteome represents one of the most complex proteomes in the human body. It contains immunoglobulin, cytokines, protein hormones, and secreted proteins indicative of infection on top of resident, hemostatic proteins. It also contains tissue leakage proteins due to the blood circulation through different tissues in the body. The blood thus contains information on the physiological state of all tissues and, combined with its accessibility, makes the blood proteome invaluable for medical purposes. Even with the recent advancements in proteomics, characterizing the proteome of blood plasma is a daunting challenge.

Temporal and spatial dynamics further complicate the study of human plasma proteome. The turnover of some proteins is quite faster than others and the protein content of an artery may substantially vary from that of a vein. All these differences make even the simplest proteomic task of cataloging the proteome seem out of reach. To tackle this problem, priorities need to be established. Capturing the most meaningful subset of proteins among the entire proteome to generate a diagnostic tool is one such priority. Secondly, since cancer is associated with enhanced glycosylation of proteins, methods that focus on this part of proteins will also be useful. Again: multiparameter analysis best reveals a pathological state. As these technologies improve, the disease profiles should be continually related to respective gene expression changes.

ACTIVITY-BASED PROTEOMICS

Activity-based proteomics, or activity-based protein profiling (ABPP) is a functional proteomic technology that uses chemical probes that react with mechanistically related classes of enzymes.

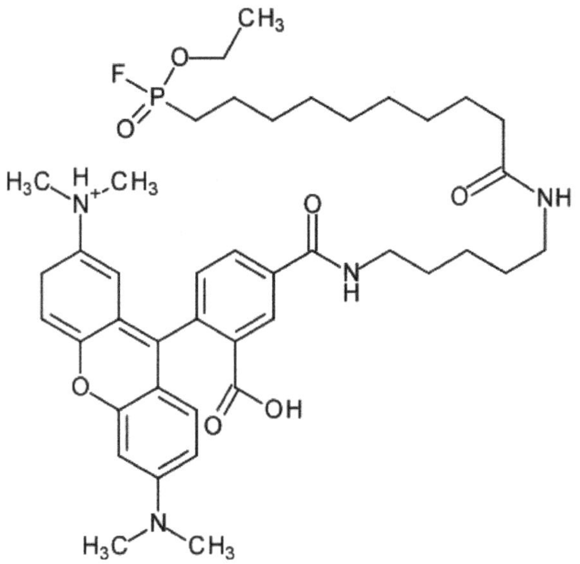

Fluorophosphonate-rhodamine (FP-Rhodamine) activity-based probe for profiling of the serine hydrolase superfamily. In this probe the fluorophosphonate is the reactive group (RG) as it binds irreversibly to the active-site serinenucleophile of serine hydrolases and the tag is rhodamine, a fluorophore for in-gel visualization.

Description

The basic unit of ABPP is the probe, which typically consists of two elements: a reactive group (RG, sometimes called a "warhead") and a tag. Additionally, some probes may contain a binding group which enhances selectivity. The reactive group usually contains a specially designed electrophile that becomes covalently-linked to a nucleophilic residue in the active site of an active enzyme. An enzyme that is inhibited or post-translationally modified will not react with an activity-based probe. The tag may be either a reporter such as a fluorophore or an affinity label such as biotin or an alkyne or azide for use with the Huisgen 1,3-dipolar cycloaddition (also known as click chemistry).

Advantages

A major advantage of ABPP is the ability to monitor the availability of the enzyme active site directly, rather than being limited to protein or mRNA abundance. With classes of enzymes such as the serine proteases and metalloproteases that often interact with endogenous inhibitors or that exist as inactive zymogens, this technique offers a valuable advantage over traditional techniques that rely on abundance rather than activity.

Multidimensional Protein Identification Technology

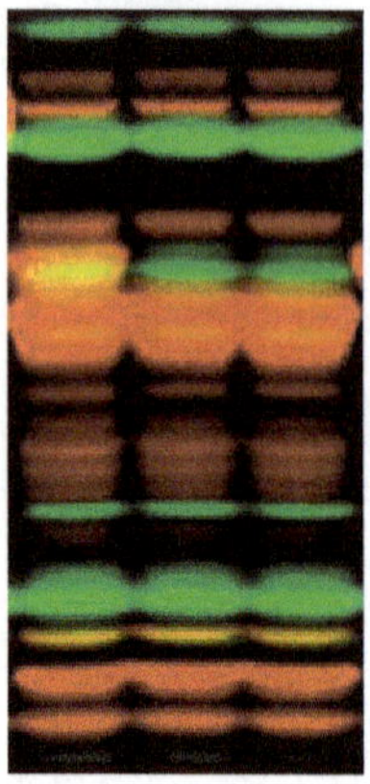

In-gel ABPP using probes with different fluorophores in the same lane to simultaneously profile differences in enzyme activities

In recent years ABPP has been combined with tandem mass spectrometry enabling the identification of hundreds of active enzymes from a single sample. This technique, known as *ABPP-MudPIT* (multidimensional protein identification technology) is especially useful for profiling inhibitor selectivity as the potency of an inhibitor can be tested against hundreds of targets simultaneously.

ABPP were first reported in the 1990s in the study of proteases.

BOTTOM-UP PROTEOMICS

Bottom-up proteomics is a common method to identify proteins and characterize their amino acid sequences and post-translational modifications by proteolytic digestion of proteins prior to analysis by mass spectrometry. The major alternative workflow used in high-throughput proteomics is called top-down proteomics and does not use proteolytic digestion.

In bottom-up proteomics, the proteins may first be purified by a method such as gel electrophoresis resulting in one or a few proteins in each proteolytic digest. Alternatively, the crude protein extract is digested directly, followed by one or more dimensions of separation of the peptides by liquid chromatography coupled to mass spectrometry, a technique known as shotgun proteomics. By comparing the masses of the proteolytic peptides or their tandem mass spectra with those predicted from a sequence database or annotated peptide spectral in a peptide spectral library, peptides can be identified and multiple peptide identifications assembled into a protein identification.

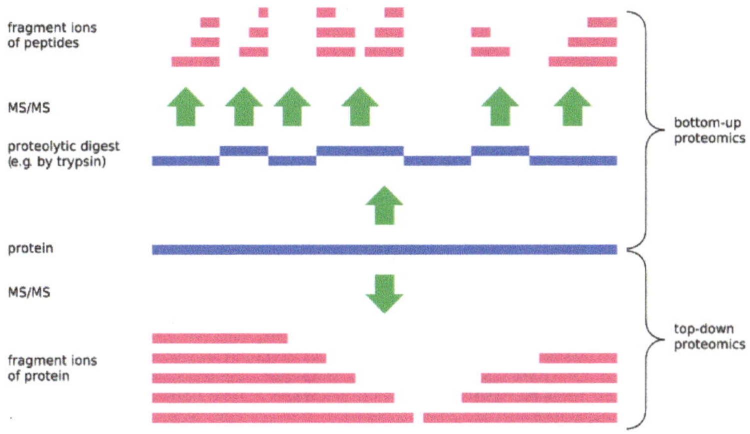

Bottom-up versus top-down proteomics.

Advantages

There is better front-end separation of peptides compared with proteins and higher sensitivity than the top-down method.

Disadvantages

There is limited protein sequence coverage by identified peptides, loss of labile PTMs, and ambiguity of the origin for redundant peptide sequences.

TOP-DOWN PROTEOMICS

Top-down proteomics is a method of protein identification that uses an ion trapping mass spectrometer to store an isolated protein ion for mass measurement and tandem mass spectrometry analysis. Top-down proteomics is capable of identifying and quantitating unique proteoforms through the analysis of intact proteins. The name is derived from the similar approach to DNA sequencing. Proteins are typically ionized by electrospray ionization and trapped in a Fourier transform ion cyclotron resonance (Penning trap) or quadrupole ion trap (Paul trap) mass spectrometer. Fragmentation for tandem mass spectrometry is accomplished by electron-capture dissociation or electron-transfer dissociation. Effective fractionation is critical for sample handling before mass-spectrometry-based proteomics. Proteome analysis routinely involves digesting intact proteins followed by inferred protein identification using mass spectrometry. Top-down proteomics interrogates protein structure through measurement of an intact mass followed by direct ion dissociation in the gas phase.

Currently the most advanced instrument used to map proteoforms is the Thermo Scientific Orbitrap Fusion Lumos Tribrid mass spectrometer. This high-performance instrument is able to give a quantitative analysis of proteoforms, identify them, and deeply characterize them with tandem MS/MS.

Advantages

- The main advantages of the top-down approach include the ability to detect degradation products, sequence variants, and combinations of post-translational modifications.
- In Top-down proteomics, researchers can feed intact full proteins directly into mass spectrometers, and are able to capture the distinct characteristics of each one-of-a-kind proteoform. In addition, Top-down proteomics allows for analysis of an entire protein molecule without digestion and also allows for low mass protein detection.
- Top-down proteomics, when accompanied with polyacrylamide gel electrophoresis, can help to complement the bottom-up proteomic approach. Top-down proteomic methods can assist in exposing large deviations from predictions and has been very successfully pursued by combining Gel Elution Liquid-based Fractionation Entrapment Electrophoresis fractionation, protein precipitation, and reverse phase HPLC with electrospray ionization and MS/MS.
- Characterization of small proteins represents a significant challenge for bottom up proteomics due to the inability to generate sufficient tryptic peptides for analysis. Top-down proteomics allows for low mass protein detection, thus increasing the repertoire of proteins known. While Bottom-up proteomics integrates cleaved products from all proteoforms produced by a gene into a single peptide map of the full-length gene product to tabulate and quantify expressed proteins, a major strength of Top-down proteomics is that it enables researchers to quantitatively track one or more proteoforms from multiple samples and to excise these proteoforms for chemical analysis.

Disadvantages

- In the recent past, the top down approach was relegated to analysis of individual proteins or simple mixtures, while complex mixtures and proteins were analyzed by more established methods such as Bottom-up proteomics. Additionally protein identification and proteoform characterization in the TDP (Top-down proteomics) approach suffer from a dynamic range challenge where the same highly abundant species are repeatedly fragmented.
- Although Top-down proteomics can be operated in relatively high output in order to successfully map proteome coverage at a large level, the rate of identifying new proteins after initial rounds reduces quite sharply.

- Top-down proteomics interrogation can overcome problems for identifying individual proteins, but has not been achieved on a large scale due to a lack of intact protein fractionation methods that are integrated with tandem mass spectrometry.

Top-down Proteomics Research and Uses

Study One: Quantitation and Identification of Thousands of Human Proteoforms below 30 kDa

- Researchers performed a study of human proteoforms below 30kDa, used primary IMR90 human fibroblasts containing a Ras function construct that were grown in medium.
- Chose to use Top-down Proteomics to characterize these proteoforms because it is currently the best method for intact proteins, as I discussed Bottom Up digests the protein and does not do a good job of providing a clear image of distinct intact proteoforms.
- Top-down Proteomics is capable of identifying and quantitating unique proteoforms through the analysis of intact proteins. The Top-down quantitation yielded changes in abundance of 1038 cytoplasmic proteoforms.

Study Two: Combining high-throughput MALDI-TOF mass spectrometry and isoelectric focusing gel electrophoresis for virtual 2D gel-based proteomics

- Researchers used top-down proteomics because could identify the exact proteoforms of intact proteins, rather than the bottom-up approach which gives fragment ions of peptides.
- This study used Virtual 2D gel along with Mass Spectrometry in order to separate protein mixtures. MALDI is a computer software that generates the intact masses of the proteins at each isoelectric point. It started with an image of an IPG-IEF (isoelectric focusing) gel selection that was then analyzed by MALDI.
- Top-down proteomics MALDI-TOF/TOF-MS is more tolerant to impurities; does not require biomarker extraction, purification, and separation; and can be directly applied to intact microorganisms.

SHOTGUN PROTEOMICS

Shotgun proteomics refers to the use of bottom-up proteomics techniques in identifying proteins in complex mixtures using a combination of high performance liquid chromatography combined with mass spectrometry. The name is derived from shotgun sequencing of DNA which is itself named after the rapidly expanding, quasi-random firing pattern of a shotgun. The most common method of shotgun proteomics starts with the proteins in the mixture being digested and the resulting peptides are separated by liquid chromatography. Tandem mass spectrometry is then used to identify the peptides.

Targeted proteomics using SRM and Data-independent acquisition methods are often considered alternatives to shotgun proteomics in the field of bottom-up proteomics. While shotgun proteomics uses data-dependent selection of precursor ions to generate fragment ion scans, the aforementioned methods use a deterministic method for acquisition of fragment ion scans.

History

Shotgun proteomics arose from the difficulties of using previous technologies to separate complex mixtures. In 1975, two-dimensional polyacrylamide gel electrophoresis (2D-PAGE) was described by O'Farrell and Klose with the ability to resolve complex protein mixtures. The development of matrix-assisted laser desorption ionization (MALDI), electrospray ionization (ESI), and database searching continued to grow the field of proteomics. However these methods still had difficulty identifying and separating low-abundance proteins, aberrant proteins, and membrane proteins. Shotgun proteomics emerged as a method that could resolve even these proteins.

Advantages

Shotgun proteomics allows global protein identification as well as the ability to systematically profile dynamic proteomes. It also avoids the modest separation efficiency and poor mass spectral sensitivity associated with intact protein analysis.

Disadvantages

The dynamic exclusion filtering that is often used in shotgun proteomics maximizes the number of identified proteins at the expense of random sampling. This problem may be exacerbated by the undersampling inherent in shotgun proteomics.

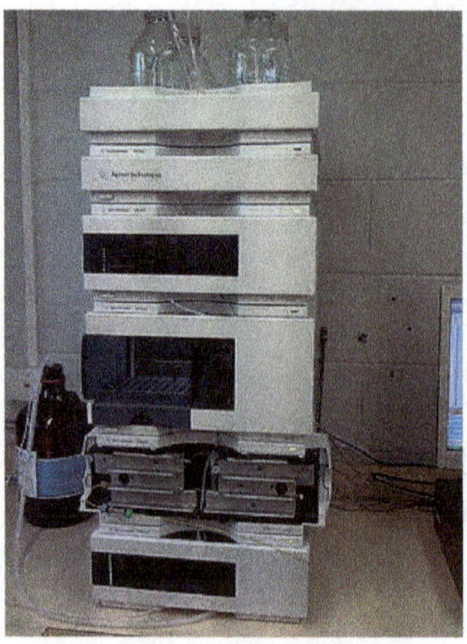

Agilent 1200 HPLC

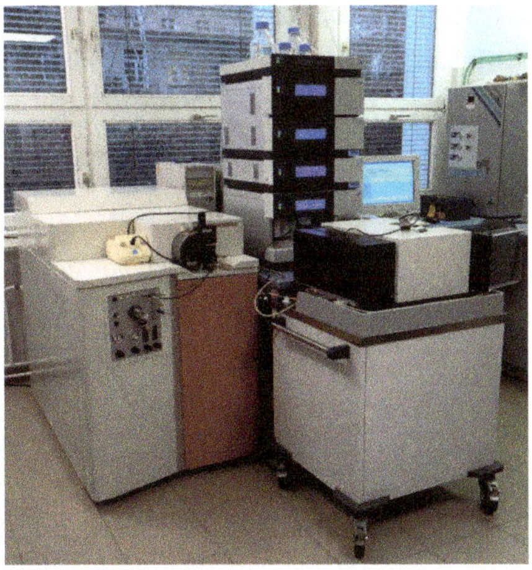

Quadrupole Time-Of-Flight tandem Mass Spectrometer (Q-TOF)

Workflow

Cells containing the protein complement desired are grown. Proteins are then extracted from the mixture and digested with a protease to produce a peptide mixture. The peptide mixture is then loaded directly onto a microcapillary column and the peptides are separated by hydrophobicity and charge. As the peptides elute from the column, they are ionized and separated by m/z in the first stage of tandem mass spectrometry. The selected ions undergo collision-induced dissociation or other process to induce fragmentation. The charged fragments are separated in the second stage of tandem mass spectrometry.

The "fingerprint" of each peptide's fragmentation mass spectrum is used to identify the protein from which they derive by searching against a sequence database with commercially available software (e.g. SEQUEST or MASCOT). Examples of sequence databases are the Genpept database or the PIR database. After the database search, each peptide-spectrum match (PSM) needs to be evaluated for validity. This analysis allows researchers to profile various biological systems.

Issues with Peptide Identification

Peptides that are degenerate (shared by two or more proteins in the database) may make it difficult to identify the protein to which they belong. Additionally, some proteome samples of vertebrates have a large number of paralogs. Finally, alternative splicing in higher eukaryotes can result in many identical protein subsequences.

Practical Applications

With the human genome sequenced, the next step is the verification and functional annotation of all predicted genes and their protein products. Shotgun proteomics can be used for functional classification or comparative analysis of these protein products. It can be used in projects ranging from large-scale whole proteome to focusing on a single protein family. It can be done in research labs or commercially.

Large-Scale Analysis

One example of this is a study by Washburn, Wolters, & Yates in which they used shotgun proteomics on the proteome of a Saccharomyces cerevisiae strain grown to mid-log phase. They were able to detect and identify 1,484 proteins as well as identify proteins rarely seen in proteome analysis, including low-abundance proteins like transcription factors and protein kinases. They were also able to identify 131 proteins with three or more predicted transmembrane domains.

Protein Family

Vaisar et al. uses shotgun proteomics to implicate protease inhibition and complement activation in the antiinflammatory properties of high-density lipoprotein. In a study by Lee et al., higher expression level of hnRNP A2/B1 and Hsp90 were observed in human hepatoma HepG2 cells than in wild type cells. This led to a search for reported functional roles mediated in concert by both these multifunctional cellular chaperones.

PROTEOMICS IDENTIFICATIONS DATABASE

The PRIDE (PRoteomics IDEntifications database) is a public data repository of mass spectrometry (MS) based proteomics data, and is maintained by the European Bioinformatics Institute as part of the Proteomics Team.

Originally designed by Lennart Martens in 2003 during a stay at the European Bioinformatics Institute as a Marie Curie fellow of the European Commission in the "Quality of Life" Programme (Contract number: QLRI-1999-50595), PRIDE was established as a production service in 2005. The original grant application document from June 2013 to start construction of PRIDE has since been published in a viewpoint article. Several similar proteomics databases have been built, including the GPMDB, PeptideAtlas, Proteinpedia and the NCBI Peptidome.

The PRIDE database constitutes a structured data repository, and stores the original experimental data from the researchers without editorial control over the submitted data.

In total, PRIDE contains data from about 60 species, the biggest fraction of it coming from human samples (including the data from the two draft human proteomes) followed by the fruit fly Drosophila melanogaster and mouse.

Formats and the Submission Process

Since detailed proteomics data currently cannot be curated from the existing literature, the source of PRIDE data is solely submissions by academic researchers.

PRIDE is a standards-compliant public repository, meaning that its own XML-based data exchange format for submissions, PRIDE XML, was built around the Proteomics

Standards Initiative mzData standard for mass spectrometry. Recently, PRIDE has been adapted to work with the modern mzML and mzIdentML standards of the Proteomics Standards Initiative. An additional format, dubbed mzTab, can be used as a simplified way to submit quantitative proteomics data.

As there are many types of different mass spectrometry instruments and software formats are currently on the market, wet-lab scientists without a strong bioinformatics background or informatics support were having problems converting their data to PRIDE XML. The development of PRIDE Converter helped to tackle this situation. PRIDE Converter is a tool, written in the Java programming language, that converts 15 different input mass spectrometry data formats into PRIDE XML via a wizard-like graphical user interface. It is freely available and is open source under the permissive Apache License. A new version of PRIDE Converter was released in 2012 as PRIDE Converter 2. This new version constituted a complete rewrite, focused on easy adaptability to different (and evolving) data sources.

Browsing, Searching & Data Mining Pride

Currently, data can be queried from PRIDE via the PRIDE web interface, through the stand-alone Java client PRIDE Inspector, or coupled directly to several search engines through PeptideShaker. Moreover, a new RESTful API allows convenient programmatic access to the PRIDE archive.

The extensive use of controlled vocabularies (CVs) and ontologies for flexible yet context-sensitive annotation of data, along with the ability to perform intelligent queries by these annotations, are key features of PRIDE.

Involvement in ProteomeXchange

The ProteomeXchange consortium has been set up to provide a coordinated submission of MS proteomics data to the main existing proteomics repositories, and to encourage optimal data dissemination. The consortium contains several member databases, including PRIDE and PeptideAtlas. The earliest conception of ProteomeXchange stems from a meeting at the HUPO 2005 conference in Munich, where the main proteomics data repositories at the time agreed in principle to exchange their data, and thus provide a means for the user to find public proteomics data at any of the participating databases. Due to the rapid development of the field, and the need to first develop suitable standards for data exchange, it took almost ten years from that meeting to actually implement this system, an effort that was funded by the 'ProteomeXchange' Coordination Action grant of the European Commission's Seventh Framework Programme (project reference 260558).

Data Recovery after the Discontinuation of Peptidome

The NCBI Peptidome database was discontinued in 2011, yet a joint effort by the PRIDE and Peptidome teams resulted in the transfer of all Peptidome data to PRIDE.

REFERENCES

1. Anderson NL, Anderson NG; Anderson (1998). "Proteome and proteomics: new technologies, new concepts, and new words". Electrophoresis. 19 (11): 1853–61. doi:10.1002/elps.1150191103. PMID 9740045.
2. Blackstock WP, Weir MP; Weir (1999). "Proteomics: quantitative and physical mapping of cellular proteins". Trends Biotechnol. 17 (3): 121–7. doi:10.1016/S0167-7799(98)01245-1. PMID 10189717.
3. P. James (1997). "Protein identification in the post-genome era: the rapid rise of proteomics". Quarterly reviews of biophysics. 30 (4): 279–331. doi:10.1017/S0033583597003399. PMID 9634650.
4. Marc R. Wilkins, Christian Pasquali, Ron D. Appel, Keli Ou, Olivier Golaz, Jean-Charles Sanchez, Jun X. Yan, Andrew. A. Gooley, Graham Hughes, Ian Humphery-Smith, Keith L. Williams & Denis F. Hochstrasser; Pasquali; Appel; Ou; Golaz; Sanchez; Yan; Gooley; Hughes; Humphery-Smith; Williams; Hochstrasser (1996). "From Proteins to Proteomes: Large Scale Protein Identification by Two-Dimensional Electrophoresis and Arnino Acid Analysis". Nature Biotechnology. 14 (1): 61–65. doi:10.1038/nbt0196-61. PMID 9636313.
5. UNSW Staff Bio: Professor Marc Wilkins Archived August 22, 2011, at the Wayback Machine.
6. Anderson, Johnathon D.; Johansson, Henrik J.; Graham, Calvin S.; Vesterlund, Mattias; Pham, Missy T.; Bramlett, Charles S.; Montgomery, Elizabeth N.; Mellema, Matt S.; Bardini, Renee L. (2016-03-01). "Comprehensive Proteomic Analysis of Mesenchymal Stem Cell Exosomes Reveals Modulation of Angiogenesis via Nuclear Factor-KappaB Signaling". Stem Cells. 34 (3): 601–613. doi:10.1002/stem.2298. ISSN 1549-4918. PMID 26782178.
7. Hood, Leroy; Rowen, Lee (2013-09-13). "The human genome project: big science transforms biology and medicine". Genome Medicine. 5 (9): 79. doi:10.1186/gm483. PMC 4066586Freely accessible. PMID 24040834.
8. Simon Rogers, Mark Girolami, Walter Kolch, Katrina M. Waters, Tao Liu, Brian Thrall and H. Steven Wiley (2008). "Investigating the correspondence between transcriptomic and proteomic expression profiles using coupled cluster models". Bioinformatics. 24 (24): 2894–2900. doi:10.1093/bioinformatics/btn553. PMC 4141638Freely accessible. PMID 18974169.
9. Vikas Dhingraa, Mukta Gupta, Tracy Andacht and Zhen F. Fu (2005). "New frontiers in proteomics research: A perspective". International Journal of Pharmaceutics. 299 (1–2): 1–18. doi:10.1016/j.ijpharm.2005.04.010. PMID 15979831.
10. Buckingham, Steven (May 2003). "The major world of microRNAs". Retrieved 2009-01-14.
11. Olsen JV, Blagoev B, Gnad F, Macek B, Kumar C, Mortensen P, Mann M; Blagoev; Gnad; Macek; Kumar; Mortensen; Mann (2006). "Global, in vivo, and site-specific phosphorylation dynamics in signaling networks". Cell. 127

(3): 635–648. doi:10.1016/j.cell.2006.09.026. PMID 17081983.

12. Srinivas, PR; Verma, M; Zhao, Y; Srivastava, S (August 2002). "Proteomics for cancer biomarker discovery". Clinical Chemistry. 48 (8): 1160–9. PMID 12142368.
13. Gygi, S. P.; Rochon, Y.; Franza, B. R.; Aebersold, R. (1999). "Correlation between protein and mRNA abundance in yeast". Molecular and Cellular Biology. 19 (3): 1720–1730. PMC 83965Freely accessible. PMID 10022859.
14. Archana Belle, Amos Tanay, Ledion Bitincka, Ron Shamir and Erin K. O'Shea (2006). "Quantification of protein half-lives in the budding yeast proteome". PNAS. 103 (35): 13004–13009. Bibcode:2006PNAS..10313004B. doi:10.1073/pnas.0605420103. PMC 1550773Freely accessible. PMID 16916930.
15. Peng, J.; Elias, J. E.; Thoreen, C. C.; Licklider, L. J.; Gygi, S. P. (2003). "Evaluation of multidimensional chromatography coupled with tandem mass spectrometry (LC/LC-MS/MS) for large-scale protein analysis: The yeast proteome". Journal of Proteome Research. 2 (1): 43–50. doi:10.1021/pr025556v. PMID 12643542.
16. Washburn, M. P.; Wolters, D.; Yates, J. R. (2001). "Large-scale analysis of the yeast proteome by multidimensional protein identification technology". Nature Biotechnology. 19 (3): 242–247. doi:10.1038/85686. PMID 11231557.
17. Tabb, DL; Vega-Montoto, L; Rudnick, PA; Variyath, AM; Ham, AJ; Bunk, DM; Kilpatrick, LE; Billheimer, DD; Blackman, RK; Cardasis, HL; Carr, SA; Clauser, KR; Jaffe, JD; Kowalski, KA; Neubert, TA; Regnier, FE; Schilling, B; Tegeler, TJ; Wang, M; Wang, P; Whiteaker, JR; Zimmerman, LJ; Fisher, SJ; Gibson, BW; Kinsinger, CR; Mesri, M; Rodriguez, H; Stein, SE; Tempst, P; Paulovich, AG; Liebler, DC; Spiegelman, C (5 February 2010). "Repeatability and reproducibility in proteomic identifications by liquid chromatography-tandem mass spectrometry". Journal of Proteome Research. 9 (2): 761–76. doi:10.1021/pr9006365. PMC 2818771Freely accessible. PMID 19921851.
18. Domon, Bruno; Aebersold, Ruedi (9 July 2010). "Options and considerations when selecting a quantitative proteomics strategy". Nature Biotechnology. 28 (7): 710–721. doi:10.1038/nbt.1661. PMID 20622845.
19. Nelson, Randall W.; Krone, Jennifer R.; Bieber, Allan L.; Williams, Peter. (1995). "Mass Spectrometric Immunoassay". Analytical Chemistry. 67 (7): 1153–1158. doi:10.1021/ac00103a003. ISSN 0003-2700. PMID 15134097.
20. https://www.broadinstitute.org/scientific-community/science/platforms/proteomics/siscapa
21. Tonge R, Shaw J, Middleton B, et al. (March 2001). "Validation and development of fluorescence two-dimensional differential gel electrophoresis proteomics technology". Proteomics. 1 (3): 377–96. doi:10.1002/1615-9861(200103)1:3<377::AID-PROT377>3.0.CO;2-6. PMID 11680884.
22. Li-Ping Wang, Jun Shen, Lin-Quan Ge, Jin-Cai Wu, Guo-Qin Yang, Gary C. Jahn; Shen; Ge; Wu; Yang; Jahn (November 2010). "Insecticide-induced increase in the protein content of male accessory glands and its effect on the fecundity of females

in the brown planthopper, Nilaparvata lugens Stål (Hemiptera: Delphacidae)". Crop Protection. 29 (11): 1280–5. doi:10.1016/j.cropro.2010.07.009.

23. Ge, Lin-Quan; Cheng, Yao; Wu, Jin-Cai; Jahn, Gary C. (2011). "Proteomic Analysis of Insecticide Triazophos-Induced Mating-Responsive Proteins ofNilaparvata lugensStål (Hemiptera: Delphacidae)". Journal of Proteome Research. 10 (10): 4597–612. doi:10.1021/pr200414g. PMID 21800909.

24. Reumann S (May 2011). "Toward a definition of the complete proteome of plant peroxisomes: Where experimental proteomics must be complemented by bioinformatics". Proteomics. 11 (9): 1764–79. doi:10.1002/pmic.201000681. PMID 21472859.

25. Uhlen M, Ponten F; Ponten (April 2005). "Antibody-based proteomics for human tissue profiling". Mol. Cell Proteomics. 4 (4): 384–93. doi:10.1074/mcp. R500009-MCP200. PMID 15695805.

26. Ole Nørregaard Jensen (2004). "Modification-specific proteomics: characterization of post-translational modifications by mass spectrometry". Current Opinion in Chemical Biology. 8 (1): 33–41. doi:10.1016/j.cbpa.2003.12.009. PMID 15036154.

27. Klopfleisch R, Klose P, Weise C, Bondzio A, Multhaup G, Einspanier R, Gruber AD.; Klose; Weise; Bondzio; Multhaup; Einspanier; Gruber (2010). "Proteome of metastatic canine mammary carcinomas: similarities to and differences from human breast cancer". J Proteome Res. 9 (12): 6380–91. doi:10.1021/pr100671c. PMID 20932060.

28. Alinejad 2015.

29. Weston, Andrea D.; Hood, Leroy (2004). "Systems Biology, Proteomics, and the Future of Health Care: Toward Predictive, Preventative, and Personalized Medicine". Journal of Proteome Research. 3 (2): 179–96. doi:10.1021/pr0499693. PMID 15113093.

30. Vaidyanathan G (March 2012). "Redefining clinical trials: the age of personalized medicine". Cell. 148 (6): 1079–80. doi:10.1016/j.cell.2012.02.041. PMID 22424218.

31. Rakwal, Randeep; Komatsu, Setsuko (2000). "Role of jasmonate in the rice (Oryza sativa L.) self-defense mechanism using proteome analysis". Electrophoresis. 21 (12): 2492–500. doi:10.1002/1522-2683(20000701)21:12<2492::AID-ELPS2492>3.0.CO;2-2. PMID 10939463.

32. Wu, Jianqiang; Baldwin, Ian T. (2010). "New Insights into Plant Responses to the Attack from Insect Herbivores". Annual Review of Genetics. 44: 1–24. doi:10.1146/annurev-genet-102209-163500. PMID 20649414.

33. Sangha J.S.; Chen Y.H.; Kaur Jatinder; Khan Wajahatullah; Abduljaleel Zainularifeen; Alanazi Mohammed S.; Mills Aaron; Adalla Candida B.; Bennett John; et al. (2013). "Proteome Analysis of Rice (Oryza sativa L.) Mutants Reveals Differentially Induced Proteins during Brown Planthopper (Nilaparvata lugens) Infestation". Int. J. Mo Sci. 14 (2): 3921–3945. doi:10.3390/ijms14023921. PMC 3588078Freely accessible. PMID 23434671.

34. de Mol, NJ (2012). "Surface plasmon resonance for proteomics". Methods in molecular biology (Clifton, N.J.). Methods in Molecular Biology. 800: 33–53. doi:10.1007/978-1-61779-349-3_4. ISBN 978-1-61779-348-6. PMID 21964781.
35. Visser, NF; Heck, AJ (June 2008). "Surface plasmon resonance mass spectrometry in proteomics.". Expert review of proteomics. 5 (3): 425–33. doi:10.1586/14789450.5.3.425. PMID 18532910.
36. Bensimon, Ariel; Heck, Albert J.R.; Aebersold, Ruedi (7 July 2012). "Mass Spectrometry–Based Proteomics and Network Biology". Annual Review of Biochemistry. 81 (1): 379–405. doi:10.1146/annurev-biochem-072909-100424.
37. Sabidó, Eduard; Selevsek, Nathalie; Aebersold, Ruedi (August 2012). "Mass spectrometry-based proteomics for systems biology". Current Opinion in Biotechnology. 23 (4): 591–597. doi:10.1016/j.copbio.2011.11.014. PMID 22169889.
38. "What is Proteomics?". ProteoConsult.[unreliable medical source?]
39. Strimbu, Kyle; Tavel, Jorge A (2010). "What are biomarkers?". Current Opinion in HIV and AIDS. 5 (6): 463–6. doi:10.1097/COH.0b013e32833ed177. PMC 3078627Freely accessible. PMID 20978388.
40. Biomarkers Definitions Working Group (2001). "Biomarkers and surrogate endpoints: preferred definitions and conceptual framework". Clinical Pharmacology & Therapeutics. 69 (3): 89–95. doi:10.1067/mcp.2001.113989. PMID 11240971.
41. Ceciliani, F; Eckersall D; Burchmore R; Lecchi C (March 2014). "Proteomics in veterinary medicine: applications and trends in disease pathogenesis and diagnostics". Veterinary Pathology. 51 (2): 351–362. doi:10.1177/0300985813502819. PMID 24045891.
42. Klopfleisch R, Gruber AD; Gruber (2009). "Increased expression of BRCA2 and RAD51 in lymph node metastases of canine mammary adenocarcinomas". Veterinary Pathology. 46 (3): 416–22. doi:10.1354/vp.08-VP-0212-K-FL. PMID 19176491.
43. Hathout, Yetrib (2007). "Approaches to the study of the cell secretome". Expert Review of Proteomics. 4 (2): 239–48. doi:10.1586/14789450.4.2.239. PMID 17425459.
44. Gupta N, Tanner S, Jaitly N, et al. (September 2007). "Whole proteome analysis of post-translational modifications: applications of mass-spectrometry for proteogenomic annotation". Genome Res. 17 (9): 1362–77. doi:10.1101/gr.6427907. PMC 1950905Freely accessible. PMID 17690205.
45. Gupta N, Benhamida J, Bhargava V, et al. (July 2008). "Comparative proteogenomics: combining mass spectrometry and comparative genomics to analyze multiple genomes". Genome Res. 18 (7): 1133–42. doi:10.1101/gr.074344.107. PMC 2493402Freely accessible. PMID 18426904.
46. Wang H, Chu C, Wang W, Pai T; Chu; Wang; Pai (April 2014). "A local average distance descriptor for flexible protein structure comparison". BMC Bioinformatics. 15 (95): 1471–2105. doi:10.1186/1471-2105-15-95. PMC 3992163Freely accessible. PMID 24694083.

47. Petrov D, Margreitter C, Gandits M, Ostenbrink C, Zagrovic B; Margreitter; Grandits; Oostenbrink; Zagrovic (July 2013). "A systematic framework for molecular dynamics simulations of protein post-translational modifications". PLoS Computational Biology. 9 (7): e1003154. Bibcode:2013PLSCB...9E3154P. doi:10.1371/journal.pcbi.1003154. PMC 3715417Freely accessible. PMID 23874192.

48. Margreitter C, Petro D, Zagrovic B; Petrov; Zagrovic (May 2013). "Vienna-PTM web server: a toolkit for MD simulations of portein post-translational modifications". Nucl. Acids Res. 41 (Web Server issue): W422–6. doi:10.1093/nar/gkt416. PMC 3692090Freely accessible. PMID 23703210.

49. Maron JL, Alterovitz G, Ramoni M, Johnson KL, Bianchi DW; Alterovitz; Ramoni; Johnson; Bianchi (December 2009). "High-throughput discovery and characterization of fetal protein trafficking in the blood of pregnant women". Proteomics: Clinical Applications. 3 (12): 1389–96. doi:10.1002/prca.200900109. PMC 2825712Freely accessible. PMID 20186258.

50. Alterovitz G, Xiang M, Liu J, Chang A, Ramoni MF; Xiang; Liu; Chang; Ramoni (2008). "System-wide peripheral biomarker discovery using information theory". Pacific Symposium on Biocomputing: 231–42. doi:10.1142/9789812776136_0024. ISBN 9789812776082. PMID 18229689.

51. Li, Jun; Lu, Yiling; Akbani, Rehan; Ju, Zhenlin; Roebuck, Paul L.; Liu, Wenbin; Yang, Ji-Yeon; Broom, Bradley M.; Verhaak, Roeland G. W. (2013-11-01). "TCPA: a resource for cancer functional proteomics data". Nature Methods. 10 (11): 1046–1047. doi:10.1038/nmeth.2650. ISSN 1548-7091. PMC 4076789Freely accessible. PMID 24037243.

CHAPTER 3

Globular Protein and Glycoproteomics

Chapter Contents

In a globular protein, the amino acid chain twists and folds in a manner that enhances the protein's solubility in water by placing polar groups of atoms at the protein's surface (where they can participate in attractive interactions with water molecules). This twisting and folding that determine the overall shape of a protein molecule (its tertiary structure) are due largely to the very complex interplay of intramolecular forces that exists among different groups of atoms within the molecule, and to intermolecular forces acting between groups of atoms on the protein and molecules in the protein's immediate surroundings. Some of the common amino acids have polar side chains; this polarity is the result of chemical bonds between atoms in these side chains that have very different electronegativities (for instance, oxygen and hydrogen). A protein's polar side chains tend to exert strong attractive forces toward other polar groups of atoms within the protein molecule, or toward polar molecules in the protein's surroundings. Similarly, nonpolar side chains exert attractive forces (of a different nature) toward other non-polar side chains within the protein. The shape assumed by a globular protein molecule tends to maximize both types of attractive forces, whereby nonpolar side chains "point" inward and interact with one another and polar side chains are oriented outward such that they are exposed to adjacent polar water molecules.

Glycoproteomics, as distinct from proteomics or glycomics, is the study of the glycosylation of proteins, a covalent modification which confers altered physico-chemical properties and functional activity on the nascent protein chain.

INTRODUCTION

Globular proteins or spheroproteins are spherical ("globe-like") proteins and are one of the common protein types (the others being fibrous, disordered and membrane proteins). Globular proteins are somewhat water-soluble (forming colloids in water), unlike the fibrous or membrane proteins. There are multiple fold classes of globular proteins, since there are many different architectures that can fold into a roughly spherical shape.

The term globin can refer more specifically to proteins including the globin fold.

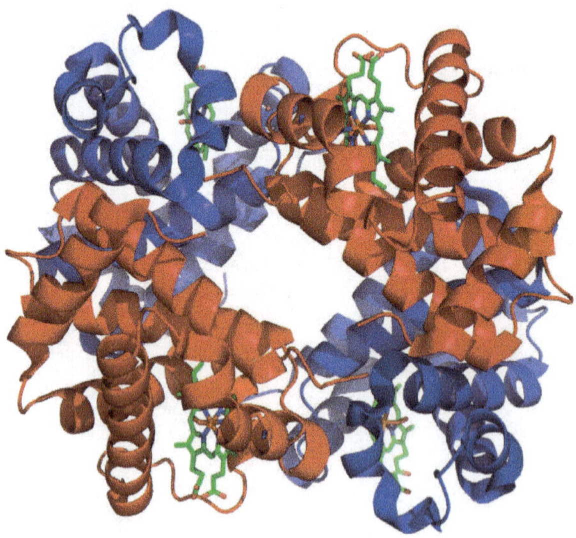

3-dimensional structure of hemoglobin, a globular protein.

GLOBULAR STRUCTURE AND SOLUBILITY

The term globular protein is quite old (dating probably from the 19th century) and is now somewhat archaic given the hundreds of thousands of proteins and more elegant and descriptive structural motif vocabulary. The globular nature of these proteins can be determined without the means of modern techniques, but only by using ultracentrifuges or dynamic light scattering techniques.

The spherical structure is induced by the protein's tertiary structure. The molecule's apolar (hydrophobic) amino acids are bounded towards the molecule's interior whereas polar (hydrophilic) amino acids are bound outwards, allowing dipole-dipole interactions with the solvent, which explains the molecule's solubility.

Globular proteins are only marginally stable because the free energy released when the protein folded into its native conformation is relatively small. This is because protein folding requires entropic cost. As a primary sequence of a polypeptide chain can form numerous conformations, native globular structure restricts its conformation to a few only. It results in a decrease in randomness, although non-covalent interactions such as hydrophobic interactions stabilize the structure.

Although it is still unknown how proteins fold up naturally, new evidence has helped advance understanding. Part of the protein folding problem is that several non-covalent, weak interactions are formed, such as hydrogen bonds and Van der Waals interactions. Via several techniques, the mechanism of protein folding is currently being studied. Even in the protein's denatured state, it can be folded into the correct structure.

Globular proteins seem to have two mechanisms for protein folding, either the diffusion-collision model or nucleation condensation model, although recent findings have shown globular proteins, such as PTP-BL PDZ2, that fold with characteristic features of both models. These new findings have shown that the transition states of proteins may affect the way they fold. The folding of globular proteins has also recently been connected to treatment of diseases, and anti-cancer ligands have been developed which bind to the folded but not the natural protein. These studies have shown that the folding of globular proteins affects its function.

By the second law of thermodynamics, the free energy difference between unfolded and folded states is contributed by enthalpy and entropy changes. As the free energy difference in a globular protein that results from folding into its native conformation is small, it is marginally stable, thus providing a rapid turnover rate and effective control of protein degradation and synthesis.

Role

Unlike fibrous proteins which only play a structural function, globular proteins can act as:

- Enzymes, by catalyzing organic reactions taking place in the organism in mild conditions and with a great specificity. Different esterases fulfill this role.
- Messengers, by transmitting messages to regulate biological processes. This function is done by hormones, i.e. insulin etc.
- Transporters of other molecules through membranes
- Stocks of amino acids.
- Regulatory roles are also performed by globular proteins rather than fibrous proteins.
- Structural proteins, e.g., actin and tubulin, which are globular and soluble as monomers, but polymerize to form long, stiff fibers

Members

Among the most known globular proteins is hemoglobin, a member of the globin protein family. Other globular proteins are the immunoglobulins (IgA, IgD, IgE, IgG and IgM), and alpha, beta and gamma globulins. See protein electrophoresis for more information on the different globulins. Nearly all enzymes with major metabolic functions are globular in shape, as well as many signal transduction proteins.

Albumins are also globular proteins, although, unlike all of the other globular proteins, they are completely soluble in water.

GLYCOPROTEOMICS

Glycoproteomics is a branch of proteomics that identifies, catalogs, and characterizes proteins containing carbohydrates as a posttranslational modification.

Phosphoproteomics

Phosphoproteomics is a branch of proteomics that identifies, catalogs, and characterizes proteins containing a phosphate group as a post-translational modification. Phosphorylation is a key reversible modification that regulates protein function, subcellular localization, complex formation, degradation of proteins and therefore cell signaling networks. With all of these modification results, it is assumed that up to 30% of all proteins may be phosphorylated, some multiple times.

Compared to expression analysis, phosphoproteomics provides two additional layers of information. First, it provides clues on what protein or pathway might be activated because a change in phosphorylation status almost always reflects a change in protein activity. Second, it indicates what proteins might be potential drug targets as exemplified by the kinase inhibitor Gleevec. While phosphoproteomics will greatly expand knowledge about the numbers and types of phosphoproteins, its greatest promise is the rapid analysis of entire phosphorylation based signalling networks.

Overview of Phosphoproteomic Analysis

A sample large-scale phosphoproteomic analysis includes

- Cultured cells undergo SILAC encoding.
- Cells are stimulated with factor of interest (e.g. growth factor, hormone).
- Stimulation can occur for various lengths of time for temporal analysis.
- Cells are lysed and enzymatically digested.
- Peptides are separated using ion exchange chromatography.
- Phosphopeptides are enriched using phosphospecific antibodies, immobilized metal affinity chromatography or titanium dioxide (TiO_2) chromatography.
- Phosphopeptides are analyzed using mass spectrometry.

- Peptides are sequenced and analyzed.

Tools and Methods

The analysis of the entire complement of phosphorylated proteins in a cell is certainly a feasible option. This is due to the optimization of enrichment protocols for phosphoproteins and phosphopeptides, better fractionation techniques using chromatography, and improvement of methods to selectively visualize phosphorylated residues using mass spectrometry. Although the current procedures for phosphoproteomic analysis are greatly improved, there is still sample loss and inconsistencies with regards to sample preparation, enrichment, and instrumentation. Bioinformatics tools and biological sequence databases are also necessary for high-throughput phosphoproteomic studies.

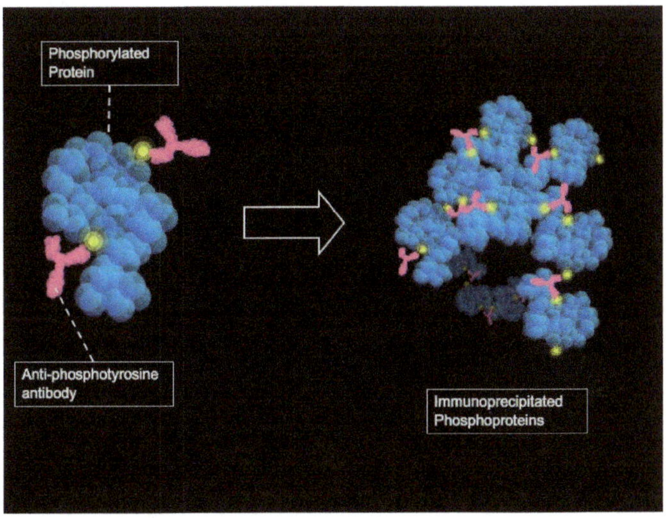

Method of phosphoprotein purification by immunoprecipitation with anti-phosohotyrosine antibodies

Enrichment Strategies

Previous procedures to isolate phosphorylated proteins included radioactive labeling with ^{32}P-labeled ATP followed by SDS polyacrylamide gel electrophoresis or thin layer chromatography. These traditional methods are inefficient because it is impossible to obtain large amounts of proteins required for phosphorylation analysis. Therefore, the current and simplest methods to enrich phosphoproteins are affinity purification using phosphospecific antibodies, immobilized metal affinity chromatography (IMAC), strong cation exchange (SCX) chromatography, or titanium dioxide chromatography. Antiphosphotyrosine antibodies have been proven very successful in purification, but fewer reports have been published using antibodies against phosphoserine- or phosphothreonine-containing proteins. IMAC enrichment is based on phosphate affinity for immobilized metal chelated to the resin. SCX separates phosphorylated from non-phosphorylated peptides based on the negatively charged phosphate group. Titanium dioxide chromatography is a newer technique that requires significantly less column preparation time. Many phosphoproteomic studies use a combination of these enrichment strategies to obtain the purest sample possible.

Mass Spectrometry Analysis

Mass spectrometry is currently the best method to adequately compare pairs of protein samples. The two main procedures to perform this task are using isotope-coded affinity tags (ICAT) and stable isotopic amino acids in cell culture (SILAC). In the ICAT procedure samples are labeled individually after isolation with mass-coded reagents that modify cysteine residues. In SILAC, cells are cultured separately in the presence of different isotopically labeled amino acids for several cell divisions allowing cellular proteins to incorporate the label. Mass spectrometry is subsequently used to identify phosphoserine, phosphothreonine, and phosphotyrosine-containing peptides.

Phosphoproteomics in the Study of Signal Transduction

Intracellular signal transduction is primarily mediated by the reversible phosphorylation of various signaling molecules by enzymes dubbed kinases. Kinases transfer phosphate groups from ATP to specific serine, threonine or tyrosine residues of target molecules. The resultant phosphorylated protein may have altered activity level, subcellular localization or tertiary structure.

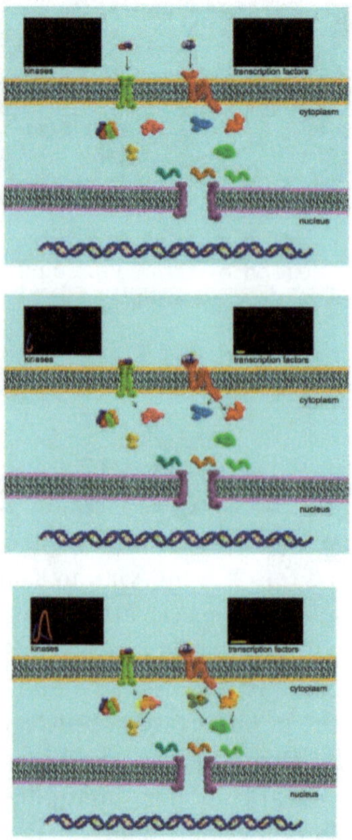

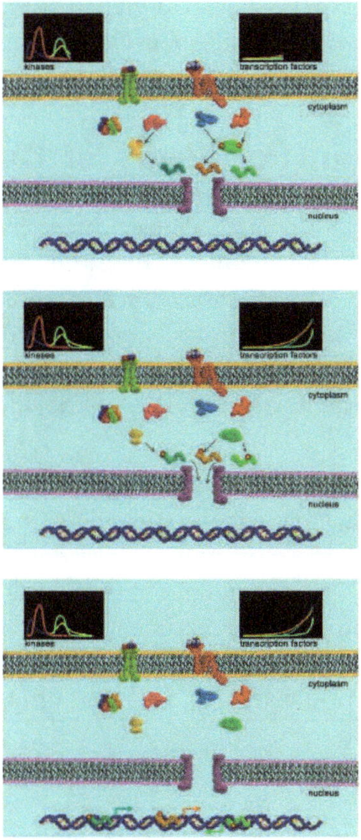

Analysis of Signal Transduction Dynamics

Phosphoproteomic analyses are ideal for the study of the dynamics of signalling networks. In one study design, cells are exposed to SILAC labelling and then stimulated by a specific growth factor. The cells are collected at various timepoints, and the lysates are combined for analysis by tandem MS. This allows experimenters to track the phosphorylation state of many phosphoproteins in the cell over time. The ability to measure the global phosphorylation state of many proteins at various time points makes this approach much more powerful than traditional biochemical methods for analyzing signalling network behavior.

One study was able to simultaneously measure the fold-change in phosphorylation state of 127 proteins between unstimulated and EphrinB1-stimulated cells. Of these 127 proteins, 40 showed increased phosphorylation with stimulation by EphrinB1. The researchers were able to use this information in combination with previously published data to construct a signal transduction network for the proteins downstream of the EphB2 receptor.

Another recent phosphoproteomic study included large-scale identification and quantification of phosphorylation events triggered by the anti-diuretic hormone vasopressin in kidney collecting duct. A total of 714 phosphorylation sites on 223 unique phosphoproteins were identified, including three novel phosphorylation sites in the vasopressin-sensitive water channel aquaporin-2 (AQP2).

Phosphoproteomics in the Study of Cancer

Since the inception of phosphoproteomics, cancer research has focused on changes to the phosphoproteome during tumor development. Phosphoproteins could be cancer markers useful to cancer diagnostics and therapeutics. In fact, research has shown that there are distinct phosphotyrosine proteomes of breast and liver tumors. There is also evidence of hyperphosphorylation at tyrosine residues in breast tumors but not in normal tissues. Findings like these suggest that it is possible to mine the tumor phosphoproteome for potential biomarkers.

Increasing amounts of data are available suggesting that distinctive phosphoproteins exist in various tumors and that phosphorylation profiling could be used to fingerprint cancers from different origins. In addition, systematic cataloguing of tumor-specific phosphoproteins in individual patients could reveal multiple causative players during cancer formation. By correlating this experimental data to clinical data such as drug response and disease outcome, potential cancer markers could be identified for diagnosis, prognosis, prediction of drug response, and potential drug targets.

Limitations

While phosphoproteomics has greatly expanded knowledge about the numbers and types of phosphoproteins, along with their role in signaling networks, there are still a few limitations to these techniques. To begin with, isolation methods such as anti-phosphotyrosine antibodies do not distinguish between isolating tyrosine-phosphorylated proteins and proteins associated with tyrosine-phosphorylated proteins. Therefore, even though phosphorylation dependent protein-protein interactions are very important, it is important to remember that a protein detected by this method is not necessarily a direct substrate of any tyrosine kinase. Only by digesting the samples before immunoprecipitation can isolation of only phosphoproteins and temporal profiles of individual phosphorylation sites be produced. Another limitation is that some relevant proteins will likely be missed since no extraction condition is all encompassing. It is possible that proteins with low stoichiometry of phosphorylation, in very low abundance, or phosphorylated as a target for rapid degradation will be lost.

GPM (PROTEOMICS)

In proteomics, GPM stands for "Global Proteome Machine". It is a web-based, open source user interface for analyzing and displaying protein identification data. It was originally designed by Rob Craig and Ron Beavis and first released in 2003. The interface creates a series of web browser page views of tandem mass spectrometry data that has been assigned to protein sequences. The underlying data documents are stored in BIOML format files.

Since its original creation, GPM has been under continuous development. Major developments include the following:

- Creation of GPMDB: a large proteomics database generated using GPM;
- Inclusion in the Human proteome project as a data analysis and information resource;
- Development of a REST API for GPMDB.

REFERENCES

1. Andreeva, A (2014). "SCOP2 prototype: a new approach to protein structure mining". Nucleic Acids Res. 42: D310–4. doi:10.1093/nar/gkt1242. PMC 3964979Freely accessible. PMID 24293656.
2. Globins at the US National Library of Medicine Medical Subject Headings (MeSH)
3. Travaglini-Allocatelli C; Ivarsson Y; Jemth P; Gianni S (Feb 2009). "Folding and stability of globular proteins and implications for function". Current Opinion in Structural Biology. 19 (1): 3–7. doi:10.1016/j.sbi.2008.12.001.
4. Lim, Y. (2005). "Mining the tumor phosphoproteome for cancer markers". Clin Cancer Res. 11 (9): 3163–3169. doi:10.1158/1078-0432.CCR-04-2243. PMID 15867208.
5. Olsen, JV; Blagoev, B; Gnad, F; Macek, B; Kumar, C; Mortensen, P; Mann, M (2006). "Global, in vivo, and site-specific phosphorylation dynamics in signaling networks". Cell. 127 (3): 635–48. doi:10.1016/j.cell.2006.09.026. PMID 17081983.
6. Kalume, D.; Molina, H; Pandey, A (2003). "Tackling the phosphoproteome: tools and strategies". Current Opinion in Chemical Biology. 7 (1): 64–69. doi:10.1016/S1367-5931(02)00009-1. PMID 12547428.
7. Schmelzle, K.; White, F. (2006). "Phosphoproteomic approaches to ellucidate cellular signaling networks". Current Opinion in Chemical Biology. 17 (4): 406–414. doi:10.1016/j.copbio.2006.06.004.
8. Mumby, M; Brekken, D (2005). "Phosphoproteomics: new insights into cellular signaling". Genome Biology. 6 (9): 230. doi:10.1186/gb-2005-6-9-230. PMC 1242200Freely accessible. PMID 16168091.
9. Zhang; Spellman, DS; Skolnik, EY; Neubert, TA (2006). "Quantitative Phosphotyrosine Proteomics of EphB2 Signaling by Stable Isotope Labeling with Amino Acids in Cell Culture (SILAC)". J. Proteome Res. 5 (3): 581–8. doi:10.1021/pr050362b. PMC 2542903Freely accessible. PMID 16512673.
10. Hoffert, JD; Pisitkun, Trairak; Wang, Guanghui; Shen, Rong-Fong; Knepper, MA (2006). "Quantitative phosphoproteomics of vasopressin-sensitive renal cells: regulation of aquaporin-2 phosphorylation at two sites". Proc Natl Acad Sci U S A. 103 (18): 7159–64. doi:10.1073/pnas.0600895103.

11. Johnson, S; Hunter, T. (2004). "Phosphoproteomics finds its timing". Nature Biotechnology. 22 (9): 1093–1094. doi:10.1038/nbt0904-1093.
12. Craig, Robertson; Cortens, John P.; Beavis, Ronald C. (2004). "Open Source System for Analyzing, Validating, and Storing Protein Identification Data". Journal of Proteome Research. 3 (6): 1234–42. doi:10.1021/pr049882h. PMID 15595733.
13. Fenyo, D (1999). "The Biopolymer Markup Language". Bioinformatics. 15 (4): 339–40. doi:10.1093/bioinformatics/15.4.339. PMID 10320402.
14. Craig, Robertson; Cortens, John P.; Beavis, Ronald C. (2004). "Open Source System for Analyzing, Validating, and Storing Protein Identification Data". Journal of Proteome Research. 3 (6): 1234–1242. doi:10.1021/pr049882h. ISSN 1535-3893. PMID 15595733.
15. Omenn, Gilbert S.; Lane, Lydie; Lundberg, Emma K.; Beavis, Ronald C.; Nesvizhskii, Alexey I.; Deutsch, Eric W. (2015). "Metrics for the Human Proteome Project 2015: Progress on the Human Proteome and Guidelines for High-Confidence Protein Identification". Journal of Proteome Research. 14 (9): 3452–3460. doi:10.1021/acs.jproteome.5b00499. ISSN 1535-3893.
16. Fenyö, David; Beavis, Ronald C. (2015). "The GPMDB REST interface". Bioinformatics. 31 (12): 2056–2058. doi:10.1093/bioinformatics/btv107. ISSN 1367-4803.

CHAPTER 4

Protein Structure Prediction and Structural Alignment

Chapter Contents

- **Introduction**
- **Protein Structure and Terminology**
- **Protein Classification**
- **Secondary Structure**
- **Tertiary Structure**
- **Quaternary Structure**
- **Structural Alignment**
- **Macromolecular Docking**

Three-dimensional structures of proteins are the key to understanding their molecular function. Most reliably protein structures are determined by experiment. Recent advances in experimental techniques have lead to a large increase in numbers of both protein sequences and 3D structures. Yet, the number of experimentally resolved proteins 3D structures is three orders of magnitude lower than that of sequences. This calls for computer support of protein structure prediction. Today several databases complement the comparatively small set of experimentally resolved protein structures with much larger sets of protein models generated by computer.

INTRODUCTION

Protein structure prediction is the inference of the three-dimensional structure of a protein from its amino acid sequence—that is, the prediction of its folding and its secondary and tertiary structure from its primary structure. Structure prediction is fundamentally different from the inverse problem of protein design. Protein structure prediction is one of the most important goals pursued by bioinformatics and theoretical chemistry; it is highly important in medicine (for example, in drug design) and biotechnology (for example, in the design of novel enzymes). Every two years, the performance of current methods is assessed in the CASP experiment (Critical Assessment of Techniques for Protein Structure Prediction). A continuous evaluation of protein structure prediction web servers is performed by the community project CAMEO3D.

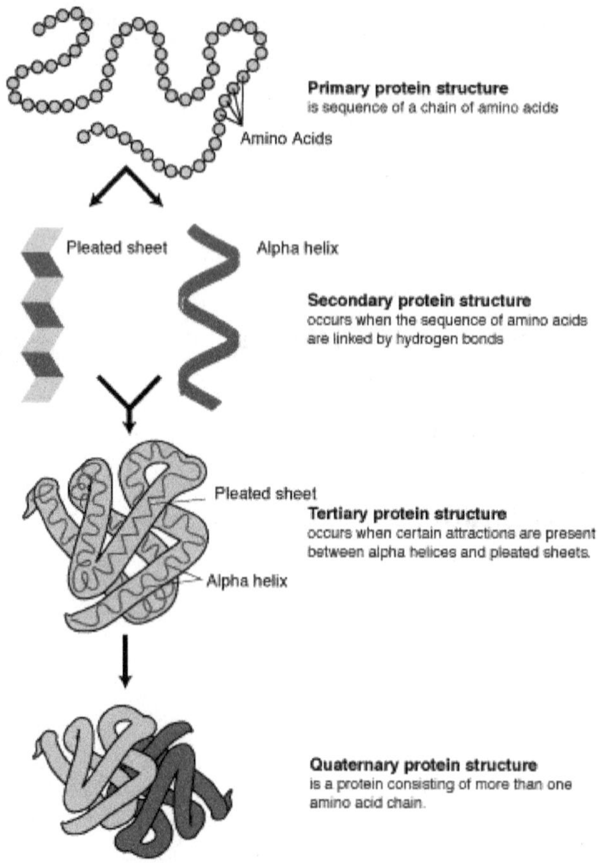

Constituent amino-acids can be analyzed to predict secondary, tertiary and quaternary protein structure.

PROTEIN STRUCTURE AND TERMINOLOGY

Proteins are chains of amino acids joined together by peptide bonds. Many conformations of this chain are possible due to the rotation of the chain about each Cα atom. It is these conformational changes that are responsible for differences in the three dimensional structure of proteins. Each amino acid in the chain is polar, i.e. it has separated positive and negative charged regions with a free C=O group, which can act as hydrogen bond acceptor and an NH group, which can act as hydrogen bond donor. These groups can therefore interact in the protein structure. The 20 amino acids can be classified according to the chemistry of the side chain which also plays an important structural role. Glycine takes on a special position, as it has the smallest side chain, only one Hydrogen atom, and therefore can increase the local flexibility in the protein structure. Cysteine on the other hand can react with another cysteine residue and thereby form a cross link stabilizing the whole structure.

The protein structure can be considered as a sequence of secondary structure elements, such as α helices and β sheets, which together constitute the overall three-dimensional configuration of the protein chain. In these secondary structures regular patterns of H bonds are formed between neighboring amino acids, and the amino acids have similar Φ and Ψ angles.

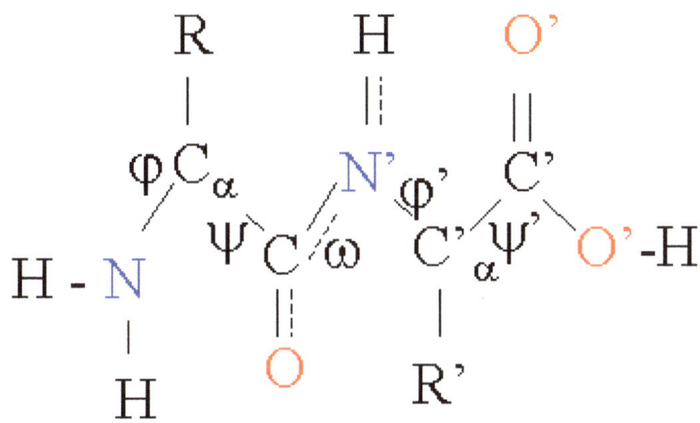

Bond angles for ψ and ω

The formation of these structures neutralizes the polar groups on each amino acid. The secondary structures are tightly packed in the protein core in a hydrophobic environment. Each amino acid side group has a limited volume to occupy and a limited number of possible interactions with other nearby side chains, a situation that must be taken into account in molecular modeling and alignments.

Alpha Helix

The alpha helix **(α-helix) is a common motif in the secondary structure of proteins and is a** righthand-coiled or spiral conformation (helix) in which every backbone N-H group donates a hydrogen bond to the backbone C=O group of the amino acid located three or four residues earlier along the protein sequence. This secondary structure is also sometimes called a classic Pauling–Corey–Branson α-helix (see below). The name 3.6_{13}-helix is also used for this type of helix, denoting the average number of residues per helical turn, with 13 atoms being involved in the ring formed by the hydrogen bond. Among types of local structure in proteins, the **α-helix** is the most regular and the most predictable from sequence, as well as the most prevalent.

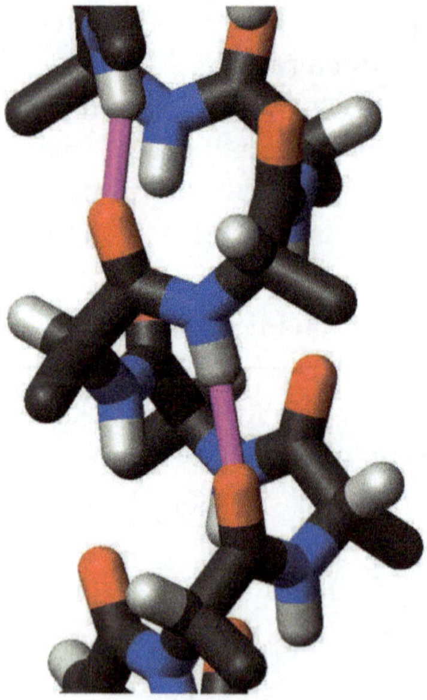

Side view of an **α-helix** of alanine residues in atomic detail. Two hydrogen bonds for the same peptide group are highlighted in magenta; the H to O distance is about 2 **Å** (0.20 nm). The protein chain runs upward here; that is, its N-terminus is at the bottom and its C-terminus at the top. Note that the sidechains (black stubs) angle slightly downward, toward the N-terminus, while the peptide oxygens (red) point up and the peptide NHs (blue with grey stubs) point down.

Discovery

In the early 1930s, William Astbury showed that there were drastic changes in the X-ray fiber diffraction of moist wool or hair fibers upon significant stretching. The data suggested that the unstretched fibers had a coiled molecular structure with a characteristic repeat of ~5.1 ångströms (0.51 nm).

Astbury initially proposed a kinked-chain structure for the fibers. He later joined other researchers (notably the American chemist Maurice Huggins) in proposing that:

- the unstretched protein molecules formed a helix (which he called the α-form)
- the stretching caused the helix to uncoil, forming an extended state (which he called the β-form).

Although incorrect in their details, Astbury›s models of these forms were correct in essence and correspond to modern elements of secondary structure, the α-helix and the β-strand (Astbury›s nomenclature was kept), which were developed by Linus Pauling, Robert Corey and Herman Branson in 1951 (see below); that paper showed both right- and left-handed helixes, although in 1960 the crystal structure of myoglobin showed that the right-handed form is the common one. Hans Neurath was the first to show that Astbury›s models could not be correct in detail, because they involved clashes of atoms. Neurath›s paper and Astbury›s data inspired H. S. Taylor,Maurice Huggins and Bragg and collaborators to propose models of keratin that somewhat resemble the modern α-helix.

Two key developments in the modeling of the modern α-helix were (1) the correct bond geometry, thanks to the crystal structure determinations of amino acids and peptides and Pauling›s prediction of *planar* peptide bonds; and (2) his relinquishing of the assumption of an integral number of residues per turn of the helix. The pivotal moment came in the early spring of 1948, when Pauling caught a cold and went to bed. Being bored, he drew a polypeptide chain of roughly correct dimensions on a strip of paper and folded it into a helix, being careful to maintain the planar peptide bonds. After a few attempts, he produced a model with physically plausible hydrogen bonds. Pauling then worked with Corey and Branson to confirm his model before publication. In 1954, Pauling was awarded his first Nobel Prize "for his research into the nature of the chemical bond and its application to the elucidation of the structure of complex substances" (such as proteins), prominently including the structure of the α-helix.

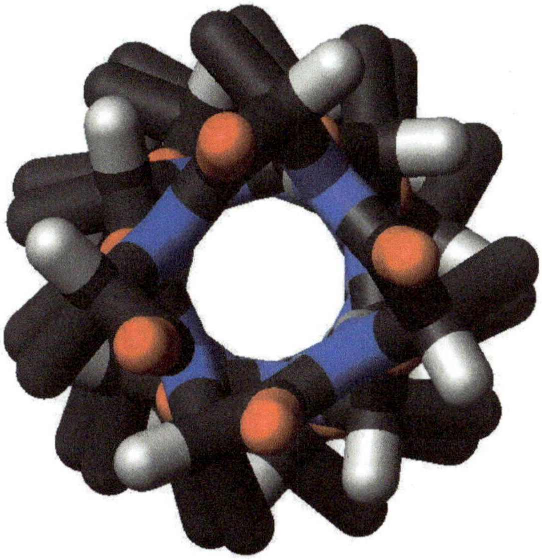

Top view of the same helix shown above. Four carbonyl groups are pointing upwards toward the viewer, spaced roughly 100° apart on the circle, corresponding to 3.6 amino-acid residues per turn of the helix.

Structure

Geometry and Hydrogen Bonding

The amino acids in an α-helix are arranged in a right-handed helical structure where each amino acid residue corresponds to a 100° turn in the helix (i.e., the helix has 3.6 residues per turn), and a translation of 1.5 Å (0.15 nm) along the helical axis. Dunitz describes how Pauling›s first article on the theme in fact shows a left-handed helix, the enantiomer of the true structure. Short pieces of left-handed helix sometimes occur with a large content of achiral glycine amino acids, but are unfavorable for the other normal, biological L-amino acids. The pitch of the alpha-helix (the vertical distance between consecutive turns of the helix) is 5.4 Å (0.54 nm), which is the product of 1.5 and 3.6. What is most important is that the N-H group of an amino acid forms a hydrogen bond with the C=O group of the amino acid *four* residues earlier; this repeated $i+4 \rightarrow i$ hydrogen bonding is the most prominent characteristic of an α-helix. Official international nomenclature specifies two ways of defining α-helices, rule 6.2 in terms of repeating φ,ψ torsion angles (see below) and rule 6.3 in terms of the combined pattern of pitch and hydrogen bonding. The alpha-helices can be identified in protein structure using several computational methods, one of which being DSSP (Dictionary of Protein Secondary Structure).

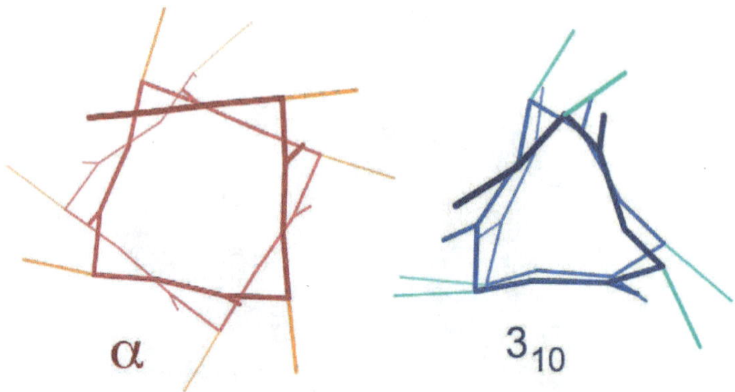

Contrast of helix end views between α (offset squarish) vs 3_{10} (triangular)

Similar structures include the 3_{10} helix ($i+3 \rightarrow i$ hydrogen bonding) and the π-helix ($i+5 \rightarrow i$ hydrogen bonding). The α-helix can be described as a 3.6_{13} helix, since the i + 4 spacing adds 3 more atoms to the H-bonded loop compared to the tighter 3_{10}helix, and on average, 3.6 amino acids are involved in one ring of α-helix. The subscripts refer to the number of atoms (including the hydrogen) in the closed loop formed by the hydrogen bond.

Residues in α-helices typically adopt backbone (φ, ψ) dihedral angles around (-60°, -45°). In more general terms, they adopt dihedral angles such that the ψ dihedral angle of one residue and the φ dihedral angle of the *next* residue sum to roughly -105°. As a consequence, α-helical dihedral angles, in general, fall on a diagonal stripe on the Ramachandran diagram (of slope -1), ranging from (-90°, -15°) to (-35°, -70°). For comparison, the sum of the dihedral angles for a 3_{10} helix is roughly -75°, whereas that for the π-helix is roughly -130°. The general formula for the rotation angle Ω per residue of any polypeptide helix with *trans* isomers is given by the equation

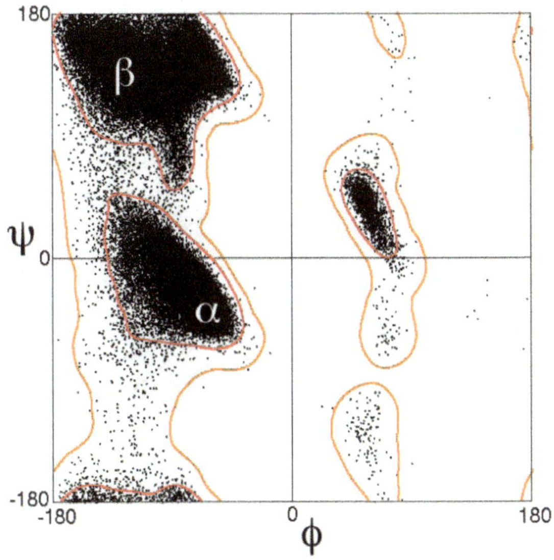

Ramachandran plot (φ,ψ plot), with data points for α-helical residues forming a dense diagonal cluster below and left of center, around the global energy minimum for backbone conformation.

$$3\cos\Omega = 1 - 4\cos^2[(\phi + \psi)/2]$$

The α-helix is tightly packed; there is almost no free space within the helix. The amino-acid side-chains are on the outside of the helix, and point roughly "downward " (i.e., toward the N-terminus), like the branches of an evergreen tree (Christmas tree effect). This directionality is sometimes used in preliminary, low-resolution electron-density maps to determine the direction of the protein backbone.

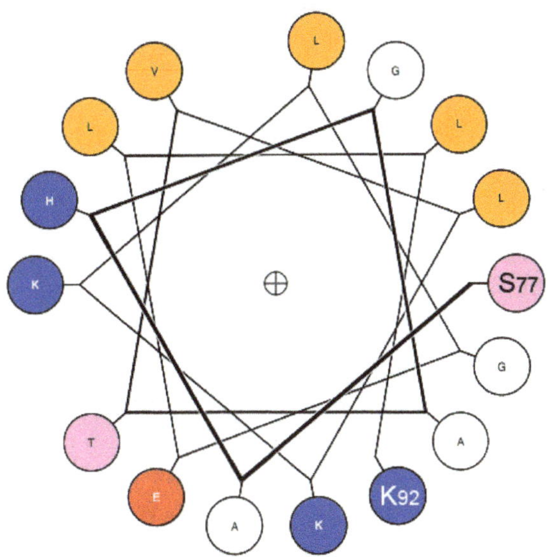

Helical wheel diagram

2D (2-Dimensional) Diagrams for Representing α-Helices

Three differently arranged styles of 2D diagrams are used to represent different aspects of the sequence and structure relationships that confer specific physical and interaction properties on individual α-helices. Two of these emphasize circular placement around the cylindrical cross-section: The first-developed such diagram is called the "helical wheel ", and a more recent version is called the "wenxiang diagram ". The latter name came from the fact that it resembles a coil-like incense used in China to repel mosquitos.

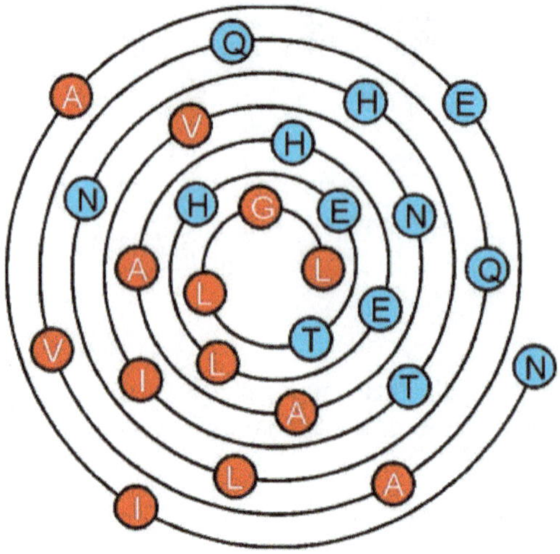

Wenxiang diagram

The helical wheel represents a helix by a projection of the Cα backbone structure down the helix axis, while the wenxiang diagram represents it more abstractly as a smooth spiral coiled on the plane of the page. Both label the sequence with one-letter amino-acid code (see amino acid) at each Cα position, using different colors or symbols to code the amino-acid properties. Hydrophobic vs hydrophilic amino acids are always distinguished, as the most important property governing helix interactions. Sometimes positively vs negatively charged hydrophilics are distinguished, and sometimes ambiguous amino acids such as glycine (G) are distinguished. Color-coding conventions are various. The helical wheel does not change representation along the helix, while the wenxiang diagram is able to show the relative locations of the amino acids in an α-helix regardless of how long it is.

Either circular style of diagram can provide an intuitive and easily visualizable 2D picture that characterizes the disposition of hydrophobic and hydrophilic residues in α-helices, and can be used to study helix-helix interactions, helix-membrane interactions as quantified by the helical hydrophobic moment, or protein-protein interactions. Various utilities and web sites are available to generate helical wheels, such as the page by Kael Fischer.

The third style of 2D diagram is called a "helical net ". It is generated by opening the cylindrical surface of each helix along a line parallel to the axis and laying the result out vertically. The helix net is not suitable for studying helix-helix packing interactions, but it has become the dominant means of representing the sequence arrangement for integral membrane proteins because it shows important relationships of the helical sequence to vertical positioning within the membrane even without knowledge of how the helices are arranged in 3D.

Stability

Helices observed in proteins can range from four to over forty residues long, but a typical helix contains about ten amino acids (about three turns). In general, short polypeptides do not exhibit much α-helical structure in solution, since the entropic cost associated with the folding of the polypeptide chain is not compensated for by a sufficient amount of stabilizing interactions. In general, the backbone hydrogen bonds of α-helices are considered slightly weaker than those found in β-sheets, and are readily attacked by the ambient water molecules. However, in more hydrophobic environments such as the plasma membrane, or in the presence of co-solvents such as trifluoroethanol (TFE), or isolated from solvent in the gas phase, oligopeptides readily adopt stable α-helical structure. Furthermore, crosslinks can be incorporated into peptides to conformationally stabilize helical folds. Crosslinks stabilize the helical state by entropically destabilizing the unfolded state and by removing enthalpically stabilized "decoy " folds that compete with the fully helical state.

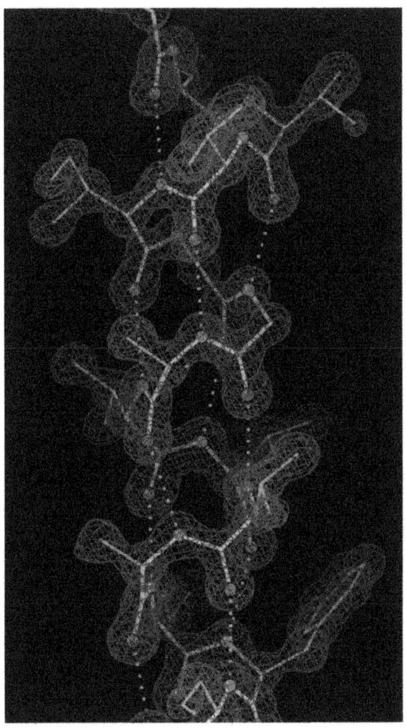

An α-helix in ultra-high-resolution electron density contours, with O atoms in red, N atoms in blue, and hydrogen bonds as green dotted lines (PDB file 2NRL, 17-32). The N-terminus is at the top, here.

Experimental Determination

Since the α-helix is defined by its hydrogen bonds and backbone conformation, the most detailed experimental evidence for α-helical structure comes from atomic-resolution X-ray crystallography.. It is clear that all the backbone carbonyl oxygens point downward (toward the C-terminus) but splay out slightly, and the H-bonds are approximately parallel to the helix axis. Protein structures from NMR spectroscopy also show helices well, with characteristic observations of nuclear Overhauser effect (NOE) couplings between atoms on adjacent helical turns. In some cases, the individual hydrogen bonds can be observed directly as a small scalar coupling in NMR.

There are several lower-resolution methods for assigning general helical structure. The NMR chemical shifts (in particular of the C^{α}, C^{β} and C' atoms) and residual dipolar couplings are often characteristic of helices. The far-UV (170-250 nm) circular dichroism spectrum of helices is also idiosyncratic, exhibiting a pronounced double minimum at ~208 nm and ~222 nm. Infrared spectroscopy is rarely used, since the α-helical spectrum resembles that of a random coil (although these might be discerned by, e.g., hydrogen-deuterium exchange). Finally, cryo electron microscopy is now capable of discerning individual α-helices within a protein, although their assignment to residues is still an active area of research.

Long homopolymers of amino acids often form helices if soluble. Such long, isolated helices can also be detected by other methods, such as dielectric relaxation, flow birefringence, and measurements of the diffusion constant. In stricter terms, these methods detect only the characteristic prolate (long cigar-like) hydrodynamic shape of a helix, or its large dipole moment.

Amino-Acid Propensities

Different amino-acid sequences have different propensities for forming α-helical structure. Methionine, alanine, leucine, glutamate, and lysine uncharged ("MALEK " in the amino-acid 1-letter codes) all have especially high helix-forming propensities, whereas proline and glycine have poor helix-forming propensities. Proline either breaks or kinks a helix, both because it cannot donate an amide hydrogen bond (having no amide hydrogen), and also because its sidechain interferes sterically with the backbone of the preceding turn - inside a helix, this forces a bend of about 30° in the helix axis. However, proline is often seen as the *first* residue of a helix, it is presumed due to its structural rigidity. At the other extreme, glycine also tends to disrupt helices because its high conformational flexibility makes it entropically expensive to adopt the relatively constrained α-helical structure.

Table of Standard Amino Acid Alpha-Helical Propensities

Estimated differences in free energy, $\Delta(\Delta G)$, estimated in kcal/mol per residue in an alpha-helical configuration, relative to Alanine arbitrarily set as zero. Higher numbers (more positive free energies) are less favoured. Significant deviations from these average numbers are possible, depending on the identities of the neighbouring residues.

Amino Acid	3-Letter	1-Letter	Helical Penalty (Kcal/mol)
Alanine	Ala	A	0
Arginine	Arg	R	0.21
Asparagine	Asn	N	0.65
Aspartic acid	Asp	D	0.69
Cysteine	Cys	C	0.68
Glutamic acid	Glu	E	0.40
Glutamine	Gln	Q	0.39
Glycine	Gly	G	1.00
Histidine	His	H	0.61
Isoleucine	Ile	I	0.41
Leucine	Leu	L	0.21
Lysine	Lys	K	0.26
Methionine	Met	M	0.24
Phenylalanine	Phe	F	0.54
Proline	Pro	P	3.16
Serine	Ser	S	0.50
Threonine	Thr	T	0.66
Tryptophan	Trp	W	0.49
Tyrosine	Tyr	Y	0.53
Valine	Val	V	0.61

Dipole Moment

A helix has an overall dipole moment due to the aggregate effect of the individual microdipoles from the carbonyl groups of the peptide bond pointing along the helix axis. The effects of this macrodipole are a matter of some controversy. α-helices often occur with the N-terminal end bound by a negatively charged group, sometimes an amino acid side chain such as glutamate or aspartate, or sometimes a phosphate ion. Some regard the helix macrodipole as interacting electrostatically with such groups. Others feel that this is misleading and it is more realistic to say that the hydrogen bond potential of the free NH groups at the N-terminus of an α-helix can be satisfied by hydrogen bonding; this can also be regarded as set of interactions between local microdipoles such as C=O...H-N.

Coiled-Coils

Coiled-coil α helices are highly stable forms in which two or more helices wrap around each other in a "supercoil " structure. Coiled coils contain a highly characteristic sequence motif known as a heptad repeat, in which the motif repeats itself every seven residues along the sequence (*amino acid* residues, not DNA base-pairs). The first and especially the fourth residues (known as the *a* and *d* positions) are almost always hydrophobic; the fourth residue is typically leucine - this gives rise to the name of the structural motif called a *leucine zipper*, which is a type of coiled-coil. These hydrophobic residues and pack together in the interior of the helix bundle. In general, the fifth and seventh residues (the *e* and *g* positions) have opposing charges and form a salt bridge stabilized by electrostatic interactions. Fibrous proteins such as keratin or the "stalks" of myosin or kinesin often adopt coiled-coil structures, as do several dimerizing proteins. A pair of coiled-coils - a four-helix bundle - is a very common structural motif in proteins. For example, it occurs in human growth hormone and several varieties of cytochrome. The Rop protein, which promotes plasmid replication in bacteria, is an interesting case in which a single polypeptide forms a coiled-coil and two monomers assemble to form a four-helix bundle.

The amino acids that make up a particular helix can be plotted on a helical wheel, a representation that illustrates the orientations of the constituent amino acids. Often in globular proteins, as well as in specialized structures such as coiled-coils and leucine zippers, an α-helix will exhibit two "faces " - one containing predominantly hydrophobic amino acids oriented toward the interior of the protein, in the hydrophobic core, and one containing predominantly polar amino acids oriented toward the solvent-exposed surface of the protein.

Larger-Scale Assemblies

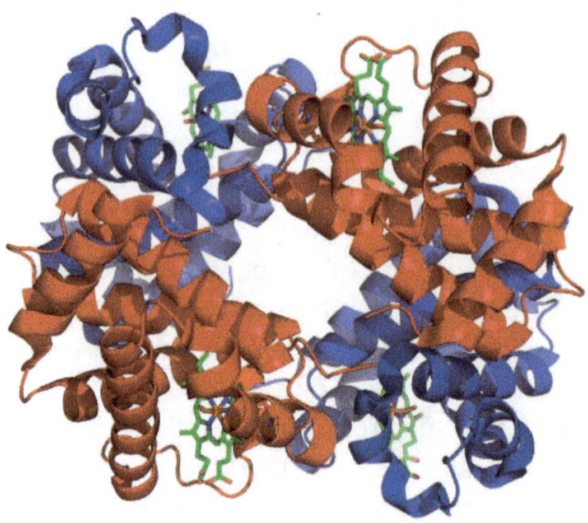

The Hemoglobin molecule has four heme-binding subunits, each made largely of α-helices.

Myoglobin and hemoglobin, the first two proteins whose structures were solved by X-ray crystallography, have very similar folds made up of about 70% α-helix, with the rest being non-repetitive regions, or "loops " that connect the helices. In classifying proteins by their dominant fold, the Structural Classification of Proteins database maintains a large category specifically for all-α proteins.

Hemoglobin then has an even larger-scale quaternary structure, in which the functional oxygen-binding molecule is made up of four subunits.

Functional Roles

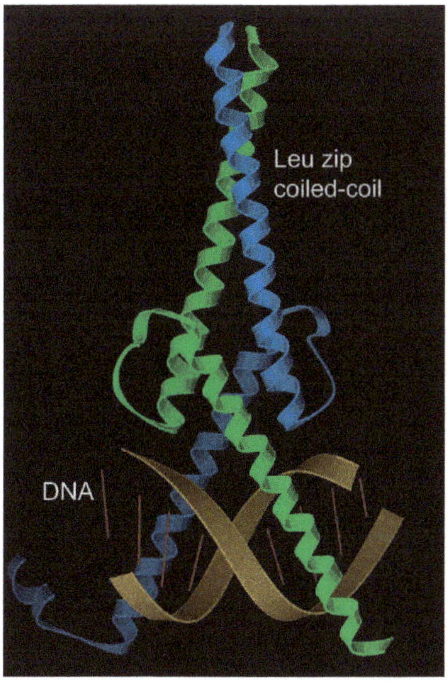

Leucine zipper coiled-coil helices & DNA-binding helices: transcription factor Max (PDB file 1HLO)

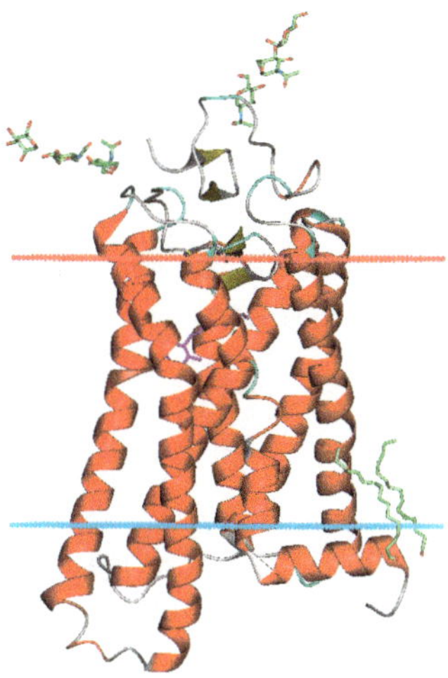

Bovine rhodopsin (PDB file 1GZM), with a bundle of seven helices crossing the membrane (membrane surfaces marked by horizontal lines)

DNA Binding

α-Helices have particular significance in DNA binding motifs, including helix-turn-helix motifs, leucine zipper motifs and zinc finger motifs. This is because of the convenient structural fact that the diameter of an α-helix is about 12Å (1.2 nm) including an average set of sidechains, about the same as the width of the major groove in B-form DNA, and also because coiled-coil (or leucine zipper) dimers of helices can readily position a pair of interaction surfaces to contact the sort of symmetrical repeat common in double-helical DNA. An example of both aspects is the transcription factor Max, which uses a helical coiled-coil to dimerize, positioning another pair of helices for interaction in two successive turns of the DNA major groove.

Membrane Spanning

α-Helices are also the most common protein structure element that crosses biological membranes (transmembrane protein) it is presumed because the helical structure can satisfy all backbone hydrogen-bonds internally, leaving no polar groups exposed to the membrane if the sidechains are hydrophobic. Proteins are sometimes anchored by a single membrane-spanning helix, sometimes by a pair, and sometimes by a helix bundle, most classically consisting of seven helices arranged up-and-down in a ring such as for rhodopsins or for [G protein–coupled receptor]s (GPCRs).

Mechanical Properties

α-Helices under axial tensile deformation, a characteristic loading condition that appears in many alpha-helix-rich filaments and tissues, results in a characteristic three-phase behavior of stiff-soft-stiff tangent modulus. Phase I corresponds to the small-deformation regime during which the helix is stretched homogeneously, followed by phase II, in which alpha-helical turns break mediated by the rupture of groups of H-bonds. Phase III is typically associated with large-deformation covalent bond stretching.

Dynamical Features

Alpha-helices in proteins may have low-frequency accordion-like motion as observed by the Raman spectroscopy and analyzed via the quasi-continuum model. Helices not stabilized by tertiary interactions show dynamic behavior, which can be mainly attributed to helix fraying from the ends.

Helix-Coil Transition

Homopolymers of amino-acids (such as poly-lysine) can adopt α-helical structure at low temperature that is "melted out " at high temperatures. This helix-coil transition was once thought to be analogous to protein denaturation. The statistical mechanics of this transition can be modeled using an elegant transfer matrix method, characterized by two parameters: the propensity to initiate a helix and the propensity to extend a helix.

The α-Helix In Art

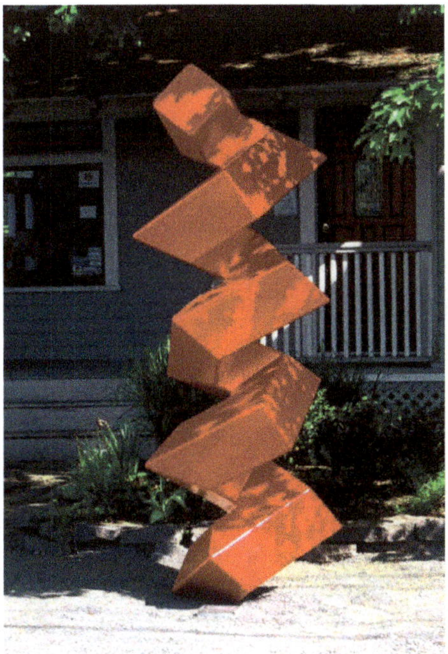

Julian Voss-Andreae's *Alpha Helix for Linus Pauling* (2004), powder coated steel, height 10 ft (3 m). The sculpture stands in front of Pauling's childhood home on 3945 SE Hawthorne Boulevard in Portland, Oregon, USA.

At least five artists have made explicit reference to the α-helix in their work: Julie Newdoll in painting and Julian Voss-Andreae, Bathsheba Grossman, Byron Rubin, and Mike Tyka in sculpture.

San Francisco area artist Julie Newdoll, who holds a degree in Microbiology with a minor in art, has specialized in paintings inspired by microscopic images and molecules since 1990. Her painting "Rise of the Alpha Helix " (2003) features human figures arranged in an α helical arrangement. According to the artist, "the flowers reflect the various types of sidechains that each amino acid holds out to the world ". It is interesting to note that this same metaphor is also echoed from the scientist›s side: "β sheets do not show a stiff repetitious regularity but flow in graceful, twisting curves, and even the α-helix is regular more in the manner of a flower stem, whose branching nodes show the influence of environment, developmental history, and the evolution of each part to match its own idiosyncratic function. "

Julian Voss-Andreae is a German-born sculptor with degrees in experimental physics and sculpture. Since 2001 Voss-Andreae creates "protein sculptures " based on protein structure with the α-helix being one of his preferred objects. Voss-Andreae has made α-helix sculptures from diverse materials including bamboo and whole trees. A monument Voss-Andreae created in 2004 to celebrate the memory of Linus Pauling, the discoverer of the α-helix, is fashioned from a large steel beam rearranged in the structure of the α-helix. The 10-foot (3 m) tall, bright-red sculpture stands in front of Pauling›s childhood home in Portland, Oregon.

Ribbon diagrams of α-helices are a prominent element in the laser-etched crystal sculptures of protein structures created by artist Bathsheba Grossman, such as those of insulin, hemoglobin, and DNA polymerase. Byron Rubin is a former protein crystallographer now professional sculptor in metal of proteins, nucleic acids, and drug molecules - many of which featuring α-helices, such as subtilisin, human growth hormone, and phospholipase A2.

Mike Tyka is a computational biochemist at the University of Washington working with David Baker. Tyka has been making sculptures of protein molecules since 2010 from copper and steel, including ubiquitin and a potassium channel tetramer.

Beta Sheet

The **β-sheet** (also **β-pleated sheet**) is a common motif of regular secondary structure in proteins. Beta sheets consist of beta strands (also **β-strand**) connected laterally by at least two or three backbone hydrogen bonds, forming a generally twisted, pleated sheet. A β-strand is a stretch of polypeptide chain typically 3 to 10 amino acids long with backbone in an extended conformation. The supramolecular association of β-sheets has been implicated in formation of the protein aggregates and fibrils observed in many human diseases, notably the amyloidoses such as Alzheimer›s disease.

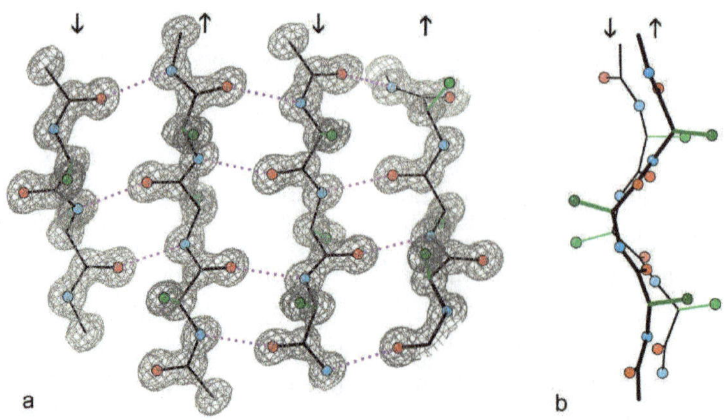

An example of a 4-stranded antiparallel β-sheet fragment from a crystal structure of the enzyme catalase (PDB file 1GWE at 0.88Å resolution). a) Front view, showing the antiparallel hydrogen bonds (dotted) between peptide NH and CO groups on adjacent strands. Arrows indicate chain direction, and electron density contours outline the non-H atoms. O atoms are red balls, N atoms are blue, and H atoms are omitted for simplicity; sidechains are shown only out to the first sidechain C atom (green). b) Edge-on view of the central two β-strands in a, showing the righthanded *twist* and the *pleat* of Cαs and sidechains that alternately stick out in opposite directions from the sheet.

History

The first β-sheet structure was proposed by William Astbury in the 1930s. He proposed the idea of hydrogen bonding between the peptide bonds of parallel or antiparallel extended β-strands. However, Astbury did not have the necessary data on the bond geometry of the amino acids in order to build accurate models, especially since he did not then know that the peptide bond was planar. A refined version was proposed by Linus Pauling and Robert Corey in 1951. Their model incorporated the planarity of the peptide bond which they previously explained as resulting from keto-enol tautomerization.

Structure and Orientation

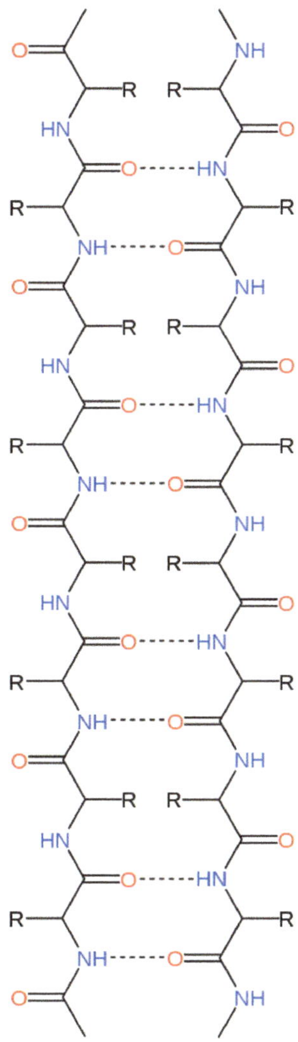

Antiparallel β-sheet hydrogen bonding patterns, represented by dotted lines. Oxygen atoms are colored red and nitrogen atoms colored **blue**.

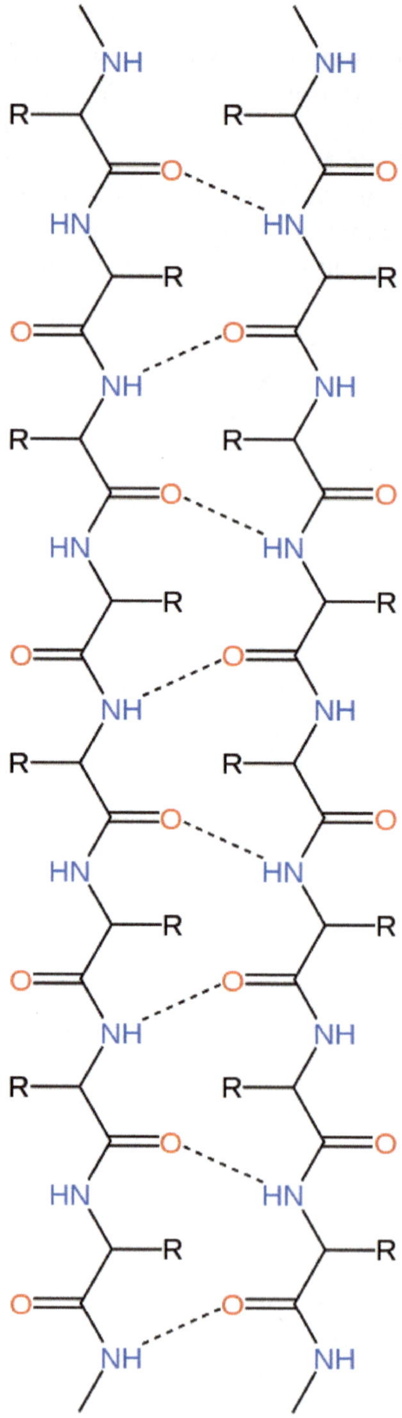

Parallel β-sheet hydrogen bonding patterns, represented by dotted lines. Oxygen atoms are colored red and nitrogen atoms colored **blue**.

Geometry

The majority of β-strands are arranged adjacent to other strands and form an extensive hydrogen bond network with their neighbors in which the N-H groups in the backbone of one strand establish hydrogen bonds with the C=O groups in the backbone of the adjacent strands. In the fully extended β-strand, successive side chains point straight up, then straight down, then straight up, etc. Adjacent β-strands in a β-sheet are aligned so that their C^{α} atoms are adjacent and their side chains point in the same direction. The "pleated " appearance of β-strands arises from tetrahedral chemical bonding at the C^{α} atom; for example, if a side chain points straight up, then the bond to the C› must point slightly downwards, since its bond angle is approximately 109.5°. The pleating causes the distance between C^{α}_{i} and C^{α}_{i+2} to be approximately 6 Å, rather than the 7.6 Å (2 × 3.8 Å) expected from two fully extended trans peptides. The "sideways " distance between adjacent C^{α} atoms in hydrogen-bonded β-strands is roughly 5 Å.

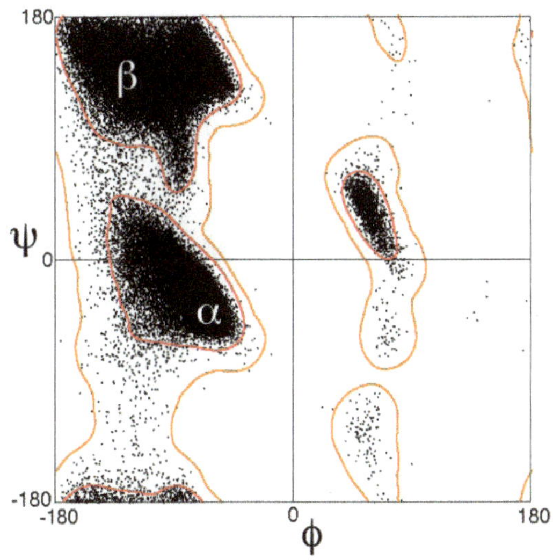

Ramachandran (φ,ψ) plot of about 100,000 high-resolution datapoints, showing the broad, favorable region around the conformation typical for β-sheet residues.

However, β-strands are rarely perfectly extended; rather, they exhibit a twist due to the chirality of their component amino acids. The energetically preferred dihedral angles near (φ, ψ) = (–135°, 135°) (broadly, the upper left region of the Ramachandran plot) diverge significantly from the fully extended conformation (φ, ψ) = (–180°, 180°). The twist is often associated with alternating fluctuations in the dihedral angles to prevent the individual β-strands in a larger sheet from splaying apart. A good example of a strongly twisted β-hairpin can be seen in the protein BPTI.

The side chains point outwards from the folds of the pleats, roughly perpendicularly to the plane of the sheet; successive residues point outwards on alternating faces of the sheet.

Hydrogen Bonding Patterns

Because peptide chains have a directionality conferred by their N-terminus and C-terminus, β-strands too can be said to be directional. They are usually represented in protein topology diagrams by an arrow pointing toward the C-terminus. Adjacent β-strands can form hydrogen bonds in antiparallel, parallel, or mixed arrangements.

In an antiparallel arrangement, the successive β-strands alternate directions so that the N-terminus of one strand is adjacent to the C-terminus of the next. This is the arrangement that produces the strongest inter-strand stability because it allows the inter-strand hydrogen bonds between carbonyls and amines to be planar, which is their preferred orientation. The peptide backbone dihedral angles (φ, ψ) are about (–140°, 135°) in antiparallel sheets. In this case, if two atoms C_i^α and C_j^α are adjacent in two hydrogen-bonded β-strands, then they form two mutual backbone hydrogen bonds to each other›s flanking peptide groups; this is known as a **close pair** of hydrogen bonds.

In a parallel arrangement, all of the N-termini of successive strands are oriented in the same direction; this orientation may be slightly less stable because it introduces nonplanarity in the inter-strand hydrogen bonding pattern. The dihedral angles (φ, ψ) are about (–120°, 115°) in parallel sheets. It is rare to find less than five interacting parallel strands in a motif, suggesting that a smaller number of strands may be unstable, however it is also fundamentally more difficult for parallel β-sheets to form because strands with N and C termini aligned necessarily must be very distant in sequence. There is also evidence that parallel β-sheet may be more stable since small amyloidogenic sequences appear to generally aggregate into β-sheet fibrils composed of primarily parallel β-sheet strands, where one would expect anti-parallel fibrils if anti-parallel were more stable.

In parallel β-sheet structure, if two atoms C_i^α and C_j^α are adjacent in two hydrogen-bonded β-strands, then they do *not* hydrogen bond to each other; rather, one residue forms hydrogen bonds to the residues that flank the other (but not vice versa). For example, residue i may form hydrogen bonds to residues $j-1$ and $j+1$; this is known as a wide **pair** of hydrogen bonds. By contrast, residue j may hydrogen-bond to different residues altogether, or to none at all.

Finally, an individual strand may exhibit a mixed bonding pattern, with a parallel strand on one side and an antiparallel strand on the other. Such arrangements are less common than a random distribution of orientations would suggest, suggesting that this pattern is less stable than the anti-parallel arrangement, however bioinformatic analysis always struggles with extracting structural thermodynamics since there are always numerous other structural features present in whole proteins. Also proteins are inherently constrained by folding kinetics as well as folding thermodynamics, so one must always be careful in concluding stability from bioinformatic analysis.

The hydrogen bonding of β-strands need not be perfect, but can exhibit localized disruptions known as β-bulges.

The hydrogen bonds lie roughly in the plane of the sheet, with the peptide carbonyl groups pointing in alternating directions with successive residues; for comparison, successive carbonyls point in the *same* direction in the alpha helix.

Amino Acid Propensities

Large aromatic residues (Tyr, Phe and Trp) and β-branched amino acids (Thr, Val, Ile) are favored to be found in β-strands in the *middle* of β-sheets. Interestingly, different types of residues (such as Pro) are likely to be found in the *edge* strands in β-sheets, presumably to avoid the "edge-to-edge " association between proteins that might lead to aggregation and amyloid formation.

Common Structural Motifs

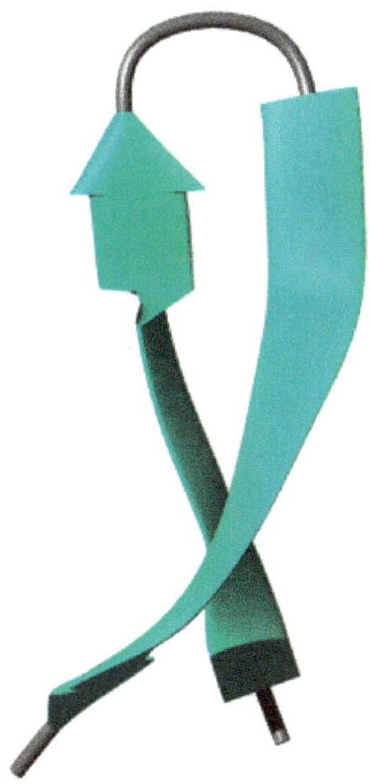

The β-hairpin motif

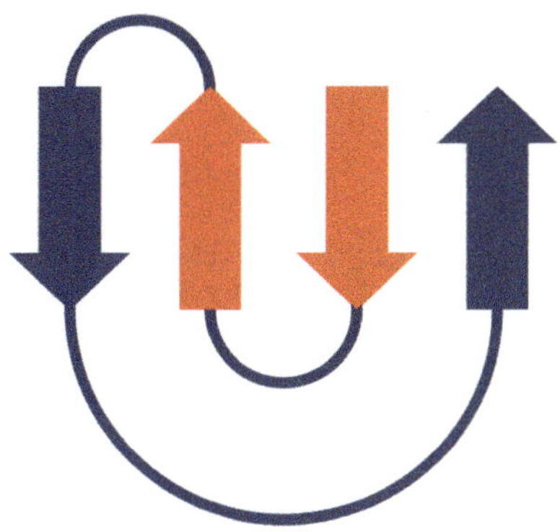

The Greek-key motif

A very simple structural motif involving β-sheets is the β-hairpin, in which two antiparallel strands are linked by a short loop of two to five residues, of which one is frequently a glycine or a proline, both of which can assume the dihedral-angle conformations required for a tight turn or a β-bulge loop. Individual strands can also be linked in more elaborate ways with longer loops that may contain α-helices.

Greek Key Motif

The Greek key motif consists of four adjacent antiparallel strands and their linking loops. It consists of three antiparallel strands connected by hairpins, while the fourth is adjacent to the first and linked to the third by a longer loop. This type of structure forms easily during the protein folding process. It was named after a pattern common to Greek ornamental artwork.

The β-α-β Motif

Due to the chirality of their component amino acids, all strands exhibit right handed twist evident in most higher-order β-sheet structures. In particular, the linking loop between two parallel strands almost always has a right-handed crossover chirality, which is strongly favored by the inherent twist of the sheet. This linking loop frequently contains a helical region, in which case it is called a β-α-β motif. A closely related motif called a β-α-β-α motif forms the basic component of the most commonly observed protein tertiary structure, the TIM barrel.

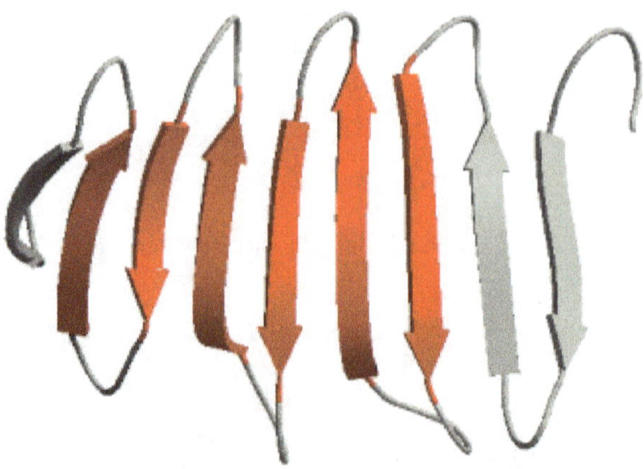

The β-meander motif from the outer surface Protein A

β-*Meander Motif*

A simple supersecondary protein topology composed of 2 or more consecutive antiparallel β-strands linked together by hairpin loops. This motif is common in β-sheets and can be found in several structural architectures including β-barrels and β-propellers.

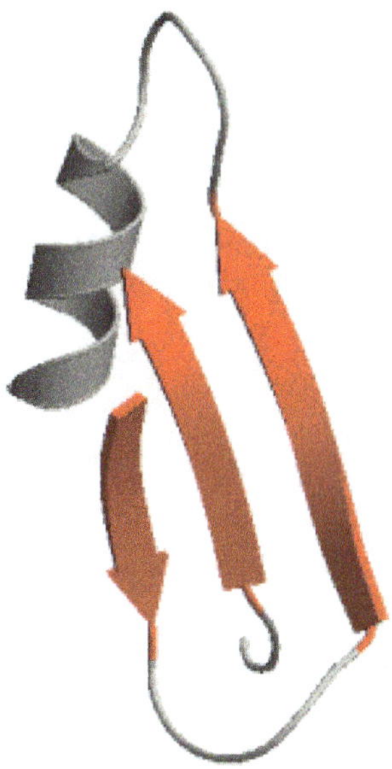

Psi-loop motif from Carboxypeptidase A

Psi-Loop Motif

The psi-loop (Ψ-loop) motif consists of two antiparallel strands with one strand in between that is connected to both by hydrogen bonds.There are four possible strand topologies for single Ψ-loops. This motif is rare as the process resulting in its formation seems unlikely to occur during protein folding. The Ψ-loop was first identified in the aspartic protease family.

Structural Architectures of Proteins with β-Sheets

β-sheets are present in all-β, α+β and α/β domains, and in many peptides or small proteins with poorly defined overall architecture. All-β domains may form β-barrels, β-sandwiches, β-prisms, β-propellers, and β-helices.

Structural Topology

The topology of a β-sheet describes the order of hydrogen-bonded β-strands along the backbone. For example, the flavodoxin fold has a five-stranded, parallel β-sheet with topology 21345; thus, the edge strands are β-strand 2 and β-strand 5 along the backbone. Spelled out explicitly, β-strand 2 is H-bonded to β-strand 1, which is H-bonded to β-strand 3, which is H-bonded to β-strand 4, which is H-bonded to β-strand 5, the other edge strand. In the same system, the Greek key motif described above has a 4123 topology.

The secondary structure of a β-sheet can be described roughly by giving the number of strands, their topology, and whether their hydrogen bonds are parallel or antiparallel.

β-sheets can be *open*, meaning that they have two edge strands (as in the flavodoxin fold or the immunoglobulin fold) or they can be *closed β-barrels* (such as the TIM barrel). β-Barrels are often described by their *stagger* or *shear*. Some open β-sheets are very curved and fold over on themselves (as in the SH3 domain) or form horseshoe shapes (as in the ribonuclease inhibitor). Open β-sheets can assemble face-to-face (such as the β-propeller domain or immunoglobulin fold) or edge-to-edge, forming one big β-sheet.

Dynamic Features

β-pleated sheet structures are made from extended β-strand polypeptide chains, with strands linked to their neighbours by hydrogen bonds. Due to this extended backbone conformation, β-sheets resist Stretching. β-sheets in proteins may carry out low-frequency accordion-like motion as observed by the Raman spectroscopy and analyzed with the quasi-continuum model.

Parallel β-Helices

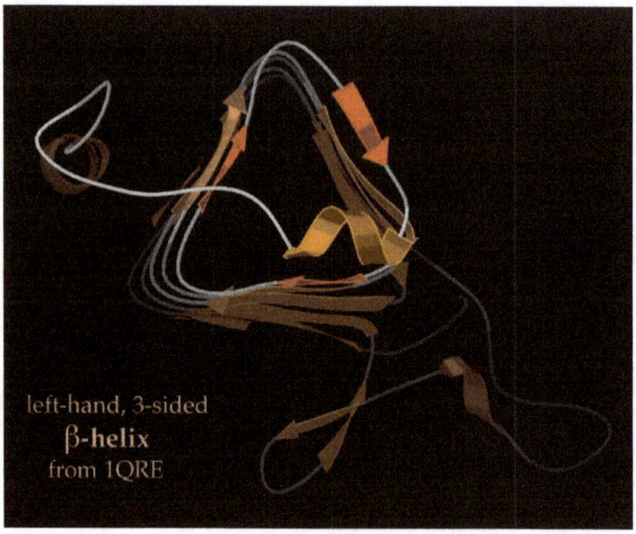

End-view of a 3-sided, left handed β-helix (PDB: 1QRE)

A β-helix is formed from repeating structural units consisting of two or three short β-strands linked by short loops. These units "stack " atop one another in a helical fashion so that successive repetitions of the same strand hydrogen-bond with each other in a parallel orientation.

In left-handed β-helices, the strands themselves are quite straight and untwisted; the resulting helical surfaces are nearly flat, forming a regular triangular prism shape, as shown for the 1QRE archaeal carbonic anhydrase at right. Other examples are the lipid A synthesis enzyme LpxA and insect antifreeze proteins with a regular array of Thr sidechains on one face that mimic the structure of ice.

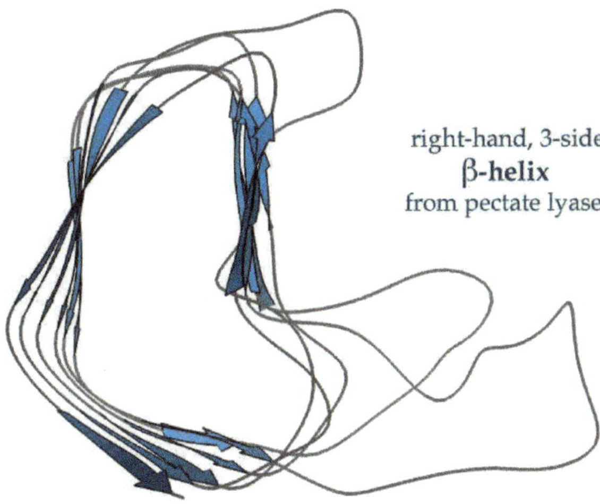

End-view of a 3-sided, right handed β-helix.

Righthanded β-helices, typified by the pectate lyase enzyme shown at left or P22 phage tailspike protein, have a less regular cross-section, longer and indented on one of the sides; of the three linker loops, one is consistently just two residues long and the others are variable, often elaborated to form a binding or active site.

A two-sided β-helix (right-handed) is found in some bacterial metalloproteases; its two loops are each six residues long and bind stabilizing calcium ions to maintain the integrity of the structure, using the backbone and the Asp side chain oxygens of a GGXGXD sequence motif. This fold is called a β-roll in the SCOP classification.

β-Sheets in Pathology

Some proteins that are disordered or helical as monomers, such as amyloid β (see amyloid plaque) can form β-sheet-rich oligomeric structures associated with pathological states. The amyloid β protein›s oligomeric form is implicated as a cause of Alzheimer›s. Its structure has yet to be determined in full, but recent data suggest that it may resemble an unusual two-strand β-helix.

The side chains from the amino acid residues found in a β-sheet structure may also be arranged such that many of the adjacent sidechains on one side of the sheet are hydrophobic, while many of those adjacent to each other on the alternate side of the sheet are polar or charged (hydrophilic), which can be useful if the sheet is to form a boundary between polar/watery and nonpolar/greasy environments.

Loop

Loops are regions of a protein chain that are (1) between α helices and β sheets, (2) of various lengths and three-dimensional configurations, and (3) on the surface of the structure. Hairpin loops that represent a complete turn in the polypeptide chain joining two antiparallel β strands may be as short as two amino acids in length. Loops interact with the surrounding aqueous environment and other proteins. Because amino acids in loops are not constrained by space and environment as are amino acids in the core region, and do not have an effect on the arrangement of secondary structures in the core, more substitutions, insertions, and deletions may occur. Thus, in a sequence alignment, the presence of these features may be an indication of a loop. The positions of introns in genomic DNA sometimes correspond to the locations of loops in the encoded protein. Loops also tend to have charged and polar amino acids and are frequently a component of active sites. A detailed examination of loop structures has shown that they fall into distinct families.

Coils

A region of secondary structure that is not a α helix, a β sheet, or a recognizable turn is commonly referred to as a coil.

PROTEIN CLASSIFICATION

Proteins may be classified according to both structural and sequence similarity. For structural classification, the sizes and spatial arrangements of secondary structures described in the above paragraph are compared in known three-dimensional structures.Classification based on sequence similarity was historically the first to be used. Initially, similarity based on alignments of whole sequences was performed. Later, proteins were classified on the basis of the occurrence of conserved amino acid patterns. Databases that classify proteins by one or more of these schemes are available. In considering protein classification schemes, it is important to keep several observations in mind. First, two entirely different protein sequences from different evolutionary origins may fold into a similar structure. Conversely, the sequence of an ancient gene for a given structure may have diverged considerably in different species while at the same time maintaining the same basic structural features. Recognizing any remaining sequence similarity in such cases may be a very difficult task. Second, two proteins that share a significant degree of sequence similarity either with each other or with a third sequence also share an evolutionary origin and should share some structural features also. However, gene duplication and genetic rearrangements during evolution may give rise to new gene copies, which can then evolve into proteins with new function and structure.

Terms Used for Classifying Protein Structures and Sequences

The more commonly used terms for evolutionary and structural relationships among proteins are listed below. Many additional terms are used for various kinds of structural features found in proteins. Descriptions of such terms may be found at the CATH Web site the Structural Classification of Proteins (SCOP) Web site and a Glaxo-Wellcome tutorial on the Swiss bioinformatics Expasy Web site.

Active Site

A localized combination of amino acid side groups within the tertiary (three-dimensional) or quaternary (protein subunit) structure that can interact with a chemically specific substrate and that provides the protein with biological activity. Proteins of very different amino acid sequences may fold into a structure that produces the same active site.

Architecture

The relative orientations of secondary structures in a three-dimensional structure without regard to whether or not they share a similar loop structure.

Fold

A type of architecture that also has a conserved loop structure.

Blocks

A conserved amino acid sequence pattern in a family of proteins. The pattern includes a series of possible matches at each position in the represented sequences, but there are not any inserted or deleted positions in the pattern or in the sequences. By way of contrast, sequence profiles are a type of scoring matrix that represents a similar set of patterns that includes insertions and deletions.

Class

A term used to classify protein domains according to their secondary structural content and organization. Four classes were originally recognized by Levitt and Chothia (1976), and several others have been added in the SCOP database. Three classes are given in the CATH database: mainly-α, mainly-β, and α–β, with the α–β class including both alternating α/β and α+β structures.

Core

The portion of a folded protein molecule that comprises the hydrophobic interior of α-helices and β-sheets. The compact structure brings together side groups of amino acids into close enough proximity so that they can interact. When comparing protein structures, as in the SCOP database, core is the region common to most of the structures that share a common fold or that are in the same superfamily. In structure prediction, core is sometimes defined as the arrangement of secondary structures that is likely to be conserved during evolutionary change.

Domain (Sequence Context)

A segment of a polypeptide chain that can fold into a three-dimensional structure irrespective of the presence of other segments of the chain. The separate domains of a given protein may interact extensively or may be joined only by a length of polypeptide chain. A protein with several domains may use these domains for functional interactions with different molecules.

Family (Sequence Context)

A group of proteins of similar biochemical function that are more than 50% identical when aligned. This same cutoff is still used by the Protein Information Resource (PIR). A protein family comprises proteins with the same function in different organisms (orthologous sequences) but may also include proteins in the same organism (paralogous sequences) derived from gene duplication and rearrangements. If a multiple sequence alignment of a protein family reveals a common level of similarity throughout the lengths of the proteins, PIR refers to the family as a homeomorphic family. The aligned region is referred to as a homeomorphic domain, and this region may comprise several smaller homology domains that are shared with other families. Families may be further subdivided into subfamilies or grouped into superfamilies based on respective higher or lower levels of sequence similarity. The SCOP database reports 1296 families and the CATH database (version 1.7 beta), reports 1846 families.

When the sequences of proteins with the same function are examined in greater detail, some are found to share high sequence similarity. They are obviously members of the same family by the above criteria. However, others are found that have very little, or even insignificant, sequence similarity with other family members. In such cases, the family relationship between two distant family members A and C can often be demonstrated by finding an additional family member B that shares significant similarity with both A and C. Thus, B provides a connecting link between A and C. Another approach is to examine distant alignments for highly conserved matches.

At a level of identity of 50%, proteins are likely to have the same three-dimensional structure, and the identical atoms in the sequence alignment will also superimpose within approximately 1 Å in the structural model. Thus, if the structure of one member of a family is known, a reliable prediction may be made for a second member of the family, and the higher the identity level, the more reliable the prediction. Protein structural modeling can be performed by examining how well the amino acid substitutions fit into the core of the three-dimensional structure.

Family (Structural Context)

As used in the FSSP database (Families of structurally similar proteins) and the DALI/

FSSP Web site, two structures that have a significant level of structural similarity but not necessarily significant sequence similarity.

Fold

Similar to structural motif, includes a larger combination of secondary structural units in the same configuration. Thus, proteins sharing the same fold have the same combination of secondary structures that are connected by similar loops. An example is the Rossman fold comprising several alternating α helices and parallel β strands. In the SCOP, CATH, and FSSP databases, the known protein structures have been classified into hierarchical levels of structural complexity with the fold as a basic level of classification.

Homologous Domain (Sequence Context)

An extended sequence pattern, generally found by sequence alignment methods, that indicates a common evolutionary origin among the aligned sequences. A homology domain is generally longer than motifs. The domain may include all of a given protein sequence or only a portion of the sequence. Some domains are complex and made up of several smaller homology domains that became joined to form a larger one during evolution. A domain that covers an entire sequence is called the homeomorphic domain by PIR (Protein Information Resource).

Module

A region of conserved amino acid patterns comprising one or more motifs and considered to be a fundamental unit of structure or function. The presence of a module has also been used to classify proteins into families.

Motif (Sequence Context)

A conserved pattern of amino acids that is found in two or more proteins. In the Prosite catalog, a motif is an amino acid pattern that is found in a group of proteins that have a similar biochemical activity, and that often is near the active site of the protein. Examples of sequence motif databases are the Prosite catalog and the Stanford Motifs Database.

Motif (Structural Context)

A combination of several secondary structural elements produced by the folding of adjacent sections of the polypeptide chain into a specific three-dimensional configuration. An example is the helix-loop-helix motif. Structural motifs are also referred to as supersecondary structures and folds.

Position-Specific Scoring Matrix (Sequence Context, Also Known As Weight or Scoring Matrix)

Represents a conserved region in a multiple sequence alignment with no gaps. Each matrix column represents the variation found in one column of the multiple sequence alignment.

Position-specific scoring matrix—3D (structural context) represents the amino acid variation found in an alignment of proteins that fall into the same structural class. Matrix columns represent the amino acid variation found at one amino acid position in the aligned structures.

Primary Structure

The linear amino acid sequence of a protein, which chemically is a polypeptide chain composed of amino acids joined by peptide bonds.

Profile (Sequence Context)

A scoring matrix that represents a multiple sequence alignment of a protein family. The profile is usually obtained from a well-conserved region in a multiple sequence alignment. The profile is in the form of a matrix with each column representing a position in the alignment and each row one of the amino acids. Matrix values give the likelihood of each amino acid at the corresponding position in the alignment. The profile is moved along the target sequence to locate the best scoring regions by a dynamic programming algorithm. Gaps are allowed during matching and a gap penalty is included in this case as a negative score when no amino acid is matched. A sequence profile may also be represented by a hidden Markov model, referred to as a profile HMM.

Profile (Structural Context)

A scoring matrix that represents which amino acids should fit well and which should fit poorly at sequential positions in a known protein structure. Profile columns represent sequential positions in the structure, and profile rows represent the 20 amino acids. As with a sequence profile, the structural profile is moved along a target sequence to find the highest possible alignment score by a dynamic programming algorithm. Gaps may be included and receive a penalty. The resulting score provides an indication as to whether or not the target protein might adopt such a structure.

Quaternary Structure

The three-dimensional configuration of a protein molecule comprising several independent polypeptide chains.

Secondary Structure

The interactions that occur between the C, O, and NH groups on amino acids in a polypeptide chain to form α-helices, β-sheets, turns, loops, and other forms, and that facilitate the folding into a three-dimensional structure.

Superfamily

A group of protein families of the same or different lengths that are related by distant yet detectable sequence similarity. Members of a given superfamily thus have a common evolutionary origin. Originally, Dayhoff defined the cutoff for superfamily status as being the chance that the sequences are not related of 10 6, on the basis of an alignment score (Dayhoff et al. 1978). Proteins with few identities in an alignment of the sequences but with a convincingly common number of structural and functional features are placed in the same superfamily. At the level of three-dimensional structure, superfamily proteins will share common structural features such as a common fold, but there may also be differences in the number and arrangement of secondary structures. The PIR resource uses the term *homeomorphic superfamilies* to refer to superfamilies that are composed of sequences that can be aligned from end to end, representing a sharing of single sequence homology domain, a region of similarity that extends throughout the alignment. This domain may also comprise smaller homology domains that are shared with other protein families and superfamilies. Although a given protein sequence may contain domains found in several superfamilies, thus indicating a complex evolutionary history, sequences will be assigned to only one homeomorphic superfamily based on the presence of similarity throughout a multiple sequence alignment. The superfamily alignment may also include regions that do not align either within or at the ends of the alignment. In contrast, sequences in the same family align well throughout the alignment.

Supersecondary Structure

A term with similar meaning to a structural motif. Tertiary structure is the three-dimensional or globular structure formed by the packing together or folding of secondary structures of a polypeptide chain.

SECONDARY STRUCTURE

Secondary structure prediction is a set of techniques in bioinformatics that aim to predict the local secondary structures of proteins based only on knowledge of their amino acid sequence. For proteins, a prediction consists of assigning regions of the amino acid sequence as likely alpha helices, beta strands (often noted as "extended" conformations), or turns. The success of a prediction is determined by comparing it to the results of the DSSP algorithm (or similar e.g. STRIDE) applied to the crystal structure of the protein. Specialized algorithms have been developed for the detection of specific well-defined patterns such as transmembrane helices and coiled coils in proteins.

The best modern methods of secondary structure prediction in proteins reach about 80% accuracy; this high accuracy allows the use of the predictions as feature improving fold recognition and ab initio protein structure prediction, classification of structural motifs, and refinement of sequence alignments. The accuracy of current protein secondary structure prediction methods is assessed in weekly benchmarks such as LiveBench and EVA.

Background

Early methods of secondary structure prediction, introduced in the 1960s and early 1970s, focused on identifying likely alpha helices and were based mainly on helix-coil transition models. Significantly more accurate predictions that included beta sheets were introduced in the 1970s and relied on statistical assessments based on probability parameters derived from known solved structures. These methods, applied to a single sequence, are typically at most about 60-65% accurate, and often underpredict beta sheets. The evolutionary conservation of secondary structures can be exploited by simultaneously assessing many homologous sequences in a multiple sequence alignment, by calculating the net secondary structure propensity of an aligned column of amino acids. In concert with larger databases of known protein structures and modern machine learning methods such as neural nets and support vector machines, these methods can achieve up 80% overall accuracy in globular proteins. The theoretical upper limit of accuracy is around 90%, partly due to idiosyncrasies in DSSP assignment near the ends of secondary structures, where local conformations vary under native conditions but may be forced to assume a single conformation in crystals due to packing constraints. Limitations are also imposed by secondary structure prediction's inability to account for tertiary structure; for example, a sequence predicted as a likely helix may still be able to adopt a beta-strand conformation if it is located within a beta-sheet region of the protein and its side chains pack well with their neighbors. Dramatic conformational changes related to the protein's function or environment can also alter local secondary structure.

Historical Perspective

To date, over 20 different secondary structure prediction methods have been developed. One of the first algorithms was Chou-Fasman method, which relies predominantly on probability parameters determined from relative frequencies of each amino acid's appearance in each type of secondary structure. The original Chou-Fasman parameters, determined from the small sample of structures solved in the mid-1970s, produce poor results compared to modern methods, though the parameterization has been updated since it was first published. The Chou-Fasman method is roughly 50-60% accurate in predicting secondary structures.

The next notable program was the GOR method, named for the three scientists who developed it — *G*arnier, *O*sguthorpe, and *R*obson, is an information theory-based method. It uses the more powerful probabilistic technique of Bayesian inference. The GOR method takes into account not only the probability of each amino acid having a particular secondary structure, but also the conditional probability of the amino acid assuming each structure given the contributions of its neighbors (it does not assume that the neighbors have that same structure). The approach is both more sensitive and more accurate than that of Chou and Fasman because amino acid structural propensities are only strong for a small number of amino acids such as proline and glycine. Weak contributions from each of many neighbors can add up to strong effects overall. The original GOR method was roughly 65% accurate and is dramatically more successful in predicting alpha helices than beta sheets, which it frequently mispredicted as loops or disorganized regions.

Another big step forward, was using machine learning methods. First artificial neural networks methods were used. As a training sets they use solved structures to identify common sequence motifs associated with particular arrangements of secondary structures. These methods are over 70% accurate in their predictions, although beta strands are still often underpredicted due to the lack of three-dimensional structural information that would allow assessment of hydrogen bonding patterns that can promote formation of the extended conformation required for the presence of a complete beta sheet. PSIPRED and JPRED are some of the most known programs based on neural networks for protein secondary structure prediction. Next, support vector machines have proven particularly useful for predicting the locations of turns, which are difficult to identify with statistical methods.

Extensions of machine learning techniques attempt to predict more fine-grained local properties of proteins, such as backbone dihedral angles in unassigned regions. Both SVMs and neural networks have been applied to this problem. More recently, real-value torsion angles can be accurately predicted by SPINE-X and successfully employed for ab initio structure prediction.

Other Improvements

It is reported that in addition to the protein sequence, secondary structure formation depends on other factors. For example, it is reported that secondary structure tendencies depend also on local environment, solvent accessibility of residues, protein structural class, and even the organism from which the proteins are obtained. Based on such observations, some studies have shown that secondary structure prediction can be improved by addition of information about protein structural class, residue accessible surface area and also contact number information.

TERTIARY STRUCTURE

The practical role of protein structure prediction is now more important than ever. Massive amounts of protein sequence data are produced by modern large-scale DNA sequencing efforts such as the Human Genome Project. Despite community-wide efforts in structural genomics, the output of experimentally determined protein structures—typically by time-consuming and relatively expensive X-ray crystallography or NMR spectroscopy—is lagging far behind the output of protein sequences.

The protein structure prediction remains an extremely difficult and unresolved undertaking. The two main problems are calculation of protein free energy and finding the global minimum of this energy. A protein structure prediction method must explore the space of possible protein structures which is astronomically large. These problems can be partially bypassed in “comparative” or homology modeling and fold recognition methods, in which the search space is pruned by the assumption that the protein in question adopts a structure that is close to the experimentally determined structure of another homologous protein. On the other hand, the *de novo* or ab initio protein structure prediction methods must explicitly resolve these problems. The progress and challenges in protein structure prediction has been reviewed in Zhang 2008.

Energy- and Fragment-Based Methods

Ab initio- or *de novo*- protein modelling methods seek to build three-dimensional protein models "from scratch", i.e., based on physical principles rather than (directly) on previously solved structures. There are many possible procedures that either attempt to mimic protein folding or apply some stochastic method to search possible solutions (i.e., global optimization of a suitable energy function). These procedures tend to require vast computational resources, and have thus only been carried out for tiny proteins. To predict protein structure *de novo* for larger proteins will require better algorithms and larger computational resources like those afforded by either powerful supercomputers (such as Blue Gene or MDGRAPE-3) or distributed computing (such as Folding@home, the Human Proteome Folding Project and Rosetta@Home). Although these computational barriers are vast, the potential benefits of structural genomics (by predicted or experimental methods) make *ab initio* structure prediction an active research field.

As of 2009, a 50-residue protein could be simulated atom-by-atom on a supercomputer for 1 millisecond. As of 2012, comparable stable-state sampling could be done on a standard desktop with a new graphics card and more sophisticated algorithms. A much larger simulation timescales can be achieved using coarse-grained modeling.

Evolutionary Covariation to Predict 3D Contacts

As sequencing became more commonplace in the 1990s several groups used protein sequence alignments to predict correlated mutations and it was hoped that these coevolved residues could be used to predict tertiary structure (using the analogy to distance constraints from experimental procedures such as NMR). The assumption is when single residue mutations are slightly deleterious, compensatory mutations may occur to restabilize residue-residue interactions. This early work used what are known as *local* methods to calculate correlated mutations from protein sequences, but suffered from indirect false correlations which result from treating each pair of residues as independent of all other pairs.

In 2011, a different, and this time *global* statistical approach, demonstrated that predicted coevolved residues were sufficient to predict the 3D fold of a protein, providing there are enough sequences available (>1,000 homologous sequences are needed). The method, EVfold, uses no homology modeling, threading or 3D structure fragments and can be run on a standard personal computer even for proteins with hundreds of residues. The accuracy of the contacts predicted using this and related approaches has now been demonstrated on many known structures and contact maps, including the prediction of experimentally unsolved transmembrane proteins.

Comparative Protein Modeling

Comparative protein modelling uses previously solved structures as starting points, or templates. This is effective because it appears that although the number of actual proteins is vast, there is a limited set of tertiarystructural motifs to which most proteins belong. It has been suggested that there are only around 2,000 distinct protein folds in nature, though there are many millions of different proteins.

These methods may also be split into two groups:

Homology Modeling

It is based on the reasonable assumption that two homologous proteins will share very similar structures. Because a protein's fold is more evolutionarily conserved than its amino acid sequence, a target sequence can be modeled with reasonable accuracy on a very distantly related template, provided that the relationship between target and template can be discerned through sequence alignment. It has been suggested that the primary bottleneck in comparative modelling arises from difficulties in alignment rather than from errors in structure prediction given a known-good alignment. Unsurprisingly, homology modelling is most accurate when the target and template have similar sequences.

Protein Threading

It scans the amino acid sequence of an unknown structure against a database of solved structures. In each case, a scoring function is used to assess the compatibility of the sequence to the structure, thus yielding possible three-dimensional models. This type of method is also known as 3D-1D fold recognition due to its compatibility analysis between three-dimensional structures and linear protein sequences. This method has also given rise to methods performing an inverse folding search by evaluating the compatibility of a given structure with a large database of sequences, thus predicting which sequences have the potential to produce a given fold.

Side-Chain Geometry Prediction

Accurate packing of the amino acid side chains represents a separate problem in protein structure prediction. Methods that specifically address the problem of predicting side-chain geometry include dead-end elimination and the self-consistent mean field methods. The side chain conformations with low energy are usually determined on the rigid polypeptide backbone and using a set of discrete side chain conformations known as "rotamers." The methods attempt to identify the set of rotamers that minimize the model's overall energy.

These methods use rotamer libraries, which are collections of favorable conformations for each residue type in proteins. Rotamer libraries may contain information about the conformation, its frequency, and the standard deviations about mean dihedral angles, which can be used in sampling. Rotamer libraries are derived from structural bioinformatics or other statistical analysis of side-chain conformations in known experimental structures of proteins, such as by clustering the observed conformations for tetrahedral carbons near the staggered (60°, 180°, -60°) values.

Rotamer libraries can be backbone-independent, secondary-structure-dependent, or backbone-dependent. Backbone-independent rotamer libraries make no reference to backbone conformation, and are calculated from all available side chains of a certain type (for instance, the first example of a rotamer library, done by Ponder and Richards at Yale in 1987). Secondary-structure-dependent libraries present different dihedral angles and/or rotamer frequencies for α-helix, β-sheet, or coil secondary structures. Backbone-dependent rotamer libraries present conformations and/or frequencies dependent on the local backbone conformation as defined by the backbone dihedral angles ϕ and ψ, regardless of secondary structure.

The modern versions of these libraries as used in most software are presented as multidimensional distributions of probability or frequency, where the peaks correspond to the dihedral-angle conformations considered as individual rotamers in the lists. Some versions are based on very carefully curated data and are used primarily for structure validation, while others emphasize relative frequencies in much larger data sets and are the form used primarily for structure prediction, such as the Dunbrack rotamer libraries.

Side-chain packing methods are most useful for analyzing the protein's hydrophobic core, where side chains are more closely packed; they have more difficulty addressing the looser constraints and higher flexibility of surface residues, which often occupy multiple rotamer conformations rather than just one.

Prediction of Structural Classes

Statistical methods have been developed for predicting structural classes of proteins based on their amino acid composition, pseudo amino acid composition and functional domain composition.

QUATERNARY STRUCTURE

In the case of complexes of two or more proteins, where the structures of the proteins are known or can be predicted with high accuracy, protein–protein docking methods can be used to predict the structure of the complex. Information of the effect of mutations at specific sites on the affinity of the complex helps to understand the complex structure and to guide docking methods.

Software

A great number of software tools for protein structure prediction exist. Approaches include homology modeling, protein threading, *ab initio* methods, secondary structure prediction, and transmembrane helix and signal peptide prediction. Two most successful methods based on CASP experiment are I-TASSER and HHpred.

Evaluation of Automatic Structure Prediction Servers

CASP, which stands for Critical Assessment of Techniques for Protein Structure Prediction, is a community-wide experiment for protein structure prediction taking place every two years since 1994. CASP provides with an opportunity to assess the quality of available human, non-automated methodology (human category) and automatic servers for protein structure prediction (server category, introduced in the CASP7). The official results of automated assessment in 2012 CASP10 are available at for automated servers and for human and server predictors. In December 2014 next CASP11 assessment will be publicly available.

The CAMEO3D Continuous Automated Model EvaluatiOn Server evaluates automated protein structure prediction servers on a weekly basis using blind predictions for newly release protein structures. CAMEO publishes the results on its website ().

STRUCTURAL ALIGNMENT

Structural alignment attempts to establish homology between two or more polymer structures based on their shape and three-dimensional conformation. This process is usually applied to protein tertiary structures but can also be used for large RNA molecules. In contrast to simple structural superposition, where at least some equivalent residues of the two structures are known, structural alignment requires no *a priori* knowledge of equivalent positions. Structural alignment is a valuable tool for the comparison of proteins with low sequence similarity, where evolutionary relationships between proteins cannot be easily detected by standard sequence alignment techniques. Structural alignment can therefore be used to imply evolutionary relationships between proteins that share very little common sequence. However, caution should be used in using the results as evidence for shared evolutionary ancestry because of the possible confounding effects of convergent evolution by which multiple unrelated amino acid sequences converge on a common tertiary structure.

Structural alignments can compare two sequences or multiple sequences. Because these alignments rely on information about all the query sequences' three-dimensional conformations, the method can only be used on sequences where these structures are known. These are usually found by X-ray crystallography or NMR spectroscopy. It is possible to perform a structural alignment on structures produced by structure prediction methods. Indeed, evaluating such predictions often requires a structural alignment between the model and the true known structure to assess the model's quality. Structural alignments are especially useful in analyzing data from structural genomics and proteomics efforts, and they can be used as comparison points to evaluate alignments produced by purely sequence-based bioinformatics methods.

The outputs of a structural alignment are a superposition of the atomic coordinate sets and a minimal root mean square deviation (RMSD) between the structures. The RMSD of two aligned structures indicates their divergence from one another. Structural alignment can be complicated by the existence of multiple protein domains within one or more of the input structures, because changes in relative orientation of the domains between two structures to be aligned can artificially inflate the RMSD.

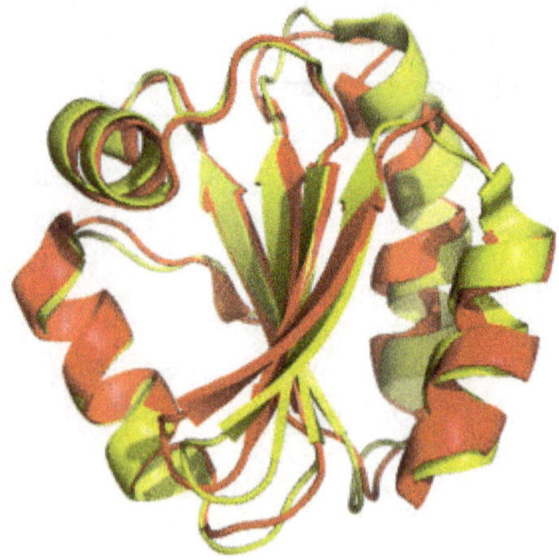

Structural alignment of thioredoxins from humans and the fly Drosophila melanogaster. The proteins are shown as ribbons, with the human protein in red, and the fly protein in yellow. Generated from PDB 3TRX and 1XWC.

Data Produced by Structural Alignment

The minimum information produced from a successful structural alignment is a set of superposed three-dimensional coordinates for each input structure. (Note that one input element may be fixed as a reference and therefore its superposed coordinates do not change.) The fitted structures can be used to calculate mutual RMSD values, as well as other more sophisticated measures of structural similarity such as the global distance test (GDT, the metric used in CASP). The structural alignment also implies a corresponding one-dimensional sequence alignment from which a sequence identity, or the percentage of residues that are identical between the input structures, can be calculated as a measure of how closely the two sequences are related.

Types of Comparisons

Because protein structures are composed of amino acids whose side chains are linked by a common protein backbone, a number of different possible subsets of the atoms that make up a protein macromolecule can be used in producing a structural alignment and calculating the corresponding RMSD values. When aligning structures with very different sequences, the side chain atoms generally are not taken into account because their identities differ between many aligned residues. For this reason it is common for structural alignment methods to use by default only the backbone atoms included in the peptide bond. For simplicity and efficiency, often only the alpha carbon positions are considered, since the peptide bond has a minimally variant planar conformation. Only when the structures to be aligned are highly similar or even identical is it meaningful to align side-chain atom positions, in which case the RMSD reflects not only the conformation of the protein backbone but also the rotameric states of the side chains. Other comparison criteria that reduce noise and bolster positive matches include secondary structure assignment, native contact maps or residue interaction patterns, measures of side chain packing, and measures of hydrogen bond retention.

Structural Superposition

The most basic possible comparison between protein structures makes no attempt to align the input structures and requires a precalculated alignment as input to determine which of the residues in the sequence are intended to be considered in the RMSD calculation. Structural superposition is commonly used to compare multiple conformations of the same protein (in which case no alignment is necessary, since the sequences are the same) and to evaluate the quality of alignments produced using only sequence information between two or more sequences whose structures are known. This method traditionally uses a simple least-squares fitting algorithm, in which the optimal rotations and translations are found by minimizing the sum of the squared distances among all structures in the superposition. More recently, maximum likelihood and Bayesian methods have greatly increased the accuracy of the estimated rotations, translations, and covariance matrices for the superposition.

Algorithms based on multidimensional rotations and modified quaternions have been developed to identify topological relationships between protein structures without the need for a predetermined alignment. Such algorithms have successfully identified canonical folds such as the four-helix bundle. The SuperPose method is sufficiently extensible to correct for relative domain rotations and other structural pitfalls.

Algorithmic Complexity

Optimal Solution

The optimal "threading" of a protein sequence onto a known structure and the production of an optimal multiple sequence alignment have been shown to be NP-complete. However, this does not imply that the structural alignment problem is NP-complete. Strictly speaking, an optimal solution to the protein structure alignment problem is only known for certain protein structure similarity measures, such as the measures used in protein structure prediction experiments, GDT_TS and MaxSub. These measures can be rigorously optimized using an algorithm capable of maximizing the number of atoms in two proteins that can be superimposed under a predefined distance cutoff. Unfortunately, the algorithm for optimal solution is not practical, since its running time depends not only on the lengths but also on the intrinsic geometry of input proteins.

Approximate Solution

Approximate polynomial-time algorithms for structural alignment that produce a family of "optimal" solutions within an approximation parameter for a given scoring function have been developed. Although these algorithms theoretically classify the approximate protein structure alignment problem as "tractable", they are still computationally too expensive for large-scale protein structure analysis. As a consequence, practical algorithms that converge to the global solutions of the alignment, given a scoring function, do not exist. Most algorithms are, therefore, heuristic, but algorithms that guarantee the convergence to at least local maximizers of the scoring functions, and are practical, have been developed.

Representation of Structures

Protein structures have to be represented in some coordinate-independent space to make them comparable. This is typically achieved by constructing a sequence-to-sequence matrix or series of matrices that encompass comparative metrics: rather than absolute distances relative to a fixed coordinate space. An intuitive representation is the distance matrix, which is a two-dimensional matrix containing all pairwise distances between some subset of the atoms in each structure (such as the alpha carbons). The matrix increases in dimensionality as the number of structures to be simultaneously aligned increases. Reducing the protein to a coarse metric such as secondary structure elements (SSEs) or structural fragments can also produce sensible alignments, despite the loss of information from discarding distances, as noise is also discarded. Choosing a representation to facilitate computation is critical to developing an efficient alignment mechanism.

Methods

Structural alignment techniques have been used in comparing individual structures or sets of structures as well as in the production of "all-to-all" comparison databases that measure the divergence between every pair of structures present in the Protein Data Bank (PDB). Such databases are used to classify proteins by their fold.

DALI

A common and popular structural alignment method is the DALI, or distance alignment matrix method, which breaks the input structures into hexapeptide fragments and calculates a distance matrix by evaluating the contact patterns between successive fragments. Secondary structure features that involve residues that are contiguous in sequence appear on the matrix's main diagonal; other diagonals in the matrix reflect spatial contacts between residues that are not near each other in the sequence. When these diagonals are parallel to the main diagonal, the features they represent are parallel; when they are perpendicular, their features are antiparallel. This representation is memory-intensive because the features in the square matrix are symmetrical (and thus redundant) about the main diagonal.

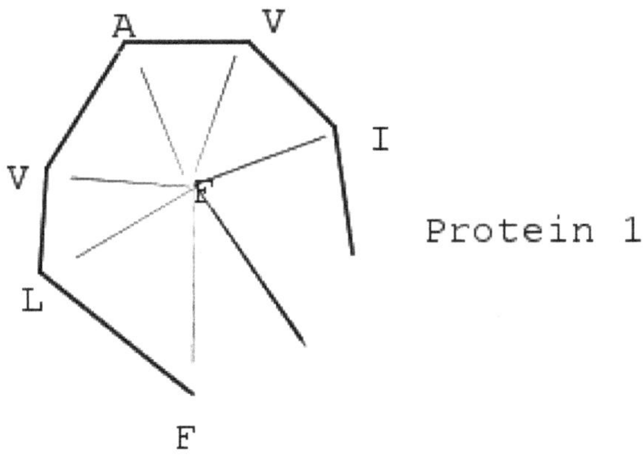

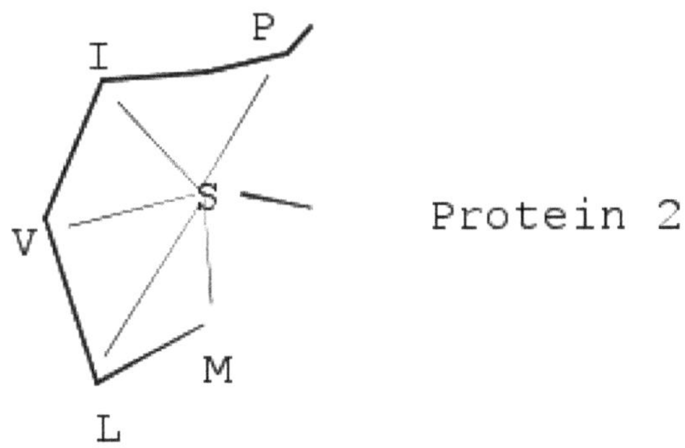

Illustration of the atom-to-atom vectors calculated in SSAP. From these vectors a series of vector differences, e.g., between (FA) in Protein 1 and (SI) in Protein 2 would be constructed. The two sequences are plotted on the two dimensions of a matrix to form a difference matrix between the two proteins. Dynamic programming is applied to all possible difference matrices to construct a series of optimal local alignment paths that are then summed to form the summary matrix, on which a second round of dynamic programming is performed.

When two proteins' distance matrices share the same or similar features in approximately the same positions, they can be said to have similar folds with similar-length loops connecting their secondary structure elements. DALI's actual alignment process requires a similarity search after the two proteins' distance matrices are built; this is normally conducted via a series of overlapping submatrices of size 6x6. Submatrix matches are then reassembled into a final alignment via a standard score-maximization algorithm — the original version of DALI used a Monte Carlo simulation to maximize a structural similarity score that is a function of the distances between putative corresponding atoms. In particular, more distant atoms within corresponding features are exponentially downweighted to reduce the effects of noise introduced by loop mobility, helix torsions, and other minor structural variations. Because DALI relies on an all-to-all distance matrix, it can account for the possibility that structurally aligned features might appear in different orders within the two sequences being compared.

The DALI method has also been used to construct a database known as FSSP (Fold classification based on Structure-Structure alignment of Proteins, or Families of Structurally Similar Proteins) in which all known protein structures are aligned with each other to determine their structural neighbors and fold classification. There is an searchable database based on DALI as well as a downloadable program and web search based on a standalone version known as DaliLite.

Combinatorial Extension

The combinatorial extension (CE) method is similar to DALI in that it too breaks each structure in the query set into a series of fragments that it then attempts to reassemble into a complete alignment. A series of pairwise combinations of fragments called aligned fragment pairs, or AFPs, are used to define a similarity matrix through which an optimal path is generated to identify the final alignment. Only AFPs that meet given criteria for local similarity are included in the matrix as a means of reducing the necessary search space and thereby increasing efficiency. A number of similarity metrics are possible; the original definition of the CE method included only structural superpositions and inter-residue distances but has since been expanded to include local environmental properties such as secondary structure, solvent exposure, hydrogen-bonding patterns, and dihedral angles.

An alignment path is calculated as the optimal path through the similarity matrix by linearly progressing through the sequences and extending the alignment with the next possible high-scoring AFP pair. The initial AFP pair that nucleates the alignment can occur at any point in the sequence matrix. Extensions then proceed with the next AFP that meets given distance criteria restricting the alignment to low gap sizes. The size of each AFP and the maximum gap size are required input parameters but are usually set to empirically determined values of 8 and 30 respectively. Like DALI and SSAP, CE has been used to construct an all-to-all fold classification database from the known protein structures in the PDB.

The RCSB PDB has recently released an updated version of CE and FATCAT as part of the RCSB PDB Protein Comparison Tool. It provides a new variation of CE that can detect circular permutations in protein structures.

SSAP

The SSAP (Sequential Structure Alignment Program) method uses double dynamic programming to produce a structural alignment based on atom-to-atom vectors in structure space. Instead of the alpha carbons typically used in structural alignment, SSAP constructs its vectors from the beta carbons for all residues except glycine, a method which thus takes into account the rotameric state of each residue as well as its location along the backbone. SSAP works by first constructing a series of inter-residue distance vectors between each residue and its nearest non-contiguous neighbors on each protein. A series of matrices are then constructed containing the vector differences between neighbors for each pair of residues for which vectors were constructed. Dynamic programming applied to each resulting matrix determines a series of optimal local alignments which are then summed into a "summary" matrix to which dynamic programming is applied again to determine the overall structural alignment.

SSAP originally produced only pairwise alignments but has since been extended to multiple alignments as well. It has been applied in an all-to-all fashion to produce a hierarchical fold classification scheme known as CATH (Class, Architecture, Topology, Homology), which has been used to construct the CATH Protein Structure Classification database.

Recent Developments

Improvements in structural alignment methods constitute an active area of research, and new or modified methods are often proposed that are claimed to offer advantages over the older and more widely distributed techniques. A recent example, TM-align, uses a novel method for weighting its distance matrix, to which standard dynamic programming is then applied. The weighting is proposed to accelerate the convergence of dynamic programming and correct for effects arising from alignment lengths. In a benchmarking study, TM-align has been reported to improve in both speed and accuracy over DALI and CE.

Other promising methods of structural alignment are local structural alignment methods. These provide comparison of pre-selected parts of proteins (e.g. binding sites, user-defined structural motifs) against binding sites or whole-protein structural databases. The MultiBind and MAPPIS servers allow the identification of common spatial arrangements of physicochemical properties such as H-bond donor, acceptor, aliphatic, aromatic or hydrophobic in a set of user provided protein binding sites defined by interactions with small molecules (MultiBind) or in a set of user-provided protein–protein interfaces (MAPPIS). Others provide comparison of entire protein structures against a number of user submitted structures or against a large database of protein structures in reasonable time (ProBiS). Unlike global alignment approaches, local structural alignment approaches are suited to detection of locally conserved patterns of functional groups, which often appear in binding sites and have significant involvement in ligand binding. As an example, comparing G-Losa, a local structure alignment tool, with TM-align, a global structure alignment based method. While G-Losa predicts drug-like ligands' positions in single-chain protein targets more precisely than TM-align, the overall success rate of TM-align is better.

However, as algorithmic improvements and computer performance have erased purely technical deficiencies in older approaches, it has become clear that there is no one universal criterion for the 'optimal' structural alignment. TM-align, for instance, is particularly robust in quantifying comparisons between sets of proteins with great disparities in sequence lengths, but it only indirectly captures hydrogen bonding or secondary structure order conservation which might be better metrics for alignment of evolutionarily related proteins. Thus recent developments have focused on optimizing particular attributes such as speed, quantification of scores, correlation to alternative gold standards, or tolerance of imperfection in structural data or ab initio structural models. An alternative methodology that is gaining popularity is to use the *consensus* of various methods to ascertain proteins structural similarities.

RNA Structural Alignment

Structural alignment techniques have traditionally been applied exclusively to proteins, as the primary biological macromolecules that assume characteristic three-dimensional structures. However, large RNA molecules also form characteristic tertiary structures, which are mediated primarily by hydrogen bonds formed between base pairs as well as base stacking. Functionally similar noncoding RNA molecules can be especially difficult to extract from genomics data because structure is more strongly conserved than sequence in RNA as well as in proteins, and the more limited alphabet of RNA decreases the information content of any given nucleotide at any given position.

However, because of the increasing interest in RNA structures and because of the growth of the number of experimentally determined 3D RNA structures, few RNA structure similarity methods have been developed recently. One of those methods is, e.g., SETTER which decomposes each RNA structure into smaller parts called general secondary structure units (GSSUs). GSSUs are subsequently aligned and these partial alignments are merged into the final RNA structure alignment and scored. The method has been implemented into the SETTER webserver.

A recent method for pairwise structural alignment of RNA sequences with low sequence identity has been published and implemented in the program FOLDALIGN. However, this method is not truly analogous to protein structural alignment techniques because it computationally predicts the structures of the RNA input sequences rather than requiring experimentally determined structures as input. Although computational prediction of the protein folding process has not been particularly successful to date, RNA structures without pseudoknots can often be sensibly predicted using free energy-based scoring methods that account for base pairing and stacking.

Software

Choosing a software tool for structural alignment can be a challenge due to the large variety of available packages that differ significantly in methodology and reliability. A partial solution to this problem was presented in and made publicly accessible through the ProCKSI webserver. A more complete list of currently available and freely distributed structural alignment software can be found in structural alignment software.

Properties of some structural alignment servers and software packages are summarized and tested with examples at Structural Alignment Tools in Proteopedia.Org.

MACROMOLECULAR DOCKING

Macromolecular docking is the computational modelling of the quaternary structure of complexes formed by two or more interacting biological macromolecules. Protein–protein complexes are the most commonly attempted targets of such modelling, followed by protein–nucleic acid complexes.

The ultimate goal of docking is the prediction of the three-dimensional structure of the macromolecular complex of interest as it would occur in a living organism. Docking itself only produces plausible candidate structures. These candidates must be ranked using methods such as scoring functions to identify structures that are most likely to occur in nature.

The term "docking" originated in the late 1970s, with a more restricted meaning; then, "docking" meant refining a model of a complex structure by optimizing the separation between the interactors but keeping their relative orientations fixed. Later, the relative orientations of the interacting partners in the modelling was allowed to vary, but the internal geometry of each of the partners was held fixed. This type of modelling is sometimes referred to as "rigid docking". With further increases in computational power, it became possible to model changes in internal geometry of the interacting partners that may occur when a complex is formed. This type of modelling is referred to as "flexible docking".

Background

The biological roles of most proteins, as characterized by which other macromolecules they interact with, are known at best incompletely. Even those proteins that participate in a well-studied biological process (e.g., the Krebs cycle) may have unexpected interaction partners or functions which are unrelated to that process.

In cases of known protein–protein interactions, other questions arise. Genetic diseases (e.g., cystic fibrosis) are known to be caused by misfolded or mutated proteins, and there is a desire to understand what, if any, anomalous protein–protein interactions a given mutation can cause. In the distant future, proteins may be designed to perform biological functions, and a determination of the potential interactions of such proteins will be essential.

For any given set of proteins, the following questions may be of interest, from the point of view of technology or natural history:

- Do these proteins bind *in vivo*?

If they do bind,

- What is the spatial configuration which they adopt in their bound state?
- How strong or weak is their interaction?

If they do not bind,

- Can they be made to bind by inducing a mutation?

Protein–protein docking is ultimately envisaged to address all these issues. Furthermore, since docking methods can be based on purely physical principles, even proteins of unknown function (or which have been studied relatively little) may be docked. The only prerequisite is that their molecular structure has been either determined experimentally, or can be estimated by a protein structure prediction technique.

Protein–nucleic acid interactions feature prominently in the living cell. Transcription factors, which regulate gene expression, and polymerases, which catalyse replication, are composed of proteins, and the genetic material they interact with is composed of nucleic acids. Modeling protein–nucleic acid complexes presents some unique challenges, as described below.

History

In the 1970s, complex modelling revolved around manually identifying features on the surfaces of the interactors, and interpreting the consequences for binding, function and activity; any computer programmes were typically used at the end of the modelling process, to discriminate between the relatively few configurations which remained after all the heuristic constraints had been imposed. The first use of computers was in a study on hemoglobin interaction in sickle-cell fibres. This was followed in 1978 by work on the trypsin-BPTI complex. Computers discriminated between good and bad models using a scoring function which rewarded large interface area, and pairs of molecules in contact but not occupying the same space. The computer used a simplified representation of the interacting proteins, with one interaction centre for each residue. Favorable electrostatic interactions, including hydrogen bonds, were identified by hand.

In the early 1990s, more structures of complexes were determined, and available computational power had increased substantially. With the emergence of bioinformatics, the focus moved towards developing generalized techniques which could be applied to an arbitrary set of complexes at acceptable computational cost. The new methods were envisaged to apply even in the absence of phylogenetic or experimental clues; any specific prior knowledge could still be introduced at the stage of choosing between the highest ranking output models, or be framed as input if the algorithm catered for it. 1992 saw the publication of the correlation method, an algorithm which used the fast Fourier transform to give a vastly improved scalability for evaluating coarse shape complementarity on rigid-body models. This was extended in 1997 to cover coarse electrostatics.

In 1996 the results of the first blind trial were published, in which six research groups attempted to predict the complexed structure of TEM-1 Beta-lactamase with Beta-lactamase inhibitor protein (BLIP). The exercise brought into focus the necessity of accommodating conformational change and the difficulty of discriminating between conformers. It also served as the prototype for the CAPRI assessment series, which debuted in 2001.

Rigid-Body Docking *vs.* Flexible Docking

If the bond angles, bond lengths and torsion angles of the components are not modified at any stage of complex generation, it is known as *rigid body docking*. A subject of speculation is whether or not rigid-body docking is sufficiently good for most docking. When substantial conformational change occurs within the components at the time of complex formation, rigid-body docking is inadequate. However, scoring all possible conformational changes is prohibitively expensive in computer time. Docking procedures which permit conformational change, or *flexible docking* procedures, must intelligently select small subset of possible conformational changes for consideration.

Methods

Successful docking requires two criteria:

- Generating a set of configurations which reliably includes at least one nearly correct one.

- Reliably distinguishing nearly correct configurations from the others.

For many interactions, the binding site is known on one or more of the proteins to be docked. This is the case for antibodies and for competitive inhibitors. In other cases, a binding site may be strongly suggested by mutagenic or phylogenetic evidence. Configurations where the proteins interpenetrate severely may also be ruled out *a priori*.

After making exclusions based on prior knowledge or stereochemical clash, the remaining space of possible complexed structures must be sampled exhaustively, evenly and with a sufficient coverage to guarantee a near hit. Each configuration must be scored with a measure that is capable of ranking a nearly correct structure above at least 100,000 alternatives. This is a computationally intensive task, and a variety of strategies have been developed.

Reciprocal Space Methods

Each of the proteins may be represented as a simple cubic lattice. Then, for the class of scores which are discrete convolutions, configurations related to each other by translation of one protein by an exact lattice vector can all be scored almost simultaneously by applying the convolution theorem. It is possible to construct reasonable, if approximate, convolution-like scoring functions representing both stereochemical and electrostatic fitness.

Reciprocal space methods have been used extensively for their ability to evaluate enormous numbers of configurations. They lose their speed advantage if torsional changes are introduced. Another drawback is that it is impossible to make efficient use of prior knowledge. The question also remains whether convolutions are too limited a class of scoring function to identify the best complex reliably.

Monte Carlo Methods

In Monte Carlo, an initial configuration is refined by taking random steps which are accepted or rejected based on their induced improvement in score, until a certain number of steps have been tried. The assumption is that convergence to the best structure should occur from a large class of initial configurations, only one of which needs to be considered. Initial configurations may be sampled coarsely, and much computation time can be saved. Because of the difficulty of finding a scoring function which is both highly discriminating for the correct configuration and also converges to the correct configuration from a distance, the use of two levels of refinement, with different scoring functions, has been proposed. Torsion can be introduced naturally to Monte Carlo as an additional property of each random move.

Monte Carlo methods are not guaranteed to search exhaustively, so that the best configuration may be missed even using a scoring function which would in theory identify it. How severe a problem this is for docking has not been firmly established.

Evaluation

Scoring Functions

To find a score which forms a consistent basis for selecting the best configuration, studies are carried out on a standard benchmark (see below) of protein–protein interaction cases. Scoring functions are assessed on the rank they assign to the best structure (ideally the best structure should be ranked 1), and on their coverage (the proportion of the benchmark cases for which they achieve an acceptable result). Types of scores studied include:

- Heuristic scores based on residue contacts.
- Shape complementarity of molecular surfaces ("stereochemistry").
- Free energies, estimated using parameters from molecular mechanics force fields such as CHARMM or AMBER.
- Phylogenetic desirability of the interacting regions.
- Clustering coefficients.

It is usual to create hybrid scores by combining one or more categories above in a weighted sum whose weights are optimized on cases from the benchmark. To avoid bias, the benchmark cases used to optimize the weights must not overlap with the cases used to make the final test of the score.

The ultimate goal in protein–protein docking is to select the ideal ranking solution according to a scoring scheme that would also give an insight into the affinity of the complex. Such a development would drive *in silico* protein engineering, computer-aided drug design and/or high-throughput annotation of which proteins bind or not (annotation of interactome). Several scoring functions have been proposed for binding affinity / free energy prediction. However the correlation between experimentally determined binding affinities and the predictions of nine commonly used scoring functions have been found to be nearly orthogonal ($R^2 \sim 0$). It was also observed that some components of the scoring algorithms may display better correlation to the experimental binding energies than the full score, suggesting that a significantly better performance might be obtained by combining the appropriate contributions from different scoring algorithms. Experimental methods for the determination of binding affinities are: surface plasmon resonance (SPR), Förster resonance energy transfer, radioligand-based techniques, isothermal titration calorimetry (ITC), microscale thermophoresis (MST) or spectroscopic measurements and other fluorescence techniques.

Benchmarks

A benchmark of 84 protein–protein interactions with known complexed structures has been developed for testing docking methods. The set is chosen to cover a wide range of interaction types, and to avoid repeated features, such as the profile of interactors' structural families according to the SCOP database. Benchmark elements are classified into three levels of difficulty (the most difficult containing the largest change in backbone conformation). The protein–protein docking benchmark contains examples of enzyme-inhibitor, antigen-antibody and homomultimeric complexes.

The latest version of protein-protein docking benchmark consists of 230 complexes. A protein-DNA docking benchmark consists of 47 test cases. A protein-RNA docking benchmark was curated as a dataset of 45 non-redundant test cases with complexes solved by X-ray crystallography only as well as an extended dataset of 71 test cases with structures derived from homology modelling as well. The protein-RNA benchmark has been updated to include more structures solved by X-ray crystallography and now it consists of 126 test cases.

A binding affinity benchmark has been based on the protein–protein docking benchmark. 81 protein–protein complexes with known experimental affinities are included; these complexes span over 11 orders of magnitude in terms of affinity. Each entry of the benchmark includes several biochemical parameters associated with the experimental data, along with the method used to determine the affinity. This benchmark was used to assess the extent to which scoring functions could also predict affinities of macromolecular complexes.

This Benchmark was post-peer reviewed and significantly expanded. The new set is diverse in terms of the biological functions it represents, with complexes that involve G-proteins and receptor extracellular domains, as well as antigen/antibody, enzyme/inhibitor, and enzyme/substrate complexes. It is also diverse in terms of the partners' affinity for each other, with K_d ranging between 10^{-5} and 10^{-14} M. Nine pairs of entries represent closely related complexes that have a similar structure, but a very different affinity, each pair comprising a cognate and a noncognate assembly. The unbound structures of the component proteins being available, conformation changes can be assessed. They are significant in most of the complexes, and large movements or disorder-to-order transitions are frequently observed. The set may be used to benchmark biophysical models aiming to relate affinity to structure in protein–protein interactions, taking into account the reactants and the conformation changes that accompany the association reaction, instead of just the final product.

The CAPRI Assessment

The Critical Assessment of PRediction of Interactions is an ongoing series of events in which researchers throughout the community try to dock the same proteins, as provided by the assessors. Rounds take place approximately every 6 months. Each round contains between one and six target protein–protein complexes whose structures have been recently determined experimentally. The coordinates and are held privately by the assessors, with the cooperation of the structural biologists who determined them. The assessment of submissions is double blind.

CAPRI attracts a high level of participation (37 groups participated worldwide in round seven) and a high level of interest from the biological community in general. Although CAPRI results are of little statistical significance owing to the small number of targets in each round, the role of CAPRI in stimulating discourse is significant. (The CASP assessment is a similar exercise in the field of protein structure prediction).

REFERENCES

1. Mount DM (2004). Bioinformatics: Sequence and Genome Analysis. 2. Cold Spring Harbor Laboratory Press. ISBN 0-87969-712-1.
2. Huang, JY.; Brutlag, DL. (Jan 2001). "The EMOTIF database". Nucleic Acids Res. 29 (1): 202–04. doi:10.1093/nar/29.1.202. PMID 11125091.
3. Pirovano, W.; Heringa, J. (2010). "Protein secondary structure prediction". Methods Mol Biol. Methods in Molecular Biology. 609: 327–48. doi:10.1007/978-1-60327-241-4_19. ISBN 978-1-60327-240-7. PMID 20221928.
4. Guzzo, AV (1965). "Influence of Amino-Acid Sequence on Protein Structure". Biophys. J. 5 (6): 809–822. Bibcode:1965BpJ.....5..809G. doi:10.1016/S0006-3495(65)86753-4. PMC 1367904Freely accessible. PMID 5884309.
5. Prothero, JW (1966). "Correlation between Distribution of Amino Acids and Alpha Helices". Biophys. J. 6 (3): 367–370. Bibcode:1966BpJ.....6..367P. doi:10.1016/S0006-3495(66)86662-6. PMC 1367951Freely accessible. PMID 5962284.
6. Schiffer, M; Edmundson AB (1967). "Use of Helical Wheels to Represent Structures of Proteins and to Identify Segments with Helical Potential". Biophys. J. 7 (2): 121–35. Bibcode:1967BpJ.....7..121S. doi:10.1016/S0006-3495(67)86579-2. PMC 1368002Freely accessible. PMID 6048867.
7. Kotelchuck, D; Scheraga HA (1969). "The Influence of Short-Range Interactions on Protein Conformation, II. A Model for Predicting the α-Helical Regions of Proteins ". Proc Natl Acad Sci USA. 62 (1): 14–21. doi:10.1073/pnas.62.1.14. PMC 285948Freely accessible. PMID 5253650.
8. Lewis, PN; Gō N; Gō M; Kotelchuck D; Scheraga HA (1970). "Helix Probability Profiles of Denatured Proteins and Their Correlation with Native Structures ". Proc Natl Acad Sci USA. 65 (4): 810–5. doi:10.1073/pnas.65.4.810. PMC 282987Freely accessible. PMID 5266152.
9. Froimowitz M, Fasman GD; Fasman (1974). "Prediction of the secondary structure of proteins using the helix-coil transition theory ". Macromolecules. 7 (5): 583–9. doi:10.1021/ma60041a009. PMID 4371089.
10. Dor O, Zhou Y; Zhou (2006). "Achieving 80% tenfold cross-validated accuracy for secondary structure prediction by large-scale training ". Proteins. 66 (4): 838–45. doi:10.1002/prot.21298. PMID 17177203.
11. Chou PY, Fasman GD; Fasman (1974). "Prediction of protein conformation ". Biochemistry. 13 (2): 222–245. doi:10.1021/bi00699a002. PMID 4358940.
12. Garnier J, Osguthorpe DJ, Robson B; Osguthorpe; Robson (1978). "Analysis of the accuracy and implications of simple methods for predicting the secondary structure of globular proteins ". J Mol Biol. 120 (1): 97–120. doi:10.1016/0022-2836(78)90297-8. PMID 642007.
13. Pham TH, Satou K, Ho TB; Satou; Ho (2005). "Support vector machines for prediction and analysis of beta and gamma-turns in proteins ". J Bioinform Comput Biol. 3 (2): 343–358. doi:10.1142/S0219720005001089. PMID 15852509.
14. Zhang Q, Yoon S, Welsh WJ; Yoon; Welsh (2005). "Improved method for

predicting beta-turn using support vector machine ". Bioinformatics. 21 (10): 2370–4. doi:10.1093/bioinformatics/bti358. PMID 15797917.

15. Zimmermann O, Hansmann UH; Hansmann (2006). "Support vector machines for prediction of dihedral angle regions ". Bioinformatics. 22 (24): 3009–15. doi:10.1093/bioinformatics/btl489. PMID 17005536.
16. Kuang R, Leslie CS, Yang AS; Leslie; Yang (2004). "Protein backbone angle prediction with machine learning approaches ". Bioinformatics. 20 (10): 1612–21. doi:10.1093/bioinformatics/bth136. PMID 14988121.
17. Faraggi E, Yang Y, Zhou Y; Yang; Zhang; Zhou (2009). "Predicting continuous local structure and the effect of its substitution for secondary structure in fragment-free protein structure prediction ". Structure. 17 (11): 1515–1527. doi:10.1016/j.str.2009.09.006. PMC 2778607Freely accessible. PMID 19913486.
18. Zhong L, Johnson WC Jr; Johnson Jr (1992). "Environment affects amino acid preference for secondary structure ". Proc Natl Acad Sci USA. 89 (10): 4462–5. doi:10.1073/pnas.89.10.4462. PMC 49102Freely accessible. PMID 1584778.
19. Macdonald JR, Johnson WC Jr; Johnson Jr (2001). "Environmental features are important in determining protein secondary structure ". Protein Sci. 10 (6): 1172–7. doi:10.1110/ps.420101. PMC 2374018Freely accessible. PMID 11369855.
20. Costantini S, Colonna G, Facchiano AM; Colonna; Facchiano (2006). "Amino acid propensities for secondary structures are influenced by the protein structural class ". Biochem Biophys Res Commun. 342 (2): 441–451. doi:10.1016/j.bbrc.2006.01.159. PMID 16487481.
21. Marashi SA; et al. (2007). "Adaptation of proteins to different environments: a comparison of proteome structural properties in Bacillus subtilis and Escherichia coli ". J Theor Biol. 244 (1): 127–132. doi:10.1016/j.jtbi.2006.07.021. PMID 16945389.
22. Costantini S, Colonna G, Facchiano AM; Colonna; Facchiano (2007). "PreSSAPro: a software for the prediction of secondary structure by amino acid properties ". Comput Biol Chem. 31 (5–6): 389–392. doi:10.1016/j.compbiolchem.2007.08.010. PMID 17888742.
23. Momen-Roknabadi A; et al. (2008). "Impact of residue accessible surface area on the prediction of protein secondary structures ". BMC Bioinformatics. 9: 357. doi:10.1186/1471-2105-9-357. PMC 2553345Freely accessible. PMID 18759992.
24. Adamczak R, Porollo A, Meller J; Porollo; Meller (2005). "Combining prediction of secondary structure and solvent accessibility in proteins ". Proteins. 59 (3): 467–475. doi:10.1002/prot.20441. PMID 15768403.
25. Lakizadeh A, Marashi SA (2009). "Addition of contact number information can improve protein secondary structure prediction by neural networks " (PDF). Excli J. 8: 66–73.
26. Zhang Y (2008). "Progress and challenges in protein structure prediction ". Curr Opin Struct Biol. 18 (3): 342–8. doi:10.1016/j.sbi.2008.02.004. PMC 2680823Freely accessible. PMID 18436442.

27. Shaw, David E.; Bowers, Kevin J.; Chow, Edmond; Eastwood, Michael P.; Ierardi, Douglas J.; Klepeis, John L.; Kuskin, Jeffrey S.; Larson, Richard H.; Lindorff-Larsen, Kresten; Maragakis, Paul; Moraes, Mark A.; Dror, Ron O.; Piana, Stefano; Shan, Yibing; Towles, Brian; Salmon, John K.; Grossman, J. P.; Mackenzie, Kenneth M.; Bank, Joseph A.; Young, Cliff; Deneroff, Martin M.; Batson, Brannon (2009). "Proceedings of the Conference on High Performance Computing Networking, Storage and Analysis - SC ‹09 ": 1. doi:10.1145/1654059.1654126. ISBN 9781605587448. |chapter= ignored (help)

28. Pierce, Levi C.T.; Salomon-Ferrer, Romelia; Augusto F. de Oliveira, Cesar; McCammon, J. Andrew; Walker, Ross C. (2012). "Routine Access to Millisecond Time Scale Events with Accelerated Molecular Dynamics ". Journal of Chemical Theory and Computation. 8 (9): 2997–3002. doi:10.1021/ct300284c. ISSN 1549-9618. PMID 22984356.

29. Kmiecik, Sebastian; Gront, Dominik; Kolinski, Michal; Wieteska, Lukasz; Dawid, Aleksandra Elzbieta; Kolinski, Andrzej (2016-06-22). "Coarse-Grained Protein Models and Their Applications ". Chemical Reviews. doi:10.1021/acs.chemrev.6b00163. ISSN 0009-2665.

30. Gobel, U.; et al. (1994). "Correlated mutations and residue contacts in proteins ". Proteins. 18 (4): 309–17. doi:10.1002/prot.340180402. PMID 8208723.

31. Taylor, W. R.; Hatrick, K. (1994). "Compensating changes in protein multiple sequence alignments ". Protein Eng. 7 (3): 341–48. doi:10.1093/protein/7.3.341. PMID 8177883.

32. Neher, E. (Jan 1994). "How frequent are correlated changes in families of protein sequences? ". Proc Natl Acad Sci U S A. 91 (1): 98–102. doi:10.1073/pnas.91.1.98. PMC 42893Freely accessible. PMID 8278414.

33. Marks, D. S.; et al. (2011). "Protein 3D structure computed from evolutionary sequence variation ". PLoS ONE. 6 (12): e28766. doi:10.1371/journal.pone.0028766. PMC 3233603Freely accessible. PMID 22163331.

34. Burger, L.; van Nimwegen, E (2010). "Disentangling direct from indirect co-evolution of residues in protein alignments ". PLoS Comput Biol. 6: e1000633. doi:10.1371/journal.pcbi.1000633.

35. Morcos, F.; Pagnani, A.; Lunt, B.; Bertolino, A.; Marks, DS.; Sander, C.; Zecchina, R.; Onuchic, JN.; et al. (Dec 2011). "Direct-coupling analysis of residue coevolution captures native contacts across many protein families ". Proc Natl Acad Sci U S A. 108 (49): E1293–1301. doi:10.1073/pnas.1111471108. PMC 3241805Freely accessible. PMID 22106262.

36. Nugent, T.; Jones, D.T. (2012). "Accurate de novo structure prediction of large transmembrane protein domains using fragment-assembly and correlated mutation analysis ". Proc Natl Acad Sci U S A. 109 (24): E1540–47. doi:10.1073/pnas.1120036109. PMID 22645369.

37. Hopf, T. A.; et al. (2012). "Three-dimensional structures of membrane proteins from genomic sequencing ". Cell. 149 (7): 1607–21. doi:10.1016/j.cell.2012.04.012. PMC 3641781Freely accessible. PMID 22579045.

38. Zhang Y & Skolnick J (2005). "The protein structure prediction problem could be solved using the current PDB library ". Proc Natl Acad Sci USA. 102 (4): 1029–34. doi:10.1073/pnas.0407152101. PMC 545829Freely accessible. PMID 15653774.

39. Bowie JU, Luthy R, Eisenberg D; Lüthy; Eisenberg (1991). "A method to identify protein sequences that fold into a known three-dimensional structure ". Science. 253 (5016): 164–170. doi:10.1126/science.1853201. PMID 1853201.

40. Dunbrack, RL (2002). "Rotamer Libraries in the 21st Century ". Curr. Opin. Struct. Biol. 12 (4): 431–440. doi:10.1016/S0959-440X(02)00344-5. PMID 12163064.

41. Ponder JW, Richards FM; Richards (1987). "Tertiary templates for proteins: use of packing criteria in the enumeration of allowed sequences for different structural classes ". J. Mol. Biol. 193 (4): 775–791. doi:10.1016/0022-2836(87)90358-5. PMID 2441069.

42. Lovell SC, Word, Richardson, Richardson (2000). "The penultimate rotamer library ". Proteins: Struc. Func. Genet. 40 (3): 389–408. doi:10.1002/1097-0134(20000815)40:3<389::AID-PROT50>3.0.CO;2-2.

43. Shapovalov MV, Dunbrack, RL; Dunbrack Jr (2011). "A smoothed backbone-dependent rotamer library for proteins derived from adaptive kernel density estimates and regressions ". Structure (Cell Press). 19 (6): 844–858. doi:10.1016/j.str.2011.03.019. PMC 3118414Freely accessible. PMID 21645855.

44. Chen, VB.; Arendall, WB.; Headd, JJ.; Keedy, DA.; Immormino, RM.; Kapral, GJ.; Murray, LW.; Richardson, JS.; Richardson, DC. (Jan 2010). "MolProbity: all-atom structure validation for macromolecular crystallography ". Acta Crystallogr D. 66 (Pt 1): 12–21. doi:10.1107/S0907444909042073. PMC 2803126Freely accessible. PMID 20057044.

45. Bower, MJ.; Cohen, FE.; Dunbrack, RL. (Apr 1997). "Prediction of protein side-chain rotamers from a backbone-dependent rotamer library: a new homology modeling tool ". J Mol Biol. 267 (5): 1268–82. doi:10.1006/jmbi.1997.0926. PMID 9150411.

46. Voigt CA, Gordon DB, Mayo SL; Gordon; Mayo (2000). "Trading accuracy for speed: A quantitative comparison of search algorithms in protein sequence design ". J Mol Biol. 299 (3): 789–803. doi:10.1006/jmbi.2000.3758. PMID 10835284.

47. Krivov GG, Shapovalov MV, Dunbrack, RL; Shapovalov; Dunbrack Jr (2009). "Improved prediction of protein side-chain conformations with SCWRL4 ". Proteins. 77 (3): 778–795. doi:10.1002/prot.22488. PMC 2885146Freely accessible. PMID 19603484.

48. Chou KC, Zhang CT; Zhang (1995). "Prediction of protein structural classes ". Crit. Rev. Biochem. Mol. Biol. 30 (4): 275–349. doi:10.3109/10409239509083488. PMID 7587280.

49. Chen C, Zhou X, Tian Y, Zou X, Cai P; Zhou; Tian; Zou; Cai (October 2006). "Predicting protein structural class with pseudo-amino acid composition and support vector machine fusion network ". Anal. Biochem. 357 (1): 116–21.

doi:10.1016/j.ab.2006.07.022. PMID 16920060.

50. Chen C, Tian YX, Zou XY, Cai PX, Mo JY; Tian; Zou; Cai; Mo (December 2006). "Using pseudo-amino acid composition and support vector machine to predict protein structural class ". J. Theor. Biol. 243 (3): 444–8. doi:10.1016/j.jtbi.2006.06.025. PMID 16908032.
51. Lin H, Li QZ; Li (July 2007). "Using pseudo amino acid composition to predict protein structural class: approached by incorporating 400 dipeptide components ". J Comput Chem. 28 (9): 1463–6. doi:10.1002/jcc.20554. PMID 17330882.
52. Xiao X, Wang P, Chou KC; Wang; Chou (October 2008). "Predicting protein structural classes with pseudo amino acid composition: an approach using geometric moments of cellular automaton image ". J. Theor. Biol. 254 (3): 691–6. doi:10.1016/j.jtbi.2008.06.016. PMID 18634802.
53. Chou KC, Cai YD; Cai (September 2004). "Predicting protein structural class by functional domain composition ". Biochem. Biophys. Res. Commun. 321 (4): 1007–9. doi:10.1016/j.bbrc.2004.07.059. PMID 15358128.
54. Battey JN, Kopp J, Bordoli L, Read RJ, Clarke ND, Schwede T; Kopp; Bordoli; Read; Clarke; Schwede (2007). "Automated server predictions in CASP7 ". Proteins. 69 (Suppl 8): 68–82. doi:10.1002/prot.21761. PMID 17894354.
55. Zhang Y, Skolnick J (2005). "The protein structure prediction problem could be solved using the current PDB library ". Proc Natl Acad Sci USA. 102 (4): 1029–34. doi:10.1073/pnas.0407152101. PMC 545829Freely accessible. PMID 15653774.
56. Zemla A. (2003). "LGA — A Method for Finding 3-D Similarities in Protein Structures ". Nucleic Acids Research. 31 (13): 3370–3374. doi:10.1093/nar/gkg571. PMC 168977Freely accessible. PMID 12824330.
57. Godzik A (1996). "The structural alignment between two proteins: Is there a unique answer? ". Protein science : a publication of the Protein Society. 5 (7): 1325–38. doi:10.1002/pro.5560050711. PMC 2143456Freely accessible. PMID 8819165.
58. Martin ACR (1982). "Rapid Comparison of Protein Structures ". Acta Crystallogr A. 38 (6): 871–873. doi:10.1107/S0567739482001806.
59. Theobald DL, Wuttke DS (2006). "Empirical Bayes hierarchical models for regularizing maximum likelihood estimation in the matrix Gaussian Procrustes problem ". Proceedings of the National Academy of Sciences. 103 (49): 18521–18527. doi:10.1073/pnas.0508445103.
60. Theobald DL, Wuttke DS (2006). "THESEUS: Maximum likelihood superpositioning and analysis of macromolecular structures ". Bioinformatics. 22 (17): 2171–2172. doi:10.1093/bioinformatics/btl332. PMC 2584349Freely accessible. PMID 16777907.
61. Diederichs K. (1995). "Structural superposition of proteins with unknown alignment and detection of topological similarity using a six-dimensional search algorithm ". Proteins. 23 (2): 187–95. doi:10.1002/prot.340230208. PMID 8592700.

62. Maiti R, Van Domselaar GH, Zhang H, Wishart DS (2004). "SuperPose: a simple server for sophisticated structural superposition ". Nucleic Acids Res. 32 (Web Server issue): W590–4. doi:10.1093/nar/gkh477. PMC 441615Freely accessible. PMID 15215457.

63. Lathrop RH. (1994). "The protein threading problem with sequence amino acid interaction preferences is NP-complete ". Protein Eng. 7 (9): 1059–68. doi:10.1093/protein/7.9.1059. PMID 7831276.

64. Wang L, Jiang T (1994) On the complexity of multiple sequence alignment). "On the complexity of multiple sequence alignment ". J Comput Biol. 1 (4): 337–348. doi:10.1089/cmb.1994.1.337. PMID 8790475. Check date values in: |date= (help)

65. Siew N, Elofsson A, Rychlewsk L, Fischer D (2000). "MaxSub: an automated measure for the assessment of protein structure prediction quality ". Bioinformatics. 16 (9): 776–85. doi:10.1093/bioinformatics/16.9.776. PMID 11108700.

66. Poleksic A (2009). "Algorithms for optimal protein structure alignment ". Bioinformatics. 25 (21): 2751–2756. doi:10.1093/bioinformatics/btp530. PMID 19734152.

67. Kolodny R, Linial N (2004). "Approximate protein structural alignment in polynomial time ". PNAS. 101 (33): 12201–12206. doi:10.1073/pnas.0404383101. PMC 514457Freely accessible. PMID 15304646.

68. Martinez L, Andreani, R, Martinez, JM. (2007). "Convergent algorithms for protein structural alignment ". BMC Bioinformatics. 8: 306. doi:10.1186/1471-2105-8-306. PMC 1995224Freely accessible. PMID 17714583.

69. Mount DM. (2004). Bioinformatics: Sequence and Genome Analysis 2nd ed. Cold Spring Harbor Laboratory Press: Cold Spring Harbor, NY ISBN 0879697121

70. Holm L, Sander C (1996). "Mapping the protein universe ". Science. 273 (5275): 595–603. doi:10.1126/science.273.5275.595. PMID 8662544.

71. Shindyalov, I.N.; Bourne P.E. (1998). "Protein structure alignment by incremental combinatorial extension (CE) of the optimal path ". Protein Engineering. 11 (9): 739–747. doi:10.1093/protein/11.9.739. PMID 9796821.

72. Prlic A, Bliven S, Rose PW, Bluhm WF, Bizon C, Godzik A, Bourne PE (2010). "Pre-calculated protein structure alignments at the RCSB PDB website ". Bioinformatics (Oxford, England). 26 (23): 2983–2985. doi:10.1093/bioinformatics/btq572. PMC 3003546Freely accessible. PMID 20937596.

73. Taylor WR, Flores TP, Orengo CA (1994). "Multiple protein structure alignment ". Protein Sci. 3 (10): 1858–70. doi:10.1002/pro.5560031025. PMC 2142613Freely accessible. PMID 7849601.

74. Orengo CA, Michie AD, Jones S, Jones DT, Swindells MB, Thornton JM (1997). "CATH: A hierarchical classification of protein domain structures ". Structure. 5 (8): 1093–1108. doi:10.1016/S0969-2126(97)00260-8. PMID 9309224.

75. Zhang Y, Skolnick J (2005) TM–align: A protein structure alignment algorithm based on TM–score). "TM-align: A protein structure alignment algorithm based

on the TM-score ". Nucleic Acids Research. 33 (7): 2302–2309. doi:10.1093/nar/gki524. PMC 1084323Freely accessible. PMID 15849316. Check date values in: |date= (help)

76. Zhang Y, Skolnick J (2004) Scoring function for automated assessment of protein structure template quality). "Scoring function for automated assessment of protein structure template quality ". Proteins. 57 (4): 702–710. doi:10.1002/prot.20264. PMID 15476259. Check date values in: |date= (help)
77. Stefano Angaran; Mary Ellen Bock; Claudio Garutti; Concettina Guerral (2009). "MolLoc: a web tool for the local structural alignment of molecular surfaces ". Nucleic Acids Research. 37: W565–70. doi:10.1093/nar/gkp405. PMC 2703929Freely accessible. PMID 19465382.
78. Gaëlle Debret; Arnaud Martel; Philippe Cuniasse (2009). "RASMOT-3D PRO: a 3D motif search webserver ". Nucleic Acids Research. 37: W459–64. doi:10.1093/nar/gkp304. PMC 2703991Freely accessible. PMID 19417073.
79. Alexandra Shulman-Peleg; Maxim Shatsky; Ruth Nussinov; Haim J. Wolfson (2008). "MultiBind and MAPPIS: webservers for multiple alignment of protein 3D-binding sites and their interactions ". Nucleic Acids Research. 36: W260–4. doi:10.1093/nar/gkn185. PMC 2447750Freely accessible. PMID 18467424.
80. Alexandra Shulman-Peleg; Maxim Shatsky; Ruth Nussinov; Haim J Wolfson (2007). "Spatial chemical conservation of hot spot interactions in protein-protein complexes ". BMC Biology Research. 5 (43).
81. Gabriele Ausiello; Pier Federico Gherardini; Paolo Marcatili; Anna Tramontano; Allegra Via; Manuela Helmer-Citterich (2008). "FunClust: a web server for the identification of structural motifs in a set of non-homologous protein structures ". BMC Biology Research. 9.
82. Janez Konc; Dušanka Janežič (2010). "ProBiS algorithm for detection of structurally similar protein binding sites by local structural alignment " (PDF). Bioinformatics. 26 (9): 1160–1168. doi:10.1093/bioinformatics/btq100. PMC 2859123Freely accessible. PMID 20305268.
83. Hui Sun Lee; Wonpil Im (2012). "Identification of Ligand Templates using Local Structure Alignment for Structure-Based Drug Design ". Journal of Chemical Information and Modeling. 52 (10): 2784–2795. doi:10.1021/ci300178e.
84. Hui Sun Lee; Wonpil Im (2013). "Ligand Binding Site Detection by Local Structure Alignment and Its Performance Complementarity ". Journal of Chemical Information and Modeling. 53 (9): 2462–2470. doi:10.1021/ci4003602.
85. Barthel D., Hirst J.D., Blazewicz J., Burke E.K. and Krasnogor N. (2007). "ProCKSI: a decision support system for Protein (Structure) Comparison, Knowledge, Similarity and Information ". BMC Bioinformatics. 8: 416. doi:10.1186/1471-2105-8-416. PMC 2222653Freely accessible. PMID 17963510.
86. Sippl, M.; Wiederstein, M. (2012). "Detection of spatial correlations in protein structures and molecular complexes ". Structure. 20 (4): 718–728. doi:10.1016/j.str.2012.01.024. PMC 3320710Freely accessible. PMID 22483118.
87. Torarinsson E, Sawera M, Havgaard JH, Fredholm M, Gorodkin J (2006).

"Torarinsson E, Sawera M, Havgaard JH, Fredholm M, Gorodkin J ". Genome Res. 16 (7): 885–9. doi:10.1101/gr.5226606. PMC 1484455Freely accessible. PMID 16751343.

88. Hoksza D, Svozil D (2012). "Efficient RNA pairwise structure comparison by SETTER method ". Bioinformatics. 28 (14): 1858–1864. doi:10.1093/bioinformatics/bts301. PMID 22611129.
89. Cech P, Svozil D, Hoksza D (2012). "SETTER: web server for RNA structure comparison ". Nucleic Acids Research. 40 (W1): W42–W48. doi:10.1093/nar/gks560.
90. Havgaard JH, Lyngso RB, Stormo GD, Gorodkin J (2005). "Pairwise local structural alignment of RNA sequences with sequence similarity less than 40% ". Bioinformatics. 21 (9): 1815–24. doi:10.1093/bioinformatics/bti279. PMID 15657094.
91. Mathews DH, Turner DH (2006). "Prediction of RNA secondary structure by free energy minimization ". Curr Opin Struct Biol. 16 (3): 270–8. doi:10.1016/j.sbi.2006.05.010. PMID 16713706.
92. Levinthal C, Wodak SJ, Kahn P, Dadivanian AK (1975). "Hemoglobin Interactions in Sickle Cell Fibers: I. Theoretical Approaches to the Molecular Contacts ". Proceedings of the National Academy of Sciences. 72 (4): 1330–1334. doi:10.1073/pnas.72.4.1330. PMC 432527Freely accessible. PMID 1055409.
93. Wodak SJ, Janin J (1978). "Computer Analysis of Protein-Protein Interactions ". Journal of Molecular Biology. 124 (2): 323–342. doi:10.1016/0022-2836(78)90302-9. PMID 712840.
94. Wodak SJ, De Crombrugghe M, Janin J (1987). "Computer Studies of Interactions between Macromolecules ". Progress in Biophysics and Molecular Biology. 49 (1): 29–63. doi:10.1016/0079-6107(87)90008-3. PMID 3310103.
95. Katchalski-Katzir E, Shariv I, Eisenstein M, Friesem AA, Aflalo C, Vakser IA (1992). "Molecular surface recognition: determination of geometric fit between proteins and their ligands by correlation techniques ". Proc. Natl. Acad. Sci. U.S.A. 89 (6): 2195–2199. doi:10.1073/pnas.89.6.2195. PMC 48623Freely accessible. PMID 1549581.
96. Gabb HA, Jackson RM, Sternberg MJ (September 1997). "Modelling protein docking using shape complementarity, electrostatics and biochemical information ". J. Mol. Biol. 272 (1): 106–120. doi:10.1006/jmbi.1997.1203. PMID 9299341.
97. Strynadka NC, Eisenstein M, Katchalski-Katzir E, Shoichet BK, Kuntz ID, Abagyan R, Totrov M, Janin J, Cherfils J, Zimmerman F, Olson A, Duncan B, Rao M, Jackson R, Sternberg M, James MN (1996). "Molecular Docking Programs Successfully Predict the Binding of a Beta-lactamase Inhibitory Protein to TEM-1 Beta-Lactamase ". Nature Structural & Molecular Biology. 3 (3): 233–239. doi:10.1038/nsb0396-233. PMID 8605624.
98. Gray JJ, Moughon S, Wang C, Schueler-Furman O, Kuhlman B, Rohl CA, Baker D (2003). "Protein–protein docking with simultaneous optimization of rigid-body displacement and side-chain conformations ". J. Mol. Biol. 331 (1):

281–299. doi:10.1016/S0022-2836(03)00670-3. PMID 12875852.

99. Camacho CJ, Vajda S (2008). "Protein docking along smooth association pathways ". Proceedings of the National Academy of Sciences. 98 (19): 10636–10641. doi:10.1073/pnas.181147798. PMC 58518Freely accessible. PMID 11517309.
100. Camacho CJ, Vajda S (2007). "In silico screening of mutational effects on enzyme-proteic inhibitor affinity: a docking-based approach ". BMC structural biology. 7: 37. doi:10.1186/1472-6807-7-37. PMC 1913526Freely accessible. PMID 17559675.
101. Zhang C, Liu S, Zhu Q, Zhou Y (2005). "A knowledge-based energy function for protein–ligand, protein–protein, and protein–DNA complexes ". Journal of Medicinal chemistry. 7 (48): 2325–2335. doi:10.1021/jm049314d. PMID 15801826.
102. Esmaielbeiki R, Nebel JC (2014). "Scoring docking conformations using predicted protein interfaces ". BMC Bioinformatics. 15: 171. doi:10.1186/1471-2105-15-171. PMC 4057934Freely accessible. PMID 24906633.
103. Kastritis PL, Bonvin AM (May 2010). "Are scoring functions in protein–protein docking ready to predict interactomes? Clues from a novel binding affinity benchmark ". J. Proteome Res. 9 (5): 2216–2225. doi:10.1021/pr9009854. PMID 20329755.
104. Rosato A, Fuentes G, Verma C (2010). "Faculty of 1000 Biology: evaluations for Kastritis PL & Bonvin AM J Proteome Res 2010 May 7 9 (5) :2216-25 ". Faculty of 1000 Biology.
105. Mintseris J, Wiehe K, Pierce B, Anderson R, Chen R, Janin J, Weng Z (2005). "Protein-Protein Docking Benchmark 2.0: an update ". Proteins. 60 (2): 214–216. doi:10.1002/prot.20560. PMID 15981264.
106. Vreven T, Moal IH, Vangone A, Pierce BG, Kastritis PL, Torchala M, Chaleil R, Jiménez-García B, Bates PA, Fernandez-Recio J, Bonvin AM, Weng Z (September 2015). "Updates to the Integrated Protein-Protein Interaction Benchmarks: Docking Benchmark Version 5 and Affinity Benchmark Version 2 ". Journal of Molecular Biology. 427 (19): 3031–41. doi:10.1016/j.jmb.2015.07.016. PMC 4677049Freely accessible. PMID 26231283.
107. van Dijk M, Bonvin AM (August 2008). "A protein-DNA docking benchmark ". Nucleic Acids Research. 36 (14): e88. doi:10.1093/nar/gkn386. PMC 2504314Freely accessible. PMID 18583363.
108. Barik A, C N, P M, Bahadur RP (July 2012). "A protein-RNA docking benchmark (I): nonredundant cases ". Proteins. 80 (7): 1866–71. doi:10.1002/prot.24083. PMID 22488669.
109. Pérez-Cano L, Jiménez-García B, Fernández-Recio J (July 2012). "A protein-RNA docking benchmark (II): extended set from experimental and homology modeling data ". Proteins. 80 (7): 1872–82. doi:10.1002/prot.24075. PMID 22488990.

110. Nithin C, Mukherjee S, Bahadur RP (November 2016). "A non-redundant protein-RNA docking benchmark version 2.0 ". Proteins: n/a–n/a. doi:10.1002/prot.25211. PMID 27862282.

111. Kastritis PL, Moal IH, Hwang H, Weng Z, Bates PA, Bonvin AM, Janin J (March 2011). "A structure-based benchmark for protein-protein binding affinity ". Protein Science. 20 (3): 482–491. doi:10.1002/pro.580. PMC 3064828Freely accessible. PMID 21213247.

112. Janin J, Henrick K, Moult J, Eyck LT, Sternberg MJ, Vajda S, Vakser I, Wodak SJ (2003). "CAPRI: a Critical Assessment of PRedicted Interactions ". Proteins. 52 (1): 2–9. doi:10.1002/prot.10381. PMID 12784359.

CHAPTER 5

Protein Microarray and Protein Sequencing

Chapter Contents

- **Introduction**
- **Motivation for Development**
- **Protein Sequencing**
- **Protein–Protein Interaction**

Protein microarray is an emerging technology that provides a versatile platform for characterization of hundreds of thousands of proteins in a highly parallel and high-throughput way. Protein microarrays are potentially powerful tools in biochemistry and molecular biology. Two types of protein microarrays are defined. One, termed a protein function array, will consist of thousands of native proteins immobilized in a defined pattern. Such arrays can be utilized for massively parallel testing of protein function, hence the name. The other type is termed a protein-detecting array. This will consist of large numbers of arrayed protein-binding agents. These arrays will allow for expression profiling to be done at the protein level.

INTRODUCTION

A protein microarray (or protein chip) is a high-throughput method used to track the interactions and activities of proteins, and to determine their function, and determining function on a large scale. Its main advantage lies in the fact that large numbers of proteins can be tracked in parallel. The chip consists of a support surface such as a glass slide, nitrocellulose membrane, bead, or microtitre plate, to which an array of capture proteins is bound. Probe molecules, typically labeled with a fluorescent dye, are added to the array. Any reaction between the probe and the immobilised protein emits a fluorescent signal that is read by a laser scanner. Protein microarrays are rapid, automated, economical, and highly sensitive, consuming small quantities of samples and reagents. The concept and methodology of protein microarrays was first introduced and illustrated in antibody microarrays (also referred to as antibody matrix) in 1983 in a scientific publication and a series of patents. The high-throughput technology behind the protein microarray was relatively easy to develop since it is based on the technology developed for DNA microarrays, which have become the most widely used microarrays.

MOTIVATION FOR DEVELOPMENT

Protein microarrays were developed due to the limitations of using DNA microarrays for determining gene expression levels in proteomics. The quantity of mRNA in the cell often doesn't reflect the expression levels of the proteins they correspond to. Since it is usually the protein, rather than the mRNA, that has the functional role in cell response, a novel approach was needed. Additionally post-translational modifications, which are often critical for determining protein function, are not visible on DNA microarrays. Protein microarrays replace traditional proteomics techniques such as 2D gel electrophoresis or chromatography, which were time consuming, labor-intensive and ill-suited for the analysis of low abundant proteins.

Making the Array

The proteins are arrayed onto a solid surface such as microscope slides, membranes, beads or microtitre plates. The function of this surface is to provide a support onto which proteins can be immobilized. It should demonstrate maximal binding properties, whilst maintaining the protein in its native conformation so that its binding ability is retained. Microscope slides made of glass or silicon are a popular choice since they are compatible with the easily obtained robotic arrayers and laser scanners that have been developed for DNA microarray technology. Nitrocellulose film slides are broadly accepted as the highest protein binding substrate for protein microarray applications.

The chosen solid surface is then covered with a coating that must serve the simultaneous functions of immobilizing the protein, preventing its denaturation, orienting it in the appropriate direction so that its binding sites are accessible, and providing a hydrophilic environment in which the binding reaction can occur. In addition, it also needs to display minimal non-specific binding in order to minimize background noise in the detection systems. Furthermore, it needs to be compatible with different detection systems. Immobilising agents include layers of aluminium or gold, hydrophilic polymers, and polyacrylamide gels, or treatment with amines, aldehyde or epoxy. Thin-film technologies like physical vapor deposition (PVD) and chemical vapor deposition (CVD) are employed to apply the coating to the support surface.

An aqueous environment is essential at all stages of array manufacture and operation to prevent protein denaturation. Therefore, sample buffers contain a high percent of glycerol(to lower the freezing point), and the humidity of the manufacturing environment is carefully regulated. Microwells have the dual advantage of providing an aqueous environment while preventing cross-contamination between samples.

In the most common type of protein array, robots place large numbers of proteins or their ligands onto a coated solid support in a pre-defined pattern. This is known as robotic contact printing or robotic spotting. Another fabrication method is ink-jetting, a drop-on-demand, non-contact method of dispersing the protein polymers onto the solid surface in the desired pattern. Piezoelectric spotting is a similar method to ink-jet printing. The printhead moves across the array, and at each spot uses electric stimulation to deliver the protein molecules onto the surface via tiny jets. This is also a non-contact process. Photolithography is a fourth method of arraying the proteins onto the surface. Light is used in association with photomasks, opaque plates with holes or transparencies that allow light to shine through in a defined pattern. A series of chemical treatments then enables deposition of the protein in the desired pattern upon the material underneath the photomask.

The capture molecules arrayed on the solid surface may be antibodies, antigens, aptamers (nucleic acid-based ligands), affibodies (small molecules engineered to mimic monoclonal antibodies), or full length proteins. Sources of such proteins include cell-based expression systems for recombinant proteins, purification from natural sources, production in vitro by cell-free translation systems, and synthetic methods for peptides. Many of these methods can be automated for high throughput production but care must be taken to avoid conditions of synthesis or extraction that result in a denatured protein which, since it no longer recognizes its binding partner, renders the array useless.

Proteins are highly sensitive to changes in their microenvironment. This presents a challenge in maintaining protein arrays in a stable condition over extended periods of time. In situ methods involve on-chip synthesis of proteins as and when required, directly from the DNA using cell-free protein expression systems. Since DNA is a highly stable molecule it does not deteriorate over time and is therefore suited to long-term storage. This approach is also advantageous in that it circumvents the laborious and often costly processes of separate protein purification and DNA cloning, since proteins are made and immobilised simultaneously in a single step on the chip surface. Examples of in situ techniques are PISA (protein in situ array), NAPPA (nucleic acid programmable protein array) and DAPA (DNA array to protein array).

Types of Arrays

There are three types of protein microarrays that are currently used to study the biochemical activities of proteins.

Analytical microarrays are also known as capture arrays. In this technique, a library of antibodies, aptamers or affibodies is arrayed on the support surface. These are used as capture molecules since each binds specifically to a particular protein. The array is probed with a complex protein solution such as a cell lysate. Analysis of the resulting binding reactions using various detection systems can provide information about expression levels of particular proteins in the sample as well as measurements of binding affinities and specificities. This type of microarray is especially useful in comparing protein expression in different solutions. For instance the response of the cells to a particular factor can be identified by comparing the lysates of cells treated with specific substances or grown under certain conditions with the lysates of control cells. Another application is in the identification and profiling of diseased tissues.

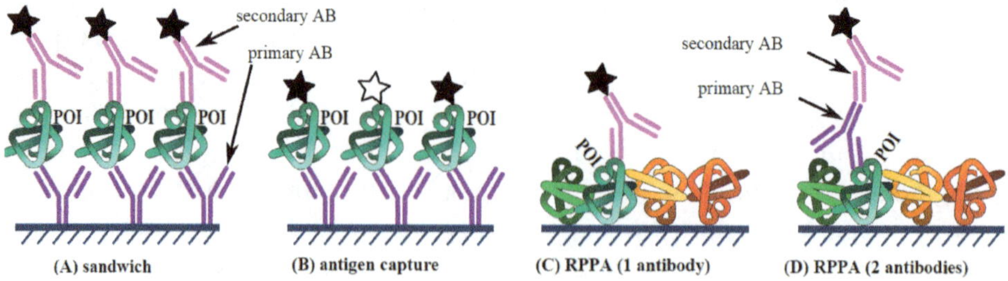

Types of protein arrays

Functional protein microarrays (also known as target protein arrays) are constructed by immobilising large numbers of purified proteins and are used to identify protein–protein, protein–DNA, protein–RNA, protein–phospholipid, and protein–small-molecule interactions, to assay enzymatic activity and to detect antibodies and demonstrate their specificity. They differ from analytical arrays in that functional protein arrays are composed of arrays containing full-length functional proteins or protein domains. These protein chips are used to study the biochemical activities of the entire proteome in a single experiment.

Reverse phase protein microarray (RPPA) involve complex samples, such as tissue lysates. Cells are isolated from various tissues of interest and are lysed. The lysate is arrayed onto the microarray and probed with antibodies against the target protein of interest. These antibodies are typically detected with chemiluminescent, fluorescent or colorimetric assays. Reference peptides are printed on the slides to allow for protein quantification of the sample lysates. RPAs allow for the determination of the presence of altered proteins or other agents that may be the result of disease. Specifically, post-translational modifications, which are typically altered as a result of disease can be detected using RPAs.

Detection

Protein array detection methods must give a high signal and a low background. The most common and widely used method for detection is fluorescence labeling which is highly sensitive, safe and compatible with readily available microarray laser scanners. Other labels can be used, such as affinity, photochemical or radioisotope tags. These labels are attached to the probe itself and can interfere with the probe-target protein reaction. Therefore, a number of label free detection methods are available, such as surface plasmon resonance (SPR), carbon nanotubes, carbon nanowire sensors (where detection occurs via changes in conductance) and microelectromechanical system (MEMS) cantilevers. All these label free detection methods are relatively new and are not yet suitable for high-throughput protein interaction detection; however, they do offer much promise for the future.

Protein quantitation on nitrocellulose coated glass slides can use near-IR fluorescent detection. This limits interferences due to auto-fluorescence of the nitrocellulose at the UV wavelengths used for standard fluorescent detection probes.

Applications

There are five major areas where protein arrays are being applied: diagnostics, proteomics, protein functional analysis, antibody characterization, and treatment development

Diagnostics involves the detection of antigens and antibodies in blood samples; the profiling of sera to discover new disease biomarkers; the monitoring of disease states and responses to therapy in personalized medicine; the monitoring of environment and food.

Proteomics pertains to protein expression profiling i.e. which proteins are expressed in the lysate of a particular cell.

Protein functional analysis is the identification of protein–protein interactions (e.g. identification of members of a protein complex), protein–phospholipid interactions, small molecule targets, enzymatic substrates (particularly the substrates of kinases) and receptor ligands.

Antibody characterization is characterizing cross-reactivity, specificity and mapping epitopes.

Treatment development involves the development of antigen-specific therapies for autoimmunity, cancer and allergies; the identification of small molecule targets that could potentially be used as new drugs.

Challenges

Despite the considerable investments made by several companies, proteins chips have yet to flood the market. Manufacturers have found that proteins are actually quite difficult to handle. A protein chip requires a lot more steps in its creation than does a DNA chip.

Challenges include: 1) finding a surface and a method of attachment that allows the proteins to maintain their secondary or tertiary structure and thus their biological activity and their interactions with other molecules, 2) producing an array with a long shelf life so that the proteins on the chip do not denature over a short time, 3) identifying and isolating antibodies or other capture molecules against every protein in the human genome, 4) quantifying the levels of bound protein while assuring sensitivity and avoiding background noise, 5) extracting the detected protein from the chip in order to further analyze it, 6) reducing non-specific binding by the capture agents, 7) the capacity of the chip must be sufficient to allow as complete a representation of the proteome to be visualized as possible; abundant proteins overwhelm the detection of less abundant proteins such as signaling molecules and receptors, which are generally of more therapeutic interest.

PROTEIN SEQUENCING

Protein sequencing is a technique to determine the amino acid sequence of a protein, as well as which conformation the protein adopts and the extent to which it is complexed with any non-peptide molecules. Discovering the structures and functions of proteins in living organisms is an important tool for understanding cellular processes, and allows drugs that target specific metabolic pathways to be invented more easily.

The two major direct methods of protein sequencing are mass spectrometry and the Edman degradation reaction. It is also possible to generate an amino acid sequence from the DNA or mRNA sequence encoding the protein, if this is known. However, there are many other reactions that can be used to gain more limited information about protein sequences and can be used as preliminaries to the aforementioned methods of sequencing or to overcome specific inadequacies within them.

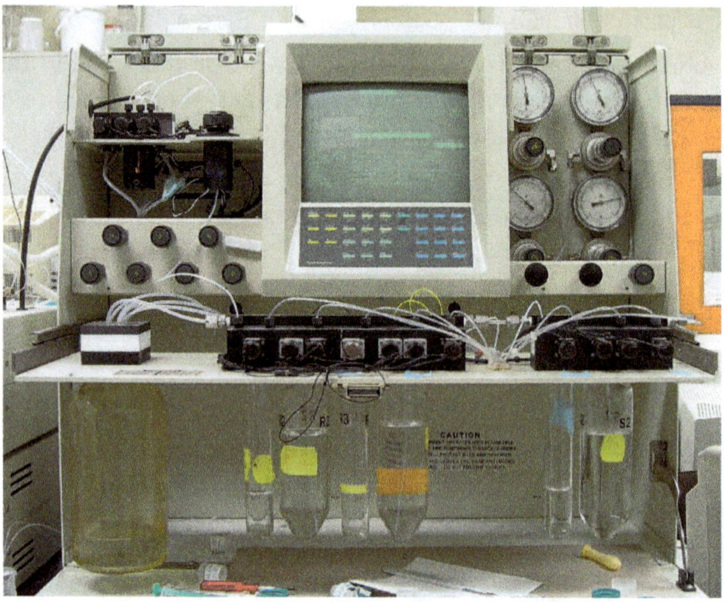

A Beckman-Coulter Porton LF3000G protein sequencing machine.

Protein Sequencer

A protein sequencer is a machine that is used to determine the sequence of amino acids in a protein.

They work by tagging and removing one amino acid at a time, which is analysed and identified. This is done repetitively for the whole polypeptide, until the whole sequence is established.

This method has generally been replaced by nucleic acid technology, and it is often easier to identify the sequence of a protein by looking at the DNA that codes for it.

Determining Amino Acid Composition

It is often desirable to know the unordered amino acid composition of a protein prior to attempting to find the ordered sequence, as this knowledge can be used to facilitate the discovery of errors in the sequencing process or to distinguish between ambiguous results. Knowledge of the frequency of certain amino acids may also be used to choose which protease to use for digestion of the protein. A generalized method often referred to as *amino acid analysis* for determining amino acid frequency is as follows:

- Hydrolyse a known quantity of protein into its constituent amino acids.
- Separate and quantify the amino acids in some way.

Hydrolysis

Hydrolysis is done by heating a sample of the protein in 6 M hydrochloric acid to 100–110 °C for 24 hours or longer. Proteins with many bulky hydrophobic groups may require longer heating periods. However, these conditions are so vigorous that some amino acids (serine, threonine, tyrosine, tryptophan, glutamine, and cysteine) are degraded. To circumvent this problem, Biochemistry Online suggests heating separate samples for different times, analysing each resulting solution, and extrapolating back to zero hydrolysis time. Rastall suggests a variety of reagents to prevent or reduce degradation, such as thiol reagents or phenol to protect tryptophan and tyrosine from attack by chlorine, and pre-oxidising cysteine. He also suggests measuring the quantity of ammonia evolved to determine the extent of amide hydrolysis.

Separation

The amino acids can be separated by ion-exchange chromatography or hydrophobic interaction chromatography. An example of the former is given by the NTRC using sulfonated polystyrene as a matrix, adding the amino acids in acid solution and passing a buffer of steadily increasing pH through the column. Amino acids will be eluted when the pH reaches their respective isoelectric points. The latter technique may be employed through the use of reversed phase chromatography. Many commercially available C8 and C18 silica columns have demonstrated successful separation of amino acids in solution in less than 40 minutes through the use of an optimized elution gradient.

Quantitative Analysis

Once the amino acids have been separated, their respective quantities are determined by adding a reagent that will form a colored derivative. If the amounts of amino acids are in excess of 10 nmol, ninhydrin can be used for this; it gives a yellow color when reacted with proline, and a vivid purple with other amino acids. The concentration of amino acid is proportional to the absorbance of the resulting solution. With very small quantities, down to 10 pmol, fluorescamine can be used as a marker: This forms a fluorescent derivative on reacting with an amino acid.

N-Terminal Amino Acid Analysis

Determining which amino acid forms the *N*-terminus of a peptide chain is useful for two reasons: to aid the ordering of individual peptide fragments' sequences into a whole chain, and because the first round of Edman degradation is often contaminated by impurities and therefore does not give an accurate determination of the *N*-terminal amino acid. A generalized method for *N*-terminal amino acid analysis follows:

- React the peptide with a reagent that will selectively label the terminal amino acid.
- Hydrolyse the protein.
- Determine the amino acid by chromatography and comparison with standards.

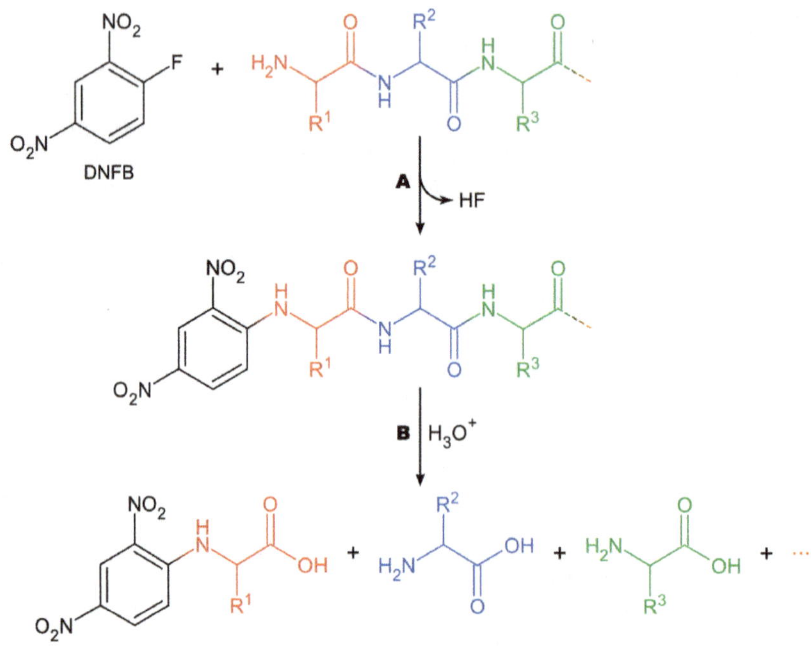

Sanger's method of peptide end-group analysis: **A** derivatization of *N*-terminal end with Sanger's reagent (DNFB), **B** total acid hydrolysis of the dinitrophenyl peptide

There are many different reagents which can be used to label terminal amino acids. They all react with amine groups and will therefore also bind to amine groups in the side chains of amino acids such as lysine - for this reason it is necessary to be careful in interpreting chromatograms to ensure that the right spot is chosen. Two of the more common reagents are Sanger's reagent (1-fluoro-2,4-dinitrobenzene) and dansyl derivatives such as dansyl chloride. Phenylisothiocyanate, the reagent for the Edman degradation, can also be used. The same questions apply here as in the determination of amino acid composition, with the exception that no stain is needed, as the reagents produce colored derivatives and only qualitative analysis is required. So the amino acid does not have to be eluted from the chromatography column, just compared with a standard. Another consideration to take into account is that, since any amine groups will have reacted with the labelling reagent, ion exchange chromatography cannot be used, and thin layer chromatography or high-pressure liquid chromatography should be used instead.

C-Terminal Amino Acid Analysis

The number of methods available for C-terminal amino acid analysis is much smaller than the number of available methods of N-terminal analysis. The most common method is to add carboxypeptidases to a solution of the protein, take samples at regular intervals, and determine the terminal amino acid by analyzing a plot of amino acid concentrations against time. This method will be very useful in the case of polypeptides and protein-blocked N termini. C-terminal sequencing would greatly help in verifying the primary structures of proteins predicted from DNA sequences and to detect any postranslational processing of gene products from known codon sequences.

Edman Degradation

The Edman degradation is a very important reaction for protein sequencing, because it allows the ordered amino acid composition of a protein to be discovered. Automated Edman sequencers are now in widespread use, and are able to sequence peptides up to approximately 50 amino acids long. A reaction scheme for sequencing a protein by the Edman degradation follows; some of the steps are elaborated on subsequently.

- Break any disulfide bridges in the protein with a reducing agent like 2-mercaptoethanol. A protecting group such as iodoacetic acid may be necessary to prevent the bonds from re-forming.
- Separate and purify the individual chains of the protein complex, if there are more than one.
- Determine the amino acid composition of each chain.
- Determine the terminal amino acids of each chain.
- Break each chain into fragments under 50 amino acids long.
- Separate and purify the fragments.
- Determine the sequence of each fragment.
- Repeat with a different pattern of cleavage.
- Construct the sequence of the overall protein.

Digestion into Peptide Fragments

Peptides longer than about 50-70 amino acids long cannot be sequenced reliably by the Edman degradation. Because of this, long protein chains need to be broken up into small fragments that can then be sequenced individually. Digestion is done either by endopeptidases such as trypsin or pepsin or by chemical reagents such as cyanogen bromide. Different enzymes give different cleavage patterns, and the overlap between fragments can be used to construct an overall sequence.

The Edman Degradation Reaction

The peptide to be sequenced is adsorbed onto a solid surface. One common substrate is glass fibre coated with polybrene, a cationic polymer. The Edman reagent, phenylisothiocyanate (PITC), is added to the adsorbed peptide, together with a mildly basic buffer solution of 12% trimethylamine. This reacts with the amine group of the N-terminal amino acid.

The terminal amino acid can then be selectively detached by the addition of anhydrous acid. The derivative then isomerises to give a substituted phenylthiohydantoin, which can be washed off and identified by chromatography, and the cycle can be repeated. The efficiency of each step is about 98%, which allows about 50 amino acids to be reliably determined.

Limitations of the Edman Degradation

Because the Edman degradation proceeds from the N-terminus of the protein, it will not work if the N-terminal amino acid has been chemically modified or if it is concealed within the body of the protein. It also requires the use of either guesswork or a separate procedure to determine the positions of disulfide bridges.

Mass Spectrometry

The other major direct method by which the sequence of a protein can be determined is mass spectrometry. This method has been gaining popularity in recent years as new techniques and increasing computing power have facilitated it. Mass spectrometry can, in principle, sequence any size of protein, but the problem becomes computationally more difficult as the size increases. Peptides are also easier to prepare for mass spectrometry than whole proteins, because they are more soluble. One method of delivering the peptides to the spectrometer is electrospray ionization, for which John Bennett Fenn won the Nobel Prize in Chemistry in 2002. The protein is digested by an endoprotease, and the resulting solution is passed through a high-pressure liquid chromatography column. At the end of this column, the solution is sprayed out of a narrow nozzle charged to a high positive potential into the mass spectrometer. The charge on the droplets causes them to fragment until only single ions remain. The peptides are then fragmented and the mass-to-charge ratios of the fragments measured. (It is possible to detect which peaks correspond to multiply charged fragments, because these will have auxiliary peaks corresponding to other isotopes - the distance between these other peaks is inversely proportional to the charge on the fragment). The mass spectrum is analysed by computer and often compared against a database of previously sequenced proteins in order to determine the sequences of the fragments. This process is then repeated with a different digestion enzyme, and the overlaps in the sequences are used to construct a sequence for the protein.

There is a fundamental issue of relying on database search to sequence the protein. The database search algorithms assume the database sequences are correct. Therefore, when comparing the spectra with the database peptides, as long as some evidences are observed, e.g. the precursor mass and the peptide mass are very close and there are some fragment ions matched, it will make the peptide spectrum assignment. But this does not mean that evidences are observed to determine each amino acid.

Predicting Protein Sequence from DNA/RNA Sequences

In organisms that do not have introns (e.g., prokaryotes) the amino acid sequence of a protein can also be determined indirectly from the mRNA or the DNA that codes for the protein. If the sequence of the gene is already known, then this is all very easy. However, it is rare that the DNA sequence of a newly isolated protein will be known, and, so, if this method is to be used, it has to be found in some way. One way that this can be done is to sequence a short section, perhaps 15 amino acids long, of the protein by one of the above methods, and then use this sequence to generate a complementary marker for the protein's RNA. This can then be used to isolate the mRNA coding for the protein, which can then be replicated in a polymerase chain reaction to yield a significant amount of DNA, which can then be sequenced relatively easily. The amino acid sequence of the protein can then be deduced from this. However, it is necessary to take into account the possibility of amino acids being removed after the mRNA has been translated.

Bioinformatics Tools for Sequencing

Bioinformatics tools exist that translate nucleic acid sequences into their corresponding polypeptide chain. Such tool takes an input of a nucleic acid sequence and will produce the corresponding amino acid sequence based on the selected settings.

Another option is to use a bioinformatics tool that takes an amino acid sequence and back-translates it into the most likely nucleic acid sequence.

PROTEIN–PROTEIN INTERACTION

Protein–protein interactions (PPIs) are the physical contacts of high specificity established between two or more protein molecules as a result of biochemical events steered by electrostatic forces including the hydrophobic effect. Many are physical contacts with molecular associations between chains that occur in a cell or in a living organism in a specific biomolecular context.

Proteins rarely act alone as their functions tend to be regulated. Many molecular processes within a cell are carried out by molecular machines that are built from a large number of protein components organized by their PPIs. These interactions make up the so-called interactomics of the organism, while aberrant PPIs are the basis of multiple aggregation-related diseases, such as Creutzfeldt–Jakob, Alzheimer's disease, and may lead to cancer.

PPIs have been studied from different perspectives: biochemistry, quantum chemistry, molecular dynamics, signal transduction, among others. All this information enables the creation of large protein interaction networks – similar to metabolic or genetic/epigenetic networks – that empower the current knowledge on biochemical cascades and molecular etiology of disease, as well as the discovery of putative protein targets of therapeutic interest.

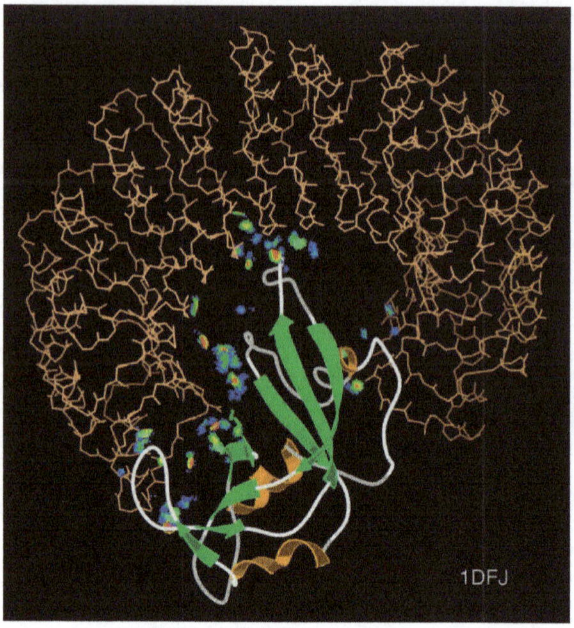

The horseshoe shaped ribonuclease inhibitor (shown as wireframe) forms a protein–protein interaction with the ribonuclease protein. The contacts between the two proteins are shown as coloured patches.

Examples

Signal Transduction

The activity of the cell is regulated by extracellular signals. Signals propagation to inside and/or along the interior of cells depends on PPIs between the various signaling molecules. The recruitment of signaling pathways through PPIs is called signal transduction and plays a fundamental role in many biological processes and in many diseases including Parkinson's disease and cancer.

Transport Across Membranes

A protein may be carrying another protein (for example, from cytoplasm to nucleus or vice versa in the case of the nuclear pore importins).

Cell Metabolism

In many biosynthetic processes enzymes interact with each other to produce small compounds or other macromolecules.

Muscle Contraction

Physiology of muscle contraction involves several interactions. Myosin filaments act as molecular motors and by binding to actin enables filament sliding. Furthermore, members of the skeletal muscle lipid droplet-associated proteins family associate with other proteins, as activator of adipose triglyceride lipase and its coactivator comparative gene identification-58, to regulate lipolysis in skeletal muscle.

Types

To describe the types of protein–protein interactions (PPIs) it is important to consider that proteins can interact in a "transient" way (to produce some specific effect in a short time) or to interact with other proteins in a "stable" way to build multiprotein complexes that are molecular machines within the living systems. A protein complex assembly can result in the formation of homo-oligomeric or hetero-oligomeric complexes. In addition to the conventional complexes, as enzyme-inhibitor and antibody-antigen, interactions can also be established between domain-domain and domain-peptide. Another important distinction to identify protein-protein interactions is the way they have been determined, since there are techniques that measure direct physical interactions between protein pairs, named "binary" methods, while there are other techniques that measure physical interactions among groups of proteins, without pairwise determination of protein partners, named "co-complex" methods.

Homo-Oligomers vs. Hetero-Oligomers

Homo-oligomers are macromolecular complexes constituted by only one type of protein subunit. Protein subunits assembly is guided by the establishment of non-covalent interactions in the quaternary structure of the protein. Disruption of homo-oligomers in order to return to the initial individual monomers often requires denaturation of the complex. Several enzymes, carrier proteins, scaffolding proteins, and transcriptional regulatory factors carry out their functions as homo-oligomers. Distinct protein subunits interact in hetero-oligomers, which are essential to control several cellular functions. The importance of the communication between heterologous proteins is even more evident during cell signaling events and such interactions are only possible due to structural domains within the proteins (as described below).

Stable Interactions vs. Transient Interactions

Stable interactions involve proteins that interact for a long time, taking part of permanent complexes as subunits, in order to carry out structural or functional roles. These are usually the case of homo-oligomers (e.g. cytochrome c), and some hetero-oligomeric proteins, as the subunits of ATPase. On the other hand, a protein may interact briefly and in a reversible manner with other proteins in only certain cellular contexts – cell type, cell cycle stage, external factors, presence of other binding proteins, etc. – as it happens with most of the proteins involved in biochemical cascades. These are called transient interactions. For example, some G protein-coupled receptors only transiently bind to $G_{i/o}$ proteins when they are activated by extracellular ligands, while some G_q-coupled receptors, such as muscarinic receptor M3, pre-couple with G_q proteins prior to the receptor-ligand binding. Interactions between intrinsically disordered protein regions to globular protein domains (i.e. MoRFs) are transient interactions.

Covalent vs. Non-Covalent

Covalent interactions are those with the strongest association and are formed by disulphide bonds or electron sharing. Although being rare, these interactions are determinant in some posttranslational modifications, as ubiquitination and SUMOylation. Non-covalent bonds are usually established during transient interactions by the combination of weaker bonds, such as hydrogen bonds, ionic interactions, Van der Waals forces, or hydrophobic bonds.

Role of Water

Water molecules play a significant role in the interactions between proteins. The crystal structures of complexes, obtained at high resolution from different but homologous proteins, have shown that some interface water molecules are conserved between homologous complexes. The majority of the interface water molecules make hydrogen bonds with both partners of each complex. Some interface amino acid residues or atomic groups of one protein partner engage in both direct and water mediated interactions with the other protein partner. Doubly indirect interactions, mediated by two water molecules, are more numerous in the homologous complexes of low affinity. Carefully conducted mutagenesis experiments, e.g. changing a tyrosine residue into a phenylalanine, have shown that water mediated interactions can contribute to the energy of interaction. Thus, water molecules may facilitate the interactions and cross-recognitions between proteins.

Structure

The molecular structures of many protein complexes have been unlocked by the technique of X-ray crystallography. The first structure to be solved by this method was that of sperm whale myoglobin by Sir John Cowdery Kendrew. In this technique the angles and intensities of a beam of X-rays diffracted by crystalline atoms are detected in a film, thus producing a three-dimensional picture of the density of electrons within the crystal.

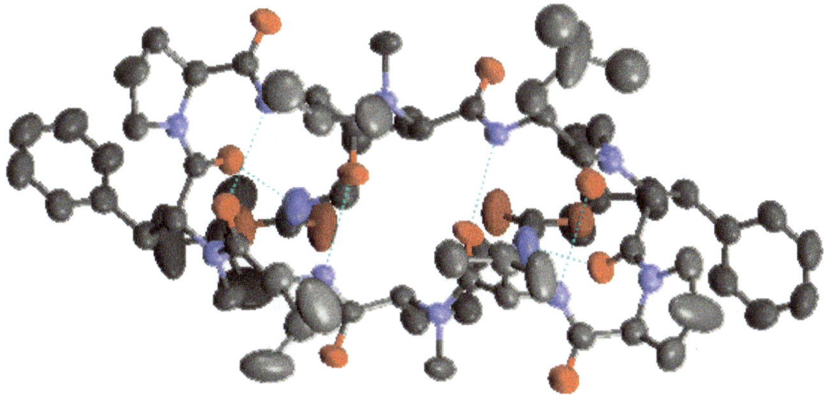

Crystal structure of modified Gramicidin S horizontally determined by X-ray crystallography

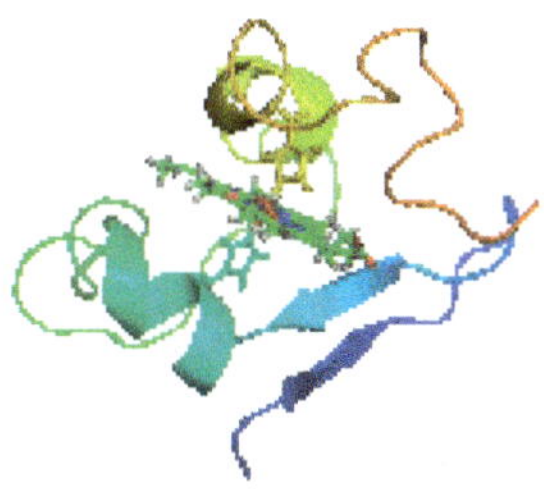

NMR structure of cytochrome C illustrating its dynamics in solution

Later, nuclear magnetic resonance also started to be applied with the aim of unravelling the molecular structure of protein complexes. One of the first examples was the structure of calmodulin-binding domains bound to calmodulin. This technique is based on the study of magnetic properties of atomic nuclei, thus determining physical and chemical properties of the correspondent atoms or the molecules. Nuclear magnetic resonance is advantageous for characterizing weak PPIs.

Domains

Proteins hold structural domains that allow their interaction with and bind to specific sequences on other proteins:

- Src homology 2 (SH2) domain

SH2 domains are structurally composed by three-stranded twisted beta sheet sandwiched flanked by two alpha-helices. The existence of a deep binding pocket with high affinity for phosphotyrosine, but not for phosphoserine or phosphothreonine, is essential for the recognition of tyrosine phosphorylated proteins, mainly autophosphorylated growth factor receptors. Growth factor receptor binding proteins and phospholipase Cγ are examples of proteins that have SH2 domains.

- Src homology 3 (SH3) domain

Structurally, SH3 domains are constituted by a beta barrel formed by two orthogonal beta sheets and three anti-parallel beta strands. These domains recognize proline enriched sequences, as polyproline type II helical structure (PXXP motifs) in cell signaling proteins like protein tyrosine kinases and the growth factor receptor bound protein 2 (Grb2).

- Phosphotyrosine-binding (PTB) domain

PTB domains interact with sequences that contain a phosphotyrosine group. These domains can be found in the insulin receptor substrate.

- LIM domain

LIM domains were initially identified in three homeodomain transcription factors (lin11, isl1, and mec3). In addition to this homeodomain proteins and other proteins involved in development, LIM domains have also been identified in non-homeodomain proteins with relevant roles in cellular differentiation, association with cytoskeleton and senescence. These domains contain a tandem cysteine-rich Zn^{2+}-finger motif and embrace the consensus sequence CX2CX16-23HX2CX2CX2CX16-21CX2C/H/D. LIM domains bind to PDZ domains, bHLH transcription factors, and other LIM domains.

- Sterile alpha motif (SAM) domain

SAM domains are composed by five helices forming a compact package with a conserved hydrophobic core. These domains, which can be found in the Eph receptor and the stromal interaction molecule (STIM) for example, bind to non-SAM domain-containing proteins and they also appear to have the ability to bind RNA.

- PDZ domain

PDZ domains were first identified in three guanylate kinases: PSD-95, DlgA and ZO-1. These domains recognize carboxy-terminal tri-peptide motifs (S/TXV), other PDZ domains or LIM domains and bind them through a short peptide sequence that has a C-terminal hydrophobic residue. Some of the proteins identified as having PDZ domains are scaffolding proteins or seem to be involved in ion receptor assembling and receptor-enzyme complexes formation.

- FERM domain

FERM domains contain basic residues capable of binding PtdIns(4,5)P_2. Talin and focal adhesion kinase (FAK) are two of the proteins that present FERM domains.

- Calponin homology (CH) domain

CH domains are mainly present in cytoskeletal proteins as parvin.

- Pleckstrin homology domain

Pleckstrin homology domains bind to phosphoinositides and acid domains in signaling proteins.

- WW domain

WW domains bind to proline enriched sequences.

- WSxWS motif

Found in cytokine receptors

Properties of the Interface

The study of the molecular structure can give fine details about the interface that enables the interaction between proteins. When characterizing PPI interfaces it is important to take into account the type of complex.

Parameters evaluated include size (measured in absolute dimensions Å^2 or in solvent-accessible surface area (SASA)), shape, complementarity between surfaces, residue interface propensities, hydrophobicity, segmentation and secondary structure, and conformational changes on complex formation.

The great majority of PPI interfaces reflects the composition of protein surfaces, rather than the protein cores, in spite of being frequently enriched in hydrophobic residues, particularly in aromatic residues. PPI interfaces are dynamic and frequently planar, although they can be globular and protruding as well. Based on three structures – insulin dimer, trypsin-pancreatic trypsin inhibitor complex, and oxyhaemoglobin – Cyrus Chothia and Joel Janin found that between 1,130 and 1,720 Å^2 of surface area was removed from contact with water indicating that hydrophobicity is a major factor of stabilization of PPIs. Later studies refined the buried surface area of the majority of interactions to 1,600±350 Å^2. However, much larger interaction interfaces were also observed and were associated with significant changes in conformation of one of the interaction partners. PPIs interfaces exhibit both shape and electrostatic complementarity.

Regulation

- Protein concentration, which in turn are affected by expression levels and degradation rates;
- Protein affinity for proteins or other binding ligands;
- Ligands concentrations (substrates, ions, etc.);
- Presence of other proteins, nucleic acids, and ions;
- Electric fields around proteins.
- Occurrence of covalent modifications;

Measurement

There are a multitude of methods to detect them. Each of the approaches has its own strengths and weaknesses, especially with regard to the sensitivity and specificity of the method. The most conventional and widely used high-throughput methods are yeast two-hybrid screening and affinity purification coupled to mass spectrometry.

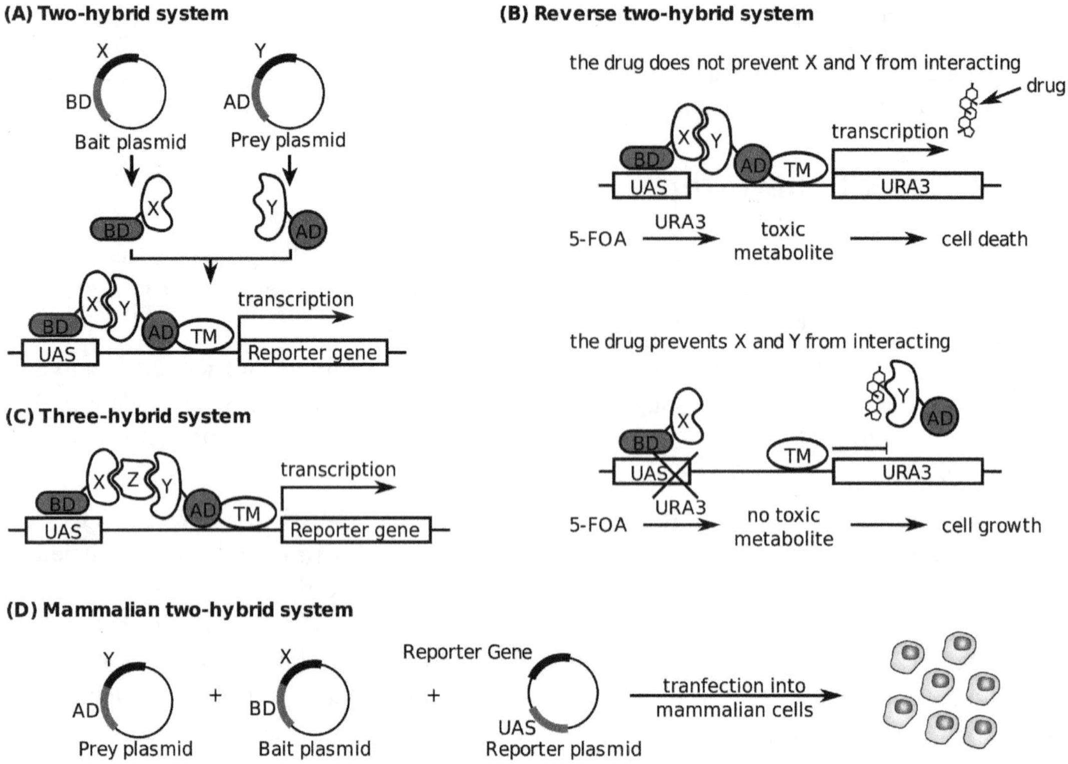

Principles of yeast and mammalian two-hybrid systems

Yeast Two-Hybrid Screening

This system was firstly described in 1989 by Fields and Song using *Saccharomyces cerevisiae* as biological model. Yeast two hybrid allows the identification of pairwise PPIs (binary method) *in vivo*, indicating non-specific tendencies towards sticky interactions.

Yeast cells are transfected with two plasmids: the bait (protein of interest fused with the DNA-binding domain of a yeast transcription factor, like Gal4), and the prey (a library of cDNA fragments linked to the activation domain of the transcription factor. Transcription of reporter genes does not occur unless bait and prey interact with each other and form a functional transcription factor. Thus, the interaction between proteins can be inferred by the presence of the products resultant of the reporter gene expression.

Despite its usefulness, the yeast two-hybrid system has limitations: specificity is relatively low; uses yeast as main host system, which can be a problem when studying other biological models; the number of PPIs identified is usually low because some transient PPIs are lost during purification steps; and, understates membrane proteins, for example. Limitations have been overcoming by the emergence of yeast two-hybrid variants, such as the membrane yeast two-hybrid (MYTH) and the split-ubiquitin system, which are not limited to interactions that occur in the nucleus; and, the bacterial two-hybrid system, performed in bacteria;

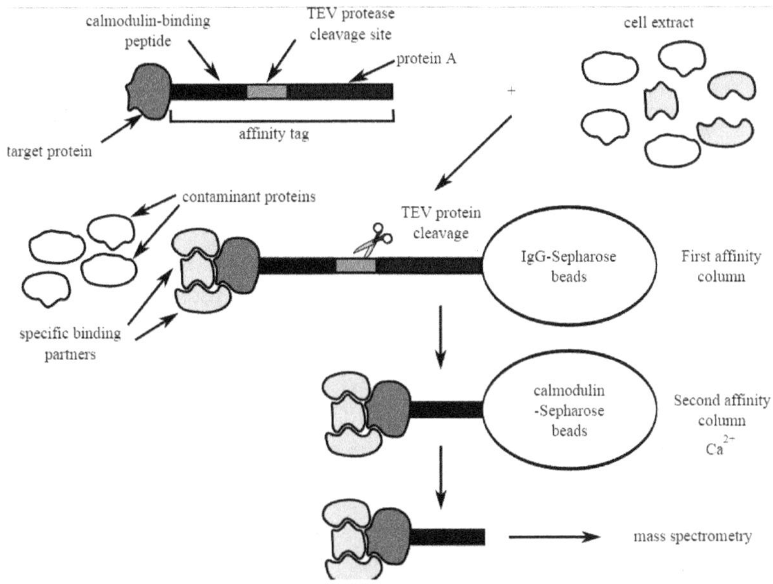

Principle of Tandem Affinity Purification

Affinity Purification Coupled to Mass Spectrometry

Affinity purification coupled to mass spectrometry mostly detects stable interactions and thus better indicates functional in vivo PPIs. This method starts by purification of the tagged protein, which is expressed in the cell usually at *in vivo* concentrations, and its interacting proteins (affinity purification). One of the most advantageous and widely used method to purify proteins with very low contaminating background is the tandem affinity purification, developed by Bertrand Seraphin and Mathias Mann and respective colleagues. PPIs can then be quantitatively and qualitatively analysed by mass spectrometry using different methods: chemical incorporation, biological or metabolic incorporation (SILAC), and label-free methods.

Other Potential Methods

Diverse techniques to identify PPIs have been emerging along with technology progression. These include co-immunoprecipitation, protein microarrays, analytical ultracentrifugation, light scattering, fluorescence spectroscopy, luminescence-based mammalian interactome mapping (LUMIER), resonance-energy transfer systems, mammalian protein–protein interaction trap, electro-switchable biosurfaces, protein-fragment complementation assay, as well as real-time label-free measurements by surface plasmon resonance, and calorimetry.

Text Mining Methods

Publicly available information from biomedical research is readily accessible through the internet and is becoming a powerful resource for predictive protein-protein interactions and protein docking. Text mining is much less time costly and consuming compared to other high-throughput techniques. Currently, these methods generally detect binary relations between interacting protein from individual sentences using machine learning and rule/pattern-based information extraction and machine learning approaches. A wide variety of text mining predicting PPIs applications are available for public use, as well as repositories which often stores manually validated and/or computationally predicted PPIs. The principal stages of text mining divides the implementation into two stages: *information retrieval*, where literature abstracts containing names of either or both proteins complexes are selected and *information extraction,* where detecting occurrences of residues are retrieved. The extraction is automated by searching for co-existing sentences, abstracts or paragraphs within textual context.

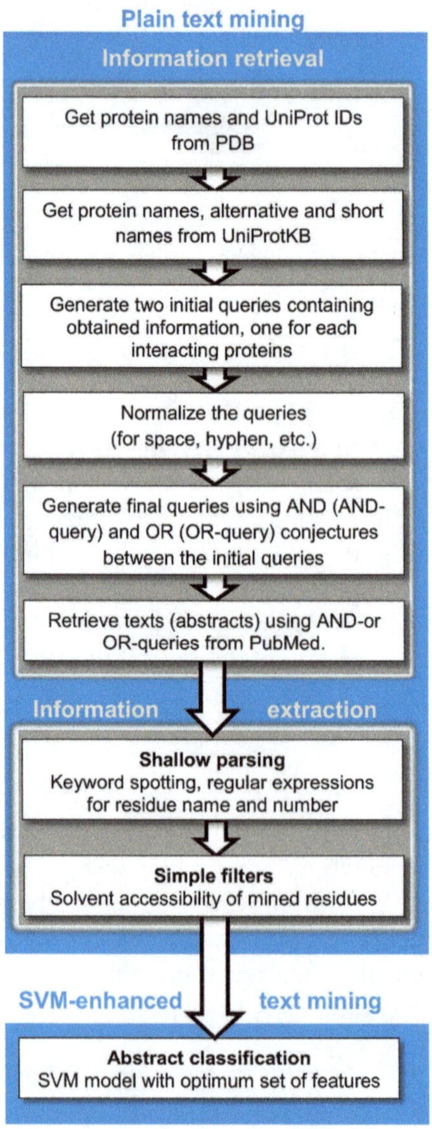

Text mining protocol.

There are also studies using phylogenetic profiling, basing their functionalities on the theory that proteins involved in common pathways co-evolve in a correlated fashion across large number of species. More complex text mining methodologies use advanced dictionaries and generate networks by Natural Language Processing (NLP) of text, considering gene names as nodes and verbs as edges, other developments involve kernel methods to predict protein interactions.

Machine Learning Methods

These methods use machine learning to distinguish how interacting protein pairs differ from non-interacting protein pairs in terms of pairwise features such as cellular colocalization, gene co-expression, how closely located on a DNA are the genes that encode the two proteins, and so on. Random Forest has been found to be most-effective machine learning method for protein interaction prediction. Such methods have been applied for discovering protein interactions on human interactome, specifically the interactome of Membrane proteins and the interactome of Schizophrenia-associated proteins.

Databases

Large scale identification of PPIs generated hundreds of thousands interactions, which were collected together in specialized biological databases that are continuously updated in order to provide complete interactomes. The first of these databases was the Database of Interacting Proteins (DIP). Since that time, the number of public databases has been increasing. Databases can be subdivided into primary databases, meta-databases, and prediction databases.

- *Primary databases* collect information about published PPIs proven to exist via small-scale or large-scale experimental methods. Examples: DIP, Biomolecular Interaction Network Database (BIND), Biological General Repository for Interaction Datasets (BioGRID), Human Protein Reference Database (HPRD), IntAct Molecular Interaction Database, Molecular Interactions Database (MINT), MIPS Protein Interaction Resource on Yeast (MIPS-MPact), and MIPS Mammalian Protein–Protein Interaction Database (MIPS-MPPI).
- *Meta-databases* normally result from the integration of primary databases information, but can also collect some original data. Examples: Agile Protein Interactomes Dataserver (APID), The Microbial Protein Interaction Database (MPIDB), and Protein Interaction Network Analysis (PINA) platform., (GPS-Prot)
- *Prediction databases* include many PPIs that are predicted using several techniques (main article). Examples: Human Protein–Protein Interaction Prediction Database (PIPs), Interlogous Interaction Database (I2D), Known and Predicted Protein–Protein Interactions (STRING), and Unified Human Interactive (UniHI).

Interaction Networks

Information found in PPIs databases supports the construction of interaction networks. Although the PPI network of a given query protein can be represented in textbooks, diagrams of whole cell PPIs are frankly complex and difficult to generate.

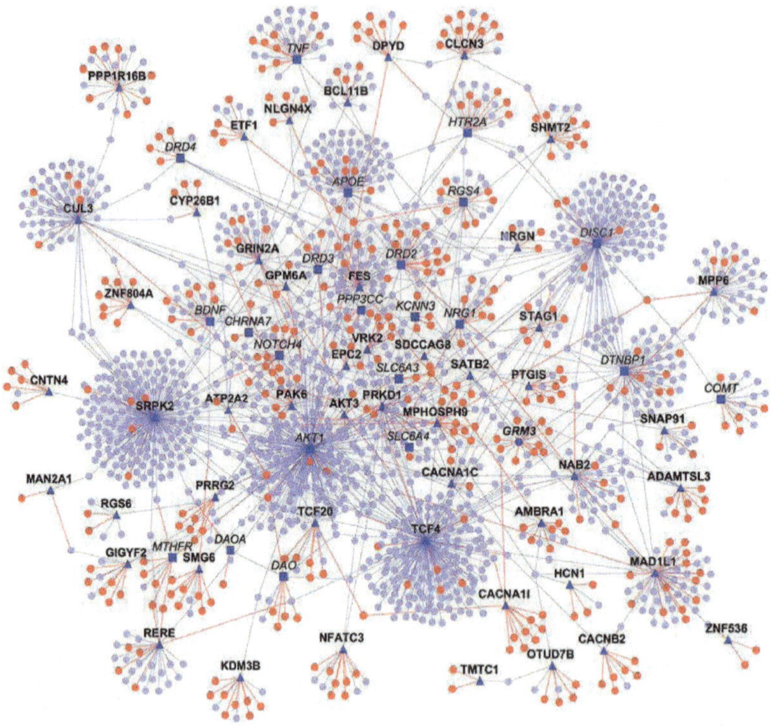

Schziophrenia PPI.

One example of a manually produced molecular interaction map is the Kurt Kohn's 1999 map of cell cycle control. Drawing on Kohn's map, Schwikowski et al. in 2000 published a paper on PPIs in yeast, linking together 1,548 interacting proteins determined by two-hybrid screening. They used a layered graph drawing method to find an initial placement of the nodes and then improved the layout using a force-based algorithm.

Bioinformatic tools have been developed to simplify the difficult task of visualizing molecular interaction networks and complement them with other types of data. For instance, Cytoscape is an open-source software widely used and lots of plugins are currently available. Pajek software is advantageous for the visualization and analysis of very large networks.

Identification of functional modules in PPI networks is an important challenge in bioinformatics. Functional modules means a set of proteins that are highly connected to each other in PPI network. It is almost similar problem as community detection in social networks. There are some methods such as Jactive modules and MoBaS. Jactive modules integrate PPI network and gene expression data where as MoBaS integrate PPI network and Genome Wide association Studies.

The awareness of the major roles of PPIs in numerous physiological and pathological processes has been driving the challenge of unravel many interactomes. Examples of published interactomes are the thyroid specific DREAM interactome and the PP1α interactome in human brain.

Protein-protein relationships are often the result of multiple types of interactions or are deduced from different approaches, including co-localization, direct interaction, suppressive genetic interaction, additive genetic interaction, physical association, and other associations.

Signed Interaction Networks

Protein–protein interactions often result in one of the interacting proteins either being 'activated' or 'repressed'. Such effects can be indicated in a PPI network by "signs" (e.g. "activation" or "inhibition"). Although such attributes have been added to networks for a long time, Vinayagam et al. (2014) coined the term *Signed network* for them. Signed networks are often expressed by labeling the interaction as either positive or negative. A positive interaction is one where the interaction results in one of the proteins being activated. Conversely a negative interaction indicates that one of the proteins being inactivated.

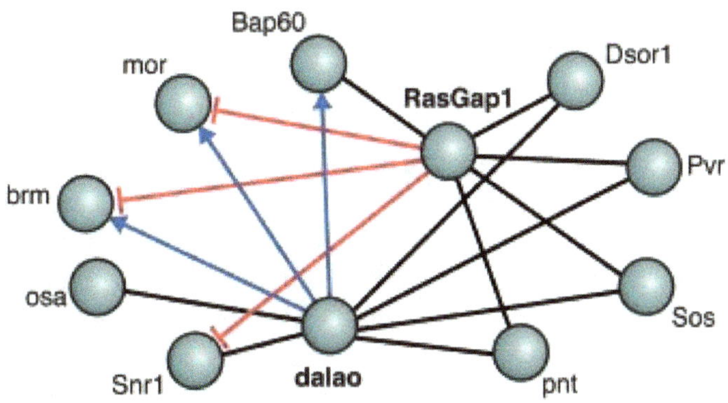

The protein protein interactions are displayed in a signed network that describes what type of interactions that are taking place

Protein–protein interaction networks are often constructed as a result of lab experiments such as yeast two hybrid screens or 'affinity purification and subsequent mass spectrometry techniques. However these methods do not provide the layer of information needed in order to determine what type of interaction is present in order to be able to attribute signs to the network diagrams.

RNA Interference Screens

RNA interference (RNAi) screens (repression of individual proteins between transcription and translation) are one method that can be utilized in the process of providing signs to the protein-protein interactions. Individual proteins are repressed and the resulting phenotypes are analyzed. A correlating phenotypic relationship (i.e. where the inhibition of either of two proteins results in the same phenotype) indicates a positive, or activating relationship. Phenotypes that do not correlate (i.e. where the inhibition of either of two proteins results in two different phenotypes) indicate a negative or inactivating relationship. If protein A is dependent on protein B for activation then the inhibition of either protein A or B will result in a cell losing the service that is provided by protein A and the phenotypes will be the same for the inhibition of either A or B. If, however, protein A is inactivated by protein B then the phenotypes will differ depending on which protein is inhibited (inhibit protein B and it can no longer inactivate protein A leaving A active however inactivate A and there is nothing for B to activate since A is inactive and the phenotype changes). Multiple RNAi screens need to be performed in order to reliably appoint a sign to a given protein-protein interaction. Vinayagam et al. who devised this technique state that a minimum of nine RNAi screens are required with confidence increasing as one carries out more screens.

As Therapeutic Targets

Modulation of PPI is challenging and is receiving increasing attention by the scientific community. Several properties of PPI such as allosteric sites and hotspots, have been incorporated into drug-design strategies.The relevance of PPI as putative therapeutic targets for the development of new treatments is particularly evident in cancer, with several ongoing clinical trials within this area. The consensus among these promising targets is, nonetheless, denoted in the already available drugs on the market to treat a multitude of diseases. Examples are Titrobifan, inhibitor of the glycoprotein IIb/IIIa, used as a cardiovascular drug, and Maraviroc, inhibitor of the CCR5-gp120 interaction, used as anti-HIV drug. Recently, Amit Jaiswal and others were able to develop 30 peptides using protein–protein interaction studies to inhibit telomerase recruitment towards telomeres.

REFERENCES

1. Melton, Lisa (2004). “Protein arrays: Proteomics in multiplex”. Nature. 429 (6987): 101–107. doi:10.1038/429101a. ISSN 0028-0836.
2. Mark Schena (2005). Protein Microarrays. Jones & Bartlett Learning. pp. 47–. ISBN 978-0-7637-3127-4.
3. Mark Schena (2005). Protein Microarrays. Jones & Bartlett Learning. pp. 322–. ISBN 978-0-7637-3127-4.
4. Mitchell, Peter (2002). “A perspective on protein microarrays”. Nature Biotechnology. 20 (3): 225–229. doi:10.1038/nbt0302-225. ISSN 1087-0156.
5. Chang TW (December 1983). “Binding of cells to matrixes of distinct antibodies coated on solid surface”. J. Immunol. Methods. 65 (1–2): 217–23.

doi:10.1016/0022-1759(83)90318-6. PMID 6606681.

6. US 4591570; US 4829010; US 5100777.
7. Hall, DA; Ptacek, J; Snyder, M (December 12, 2012). "Protein Microarray Technology". Mech. Ageing Dev. 128: 161–7. doi:10.1016/j.mad.2006.11.021. PMC 1828913Freely accessible. PMID 17126887.
8. Talapatra, Anupam; Rouse, Richard; Hardiman, Gary (2002). "Protein microarrays: challenges and promises". Pharmacogenomics. 3 (4): 527–536. doi:10.1517/14622416.3.4.527. ISSN 1462-2416.
9. Calvert, Paul (2001). "Inkjet Printing for Materials and Devices". Chemistry of Materials. 13 (10): 3299–3305. doi:10.1021/cm0101632. ISSN 0897-4756.
10. "DNA Microarrays: Techniques". Arabidopsis.info. Archived from the original on August 28, 2008. Retrieved 2013-01-19.
11. "photolithography". Phys.org. Retrieved 2013-01-19.
12. Hall, DA; Ptacek, J; Snyder, M (2007). "Protein microarray technology". Mech. Ageing Dev. 128: 161–7. doi:10.1016/j.mad.2006.11.021. PMC 1828913Freely accessible. PMID 17126887.
13. Williams, Richard J.; Narayanan, Narasimhachari.; Casay, Guillermo A.; Lipowska, Malgorzata.; Peralta, Jose Mauro.; Tsang, Victor C. W.; Strekowski, Lucjan.; Patonay, Gabor. (1994). "Instrument To Detect Near-Infrared Fluorescence in Solid-Phase Immunoassay". Analytical Chemistry. 66 (19): 3102–3107. doi:10.1021/ac00091a018. ISSN 0003-2700.
14. Fung, Eric T; Thulasiraman, Vanitha; Weinberger, Scot R; Dalmasso, Enrique A (2001). "Protein biochips for differential profiling". Current Opinion in Biotechnology. 12 (1): 65–69. doi:10.1016/S0958-1669(00)00167-1. ISSN 0958-1669.
15. Michail A. Alterman; Peter Hunziker (2 December 2011). Amino Acid Analysis: Methods and Protocols. Humana Press. ISBN 978-1-61779-444-5.
16. Coon, Joshua J. (April 13, 2009). "Collisions or Electrons? Protein Sequence Analysis in the 21st Century". Anal. Chem. 81 (9): 3208–3215. doi:10.1021/ac802330b.

CHAPTER 6

Protein Homeostasis

Chapter Contents

- **Introduction**
- **Mechanisms of Proteostasis**
- **Signaling Events in Proteostasis**
- **Diseases of Proteostasis**
- **Proteolysis**

Protein homeostasis or '**proteostasis**' is the process that regulates proteins within the cell in order to maintain the health of both the cellular proteome and the organism itself. **Proteostasis** involves a highly complex interconnection of pathways that influence the fate of a protein from synthesis to degradation.

INTRODUCTION

Proteostasis, a portmanteau of the words protein and homeostasis, is the concept that there are competing and integrated biological pathways within cells that control the biogenesis, folding, trafficking and degradation of proteins present within and outside the cell. The concept of proteostasis maintenance is central to understanding the cause of diseases associated with excessive protein misfolding and degradation leading to loss-of-function phenotypes, as well as aggregation-associated degenerative disorders. Therefore, adapting proteostasis should enable the restoration of proteostasis once its loss leads to pathology. Cellular proteostasis is key to ensuring successful development, healthy aging, resistance to environmental stresses, and to minimize homeostasis perturbations by pathogens such as viruses. Mechanisms by which proteostasis is ensured include regulated protein translation, chaperone assisted protein folding and protein degradation pathways. Adjusting each of these mechanisms to the demand for proteins is essential to maintain all cellular functions relying on a correctly folded proteome.

MECHANISMS OF PROTEOSTASIS

The Roles of the Ribosome In Proteostasis

One of the first points of regulation for proteostasis is during translation. This is accomplished via the structure of the ribosome, a complex central to translation. These two characteristics shape the way the protein folds and influences the proteins future interactions. The synthesis of a new peptide chain using the ribosome is very slow and the ribosome can even be stalled when it encounters a rare codon, a codon found at low concentrations in the cell. These pauses provide an opportunity for an individual protein domain to have the necessary time to become folded before the production of following domains. This facilitates the correct folding of multi-domain proteins. The newly synthesized peptide chain exits the ribosome into the cellular environment through the narrow ribosome exit channel (width: 10Å to 20Å, length 80Å). Due to space restriction in the exit channel the nascent chain already forms secondary and limited tertiary structures. For example, an alpha helix is one such structural property that is commonly induced in this exit channel. At the same time the exit channel also prevents premature folding by impeding large scale interactions within the peptide chain which would require more space.

Molecular Chaperones and Post-Translational Maintenance in Proteostasis

In order to maintain protein homeostasis post-translationally, the cell makes use of molecular chaperones and/or chaperonins, which aid in the assembly or disassembly of proteins. They recognize exposed segments of hydrophobic amino acids in the nascent peptide chain and then work to promote the proper formation of noncovalent interactions that lead to the desired folded state. Chaperones begin to assist in protein folding as soon as a nascent chain longer than 60 amino acids emerges from the ribosome exit channel. One of the most studied ribosome binding chaperones is trigger factor. Trigger Factor works to stabilize the peptide, promotes its folding, prevents aggregation, and promotes refolding of denatured model substrates. Trigger factor not only directly works to properly fold the protein but also recruits other chaperones to the ribosome, such as Hsp70. Hsp70 surrounds an unfolded peptide chain, thereby preventing aggregation and promoting folding.,

Chaperonins are a special class of chaperones that promote native state folding by cyclically encapsulating the peptide chain. Chaperonins are divided into two groups. Group 1 chaperonins are commonly found in bacteria, chloroplasts, and mitochondria. Group 2 chaperonins are found in both the cytosol of eukaryotic cells as well as in archaea. Group 2 chaperonins also contain an additional helical component which acts as a lid for the cylindrical protein chamber, unlike Group 1 which instead relies on an extra cochaperone to act as a lid. All chaperonins exhibit two states (open and closed), between which they can cycle. This cycling process is important during the folding of an individual polypeptide chain as it helps to avoid undesired interactions as well as to prevent the peptide from entering into kinetically trapped states.

Regulating Proteostasis by Protein Degradation

The third component of the proteostasis network is the protein degradation machinery. Protein degradation occurs in proteostasis when the cellular signals indicate the need to decrease overall cellular protein levels. The effects of protein degradation can be local, with the cell only experiencing effects from the loss of the degraded protein itself or widespread, with the entire protein landscape changing due to loss of other proteins' interactions with the degraded protein. Multiple substrates are targets for proteostatic degradation. These degradable substrates include nonfunctional protein fragments produced from ribosomal stalling during translation, misfolded or unfolded proteins, aggregated proteins, and proteins that are no longer needed to carry out cellular function. Several different pathways exist for carrying out these degradation processes. When proteins are determined to be unfolded or misfolded, they are typically degraded via the unfolded protein response (UPR) or ER associated degradation (ERAD). Substrates that are unfolded, misfolded, or no longer required for cellular function can also be ubiquitin tagged for degradation by ATP dependent proteases, such as the proteasome in eukaryotes or ClpXP in prokaryotes. Autophagy, or self engulfment, lysosomal targeting, and phagocytosis (engulfment of waste products by other cells) can also be used as proteostatic degradation mechanisms.

SIGNALING EVENTS IN PROTEOSTASIS

Protein misfolding is detected by mechanisms that are specific for the cellular compartment in which they occur. Distinct surveillance mechanisms that respond unfolded protein have been characterized in the cytoplasm, ER and mitochondria. This response acts locally in a cell autonomous fashion but can also extend to intercellular signaling to protect the organism from anticipated proteotoxic stress.

Cell-autonomous Stress Responses

Cellular stress response pathways detect and alleviate proteotoxic stress which is triggered by imbalances in proteostasis. The cell-autonomous regulation occurs through direct detection of misfolded proteins or inhibition of pathway activation by sequestering activating components in response to heat shock. Cellular responses to this stress signaling include transcriptional activation of chaperone expression, increased efficiency in protein trafficking and protein degradation and translational reduction.

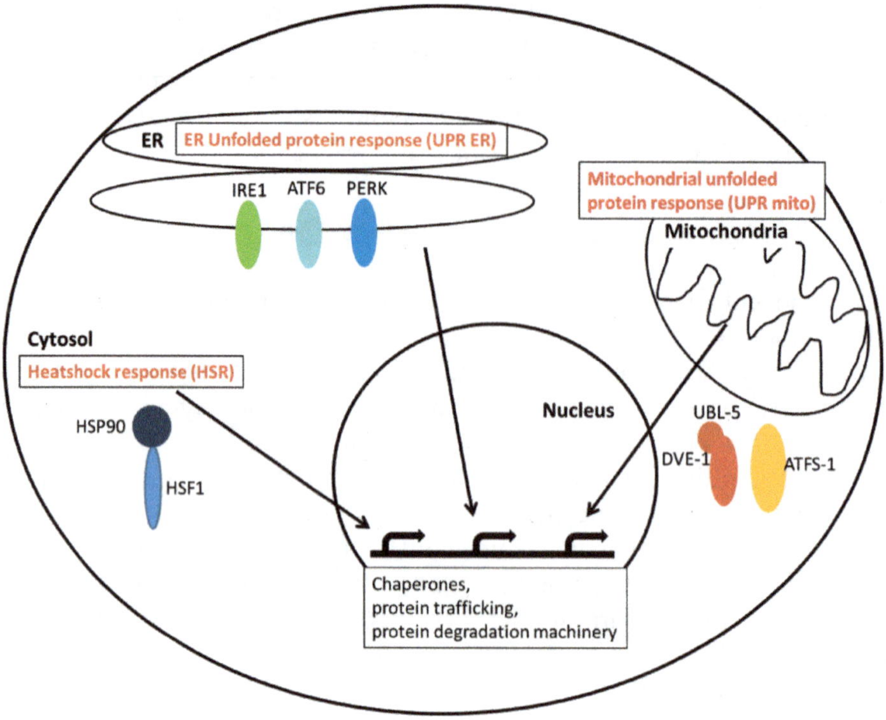

Proteostasis stress signaling response.

Cytosolic heat shock response

The cytosolic HSR is mainly mediated by the transcription factor family HSF (heat shock family). HSF is constitutively bound by Hsp90. Upon a proteotoxic stimulus Hsp90 is recruited away from HSF which can then bind to heat response elements in the DNA and upregulate gene expression of proteins involved in the maintenance of proteostasis.

ER Unfolded Protein Response

The unfolded protein response in the endoplasmatic reticulum is activated by imbalances of unfolded proteins inside the ER and the proteins mediating protein homeostasis. Different "detectors" - such as IRE1, ATF6 and PERK - can recognize misfolded proteins in the ER and mediate transcriptional responses which help alleviate the effects of ER stress.

Mitochondrial Unfolded Protein Response

The mitochondrial unfolded protein response detects imbalances in protein stoichiometry of mitochondrial proteins and misfolded proteins. The expression of mitochondrial chaperones is upregulated by the activation of the transcription factors ATF-1 and/or DVE-1 with UBL-5.

Systemic Stress Signaling

Stress responses can also be triggered in a non-cell autonomous fashion by intercellular communication. The stress that is sensed in one tissue could thereby be communicated to other tissues to protect the proteome of the organism or to regulate proteostasis systemically. Cell non-autonomous activation can occur for all three stress responses.

Work on the model organism *C. elegans* has shown that neurons play a role in this intercellular communication of cytosolic HSR. Stress induced in the neurons of the worm can in the long run protect other tissues such as muscle and intestinal cells from chronic proteotoxicity. Similarly ER and mitochondrial UPR in neurons are relayed to intestinal cells . These systemic responses have been implicated in mediating not only systemic proteostasis but also influence organismal aging.

DISEASES OF PROTEOSTASIS

Proteostasis and Diseases of Protein Folding

Dysfunction in proteostasis can arise from errors in or misregulation of protein folding. The classic examples are missense mutations and deletions that change the thermodynamic and kinetic parameters for the protein folding process. These mutations are often inherited and range in phenotypic severity from having no noticeable effect to embryonic lethality. Disease develops when these mutations render a protein significantly more susceptible to misfolding, aggregation, and degradation. If these effects only alter the mutated protein, the negative consequences will only be local loss of function. However, if these mutations occur in a chaperone or a protein that interacts with many other proteins, dramatic global alterations in the proteostasis boundary will occur. Examples of diseases resulting from proteostatic changes from errors in protein folding include cystic fibrosis, Huntington's disease, Alzheimer's disease, lysosomal storage disorders, and others.

The role of Model Systems in the Elucidation of Protein-Misfolding Diseases

Small animal model systems have been and continue to be instrumental in the identification of functional mechanisms that safeguard proteostasis. Model systems of diverse misfolding-prone disease proteins have so far revealed numerous chaperone and co-chaperone modifiers of proteotoxicity.

Proteostasis and Cancer

The unregulated cell division that marks cancer development requires increased protein synthesis for cancer cell function and survival. This increased protein synthesis is typically seen in proteins that modulate cell metabolism and growth processes. Cancer cells sometimes susceptible to drugs that inhibit chaperones and disrupt proteostasis, such as Hsp90 inhibitors or proteasome inhibitors.

Proteostasis and Obesity

A hallmark of cellular proteostatic networks is their ability to adapt to stress via protein regulation. Metabolic disease, such as that associated with obesity, alters the ability of cellular proteostasis networks adapt to stress, often with detrimental health effects. For example, when insulin production exceeds the cell's insulin secretion capacity, proteostatic collapse occurs and chaperone production is severely impaired. This disruption leads to the disease symptoms exhibited in individuals with diabetes.

Proteostasis and Aging

Over time, the proteostasis network becomes burdened with proteins modified by reactive oxygen species and metabolites that induce oxidative damage. These byproducts can react with cellular proteins to cause misfolding and aggregation (especially in nondividing cells like neurons). This risk is particularly high for intrinsically disordered proteins. The IGFR-1 pathway has been shown in *C. elegans* to protect against these harmful aggregates, and some experimental work has suggested that upregulation of insulin growth factor receptor 1 (IGFR-1) may stabilize proteostatic network and prevent detrimental effects of aging. Expression of the chaperome, the ensemble of chaperones and co-chaperones that interact in a complex network of molecular folding machines to regulate proteome function, is dramatically repressed in human aging brains and in the brains of patients with neurodegenerative diseases. Functional assays in *C. elegant* and human cells have identified a conserved chaperome sub-network of 16 chaperone genes, corresponding to 28 human orthologs as a proteostasis safeguard in aging and age-onset neurodegenerative disease.

Pharmacologic Intervention in Proteostasis

There are two main approaches that have been used for therapeutic development targeting the proteostatic network: pharmacologic chaperones and proteostasis regulators. The principle behind designing pharmacologic chaperones for intervention in diseases of proteostasis is to design small molecules that stabilize borderline proteins. Previously, this approach has been used to target and stabilize G-protein coupled receptors, neurotransmitter receptors, glycosidases, lysosomal storage proteins, and the mutant CFTR protein that causes cystic fibrosis.

The principle behind proteostasis regulators is similar, but seeks to stabilize the proteostatic boundary on a widespread scale. For example, some proteostasis regulators target chaperones such as heat shock proteins for stabilization. It has been suggested that this approach could even be applied prophylactically, such as upregulating certain protective pathways before experiencing an anticipated severe cellular stress. One theoretical mechanism for this approach includes upregulating the unfolded protein response to rescue proteins from degradation during cellular stress.

PROTEOLYSIS

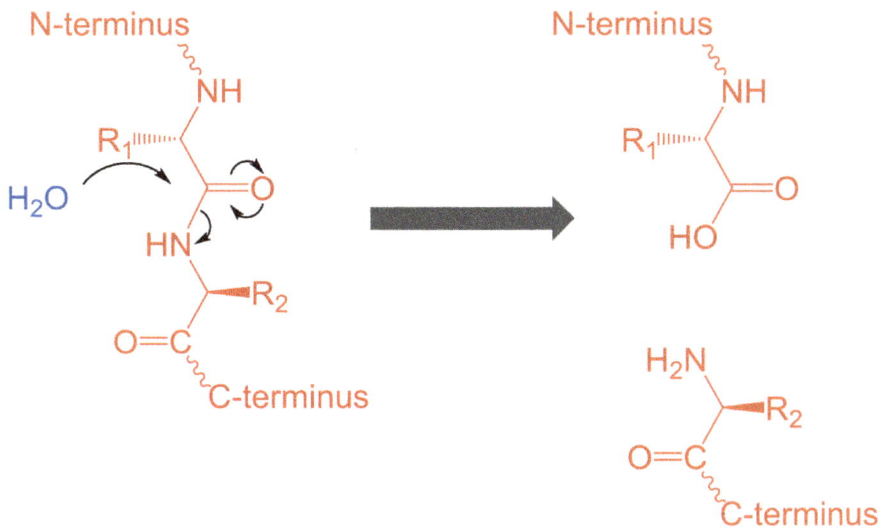

The hydrolysis of a protein (red) by the nucleophilic attack of water (blue). The uncatalysed half-life is several hundred years.

Proteolysis is the breakdown of proteins into smaller polypeptides or amino acids. Uncatalysed, the hydrolysis of peptide bonds is extremely slow, taking hundreds of years. Proteolysis is typically catalysed by cellular enzymes called proteases, but may also occur by intra-molecular digestion. Low pH or high temperatures can also cause proteolysis non-enzymatically.

Proteolysis in organisms serves many purposes; for example, digestive enzymes break down proteins in food to provide amino acids for the organism, while proteolytic processing of a polypeptide chain after its synthesis may be necessary for the production of an active protein. It is also important in the regulation of some physiological and cellular processes, as well as preventing the accumulation of unwanted or abnormal proteins in cells. Consequently, dis-regulation of proteolysis can cause diseases and is used in some venoms to damage their prey.

Proteolysis is important as an analytical tool for studying proteins in the laboratory, as well as industrially, for example in food processing and stain removal.

Biological Functions

Post-translational Proteolytic Processing

Limited proteolysis of a polypeptide during or after translation in protein synthesis often occurs for many proteins. This may involve removal of the N-terminal methionine, signal peptide, and/or the conversion of an inactive or non-functional protein to an active one. The precursor to the final functional form of protein is termed proprotein, and these proproteins may be first synthesized as preproprotein. For example, albumin is first synthesized as preproalbumin and contains an uncleaved signal peptide. This forms the proalbumin after the signal peptide is cleaved, and a further processing to remove the N-terminal 6-residue propeptide yields the mature form of the protein.

Removal of N-terminal Methionine

The initiating methionine (and, in prokaryotes, fMet) may be removed during translation of the nascent protein. For *E. coli*, fMet is efficiently removed if the second residue is small and uncharged, but not if the second residue is bulky and charged. In both prokaryotes and eukaryotes, the exposed N-terminal residue may determine the half-life of the protein according to the N-end rule.

Removal of the Signal Sequence

Proteins that are to be targeted to a particular organelle or for secretion have an N-terminal signal peptide that directs the protein to its final destination. This signal peptide is removed by proteolysis after their transport through a membrane.

Cleavage of Polyproteins

Some proteins and most eukaryotic polypeptide hormones are synthesized as a large precursor polypeptide known as a polyprotein that requires proteolytic cleavage into individual smaller polypeptide chains. The polyprotein pro-opiomelanocortin (POMC) contains many polypeptide hormones. The cleavage pattern of POMC, however, may vary between different tissues, yielding different sets of polypeptide hormones from the same polyprotein.

Many viruses also produce their proteins initially as a single polypeptide chain that were translated from a polycistronic mRNA. This polypeptide is subsequently cleaved into individual polypeptide chains.

Cleavage of Precursor Proteins

Many proteins and hormones are synthesized in the form of their precursors - zymogens, proenzymes, and prehormones. These proteins are cleaved to form their final active structures. Insulin, for example, is synthesized as preproinsulin, which yields proinsulin after the signal peptide has been cleaved. The proinsulin is then cleaved at two positions to yield two polypeptide chains linked by two disulfide bonds. Removal of two C-terminal residues from the B-chain then yields the mature insulin. Protein folding occurs in the single-chain Proinsulin form which facilitates formation of the ultimately inter-peptide disulfide bonds, and the ultimately intra-peptide disulfide bond, found in the native structure of insulin.

Proteases in particular are synthesized in the inactive form so that they may be safely stored in cells, and ready for release in sufficient quantity when required. This is to ensure that the protease is activated only in the correct location or context, as inappropriate activation of these proteases can be very destructive for an organism. Proteolysis of the zymogen yields an active protein; for example, when trypsinogen is cleaved to form trypsin, a slight rearrangement of the protein structure that completes the active site of the protease occurs, thereby activating the protein.

Proteolysis can, therefore, be a method of regulating biological processes by turning inactive proteins into active ones. A good example is the blood clotting cascade whereby an initial event triggers a cascade of sequential proteolytic activation of many specific proteases, resulting in blood coagulation. The complement system of the immune response also involves a complex sequential proteolytic activation and interaction that result in an attack on invading pathogens.

Protein Degradation

Protein degradation may take place intracellularly or extracellularly. In digestion of food, digestive enzymes may be released into the environment for extracellular digestion whereby proteolytic cleavage breaks down proteins into smaller peptides and amino acids so that they may be absorbed and used by an organism. In animals the food may be processed extracellularly in specialized digestive organs or guts, but in many bacteria the food may be internalized into the cell via phagocytosis. Microbial degradation of protein in the environment can be regulated by nutrient availability. For example, limitation for major elements in proteins (carbon, nitrogen, and sulfur) has been shown to induce proteolytic activity in the fungus *Neurospora crassa* as well as in whole communities of soil organisms.

Proteins in cells are also constantly being broken down into amino acids. This intracellular degradation of protein serves a number of functions: It removes damaged and abnormal protein and prevent their accumulation, and it also serves to regulate cellular processes by removing enzymes and regulatory proteins that are no longer needed. The amino acids may then be reused for protein synthesis.

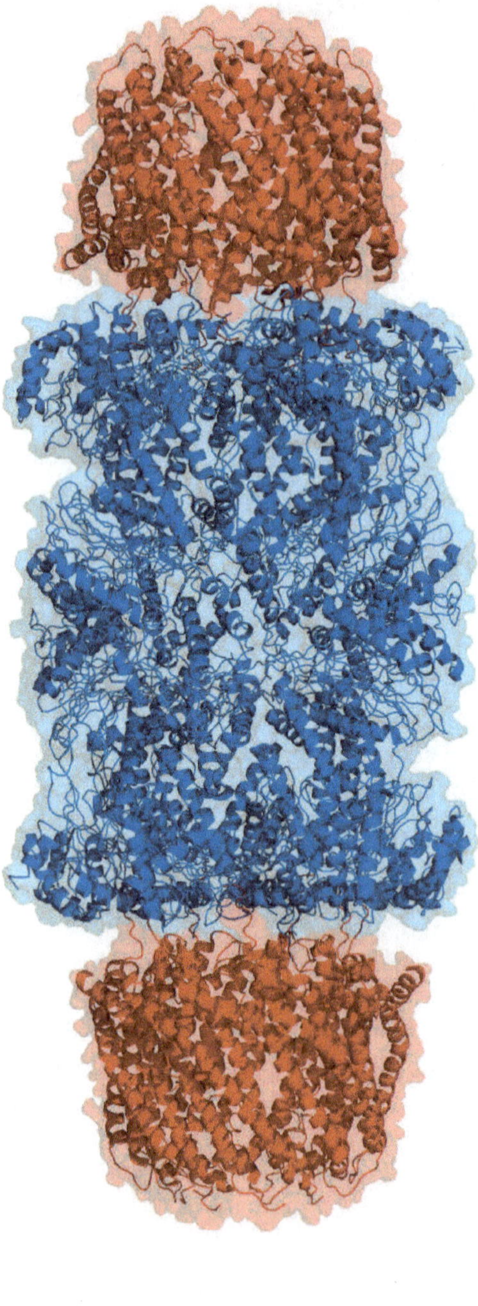

Structure of a proteasome. Its active sites are inside the tube (blue) where proteins are degraded.

Lysosome and Proteasome

The intracellular degradation of protein may be achieved in two ways - proteolysis in lysosome, or a ubiquitin-dependent process that targets unwanted proteins to proteasome.

The autophagy-lysosomal pathway is normally a non-selective process, but it may become selective upon starvation whereby proteins with peptide sequence KFERQ or similar are selectively broken down. The lysosome contains a large number of proteases such as cathepsins.

The ubiquitin-mediated process is selective. Proteins marked for degradation are covalently linked to ubiquitin. Many molecules of ubiquitin may be linked in tandem to a protein destined for degradation. The polyubiquinated protein is targeted to an ATP-dependent protease complex, the proteasome. The ubiquitin is released and reused, while the targeted protein is degraded.

Rate of Intracellular Protein Degradation

Different proteins are degraded at different rates. Abnormal proteins are quickly degraded, whereas the rate of degradation of normal proteins may vary widely depending on their functions. Enzymes at important metabolic control points may be degraded much faster than those enzymes whose activity is largely constant under all physiological conditions. One of the most rapidly degraded proteins is ornithine decarboxylase, which has a half-life of 11 minutes. In contrast, other proteins like actin and myosin have a half-life of a month or more, while, in essence, haemoglobin lasts for the entire life-time of an erythrocyte.

The N-end rule may partially determine the half-life of a protein, and proteins with segments rich in proline, glutamic acid, serine, and threonine (the so-called PEST proteins) have short half-life. Other factors suspected to affect degradation rate include the rate deamination of glutamine and asparagine and oxidation of cystein, histidine, and methionine, the absence of stabilizing ligands, the presence of attached carbohydrate or phosphate groups, the presence of free α-amino group, the negative charge of protein, and the flexibility and stability of the protein. Proteins with larger degrees of intrinsic disorder also tend to have short cellular half-life, with disordered segments having been proposed to facilitate efficient initiation of degradation by the proteasome.

The rate of proteolysis may also depend on the physiological state of the organism, such as its hormonal state as well as nutritional status. In time of starvation, the rate of protein degradation increases.

Digestion

In human digestion, proteins in food are broken down into smaller peptide chains by digestive enzymes such as pepsin, trypsin, chymotrypsin, and elastase, and into amino acids by various enzymes such as carboxypeptidase, aminopeptidase, and dipeptidase. It is necessary to break down proteins into small peptides (tripeptides and dipeptides) and amino acids so they can be absorbed by the intestines, and the absorbed tripeptides and dipeptides are also further broken into amino acids intracellularly before they enter the bloodstream. Different enzymes have different specificity for their substrate; trypsin, for example, cleaves the peptide bond after a positively charged residue (arginine and lysine); chymotrypsin cleaves the bond after an aromatic residue (phenylalanine, tyrosine, and tryptophan); elastase cleaves the bond after a small non-polar residue such as alanine or glycine.

In order to prevent inappropriate or premature activation of the digestive enzymes (they may, for example, trigger pancreatic self-digestion causing pancreatitis), these enzymes are secreted as inactive zymogen. The precursor of pepsin, pepsinogen, is secreted by the stomach, and is activated only in the acidic environment found in stomach. The pancreas secretes the precursors of a number of proteases such as trypsin and chymotrypsin. The zymogen of trypsin is trypsinogen, which is activated by a very specific protease, enterokinase, secreted by the mucosa of the duodenum. The trypsin, once activated, can also cleave other trypsinogens as well as the precursors of other proteases such as chymotrypsin and carboxypeptidase to activate them.

In bacteria, a similar strategy of employing an inactive zymogen or prezymogen is used. Subtilisin, which is produced by *Bacillus subtilis*, is produced as preprosubtilisin, and is released only if the signal peptide is cleaved and autocatalytic proteolytic activation has occurred.

Cellular regulation

Proteolysis is also involved in the regulation of many cellular processes by activating or deactivating enzymes, transcription factors, and receptors, for example in the biosynthesis of cholesterol, or the mediation of thrombin signalling through protease-activated receptors.

Some enzymes at important metabolic control points such as ornithine decarboxylase is regulated entirely by its rate of synthesis and its rate of degradation. Other rapidly degraded proteins include the protein products of proto-oncogenes, which play central roles in the regulation of cell growth.

Cell cycle Regulation

Cyclins are a group of proteins that activate kinases involved in cell division. The degradation of cyclins is the key step that governs the exit from mitosis and progress into the next cell cycle. Cyclins accumulate in the course the cell cycle, then abruptly disappear just before the anaphase of mitosis. The cyclins are removed via a ubiquitin-mediated proteolytic pathway.

Apoptosis

Caspases are an important group of proteases involved in apoptosis. The precursors of caspase, procaspase, may be activated by proteolysis through its association with a protein complex that forms apoptosome, or by granzyme B, or via the death receptor pathways.

Proteolysis and Diseases

Abnormal proteolytic activity is associated with many diseases. In pancreatitis, leakage of proteases and their premature activation in the pancreas results in the self-digestion of the pancreas. People with diabetes mellitus may have increased lysosomal activity and the degradation of some proteins can increase significantly. Chronic inflammatory diseases such as rheumatoid arthritis may involve the release of lysosomal enzymes into extracellular space that break down surrounding tissues. Abnormal proteolysis and generation of peptides that aggregate in cells and their ineffective removal may result in many age-related neurological diseases such as Alzheimer›s.

Proteases may be regulated by antiproteases or protease inhibitors, and imbalance between proteases and antiproteases can result in diseases, for example, in the destruction of lung tissues in emphysema brought on by smoking tobacco. Smoking is thought to increase the neutrophils and macrophages in the lung which release excessive amount of proteolytic enzymes such as elastase, such that they can no longer be inhibited by serpins such as α_1-antitrypsin, thereby resulting in the breaking down of connective tissues in the lung. Other proteases and their inhibitors may also be involved in this disease, for example matrix metalloproteinases (MMPs) and tissue inhibitors of metalloproteinases (TIMPs).

Other diseases linked to aberrant proteolysis include muscular dystrophy, degenerative skin disorders, respiratory and gastrointestinal diseases, and malignancy.

Non-enzymatic Proteolysis

Protein backbones are very stable in water at neutral pH and room temperature, although the rate of hydrolysis of different peptide bonds can vary. The half life of a peptide bond under normal conditions can range from 7 years to 350 years, even higher for peptides protected by modified terminus or within the protein interior. The rate of proteolysis however can be significantly increased by extremes of pH and heat.

Strong mineral acids can readily hydrolyse the peptide bonds in a protein (acid hydrolysis). The standard way to hydrolyze a protein or peptide into its constituent amino acids for analysis is to heat it to 105 °C for around 24 hours in 6M hydrochloric acid. However, some proteins are resistant to acid hydrolysis. One well-known example is ribonuclease A, which can be purified by treating crude extracts with hot sulphuric acid so that other proteins become degraded while ribonuclease A is left intact.

Certain chemicals cause proteolysis only after specific residues, and these can be used to selectively break down a protein into smaller polypeptides for laboratory analysis. For example, cyanogen bromide cleaves the peptide bond after a methionine. Similar methods may be used to specifically cleave tryptophanyl, aspartyl, cysteinyl, and asparaginyl peptide bonds. Acids such as trifluoroacetic acid and formic acid may also be used.

Like other biomolecules, proteins can also be broken down by high heat alone. At 250 °C, the peptide bond may be easily hydrolyzed, with its half-life dropping to about a minute. Protein may also be broken down without hydrolysis through pyrolysis; small heterocyclic compounds may start to form upon degradation, above 500 °C, polycyclic aromatic hydrocarbon may also form, which is of interest in the study of generation of carcinogens in tobacco smoke and cooking at high heat.

Laboratory Applications

Proteolysis is also used in research and diagnostic applications:

- Cleavage of fusion protein so that the fusion partner and protein tag used in protein expression and purification may be removed. The proteases used have high degree of specificity, such as thrombin, enterokinase, and TEV protease, so that only the targeted sequence may be cleaved.

- Complete inactivation of undesirable enzymatic activity or removal of unwanted proteins. For example, proteinase K, a broad-spectrum proteinase stable in urea and SDS, is often used in the preparation of nucleic acids to remove unwanted nuclease contaminants that may otherwise degrade the DNA or RNA.
- Partial inactivation, or changing the functionality, of specific protein. For example, treatment of DNA polymerase I with subtilisin yields the Klenow fragment, which retains its polymerase function but lacks 5›-exonuclease activity.
- Digestion of proteins in solution for proteome analysis by liquid chromatography-mass spectrometry (LC-MS). This may also be done by in-gel digestion of proteins after separation by gel electrophoresis for the identification by mass spectrometry.
- Analysis of the stability of folded domain under a wide range of conditions.
- Increasing success rate of crystallisation projects
- Production of digested protein used in growth media to culture bacteria and other organisms, e.g. tryptone in Lysogeny Broth.

Protease Enzymes

Proteases may be classified according to the catalytic group involved in its active site.

- Cysteine protease
- Serine protease
- Threonine protease
- Aspartic protease
- Glutamic protease
- Metalloprotease
- Asparagine peptide lyase

Venoms

Certain types of venom, such as those produced by venomous snakes, can also cause proteolysis. These venoms are, in fact, complex digestive fluids that begin their work outside of the body. Proteolytic venoms cause a wide range of toxic effects, including effects that are:

- cytotoxic (cell-destroying)
- hemotoxic (blood-destroying)
- myotoxic (muscle-destroying)
- hemorrhagic (bleeding)

REFERENCES

1. Thomas E Creighton (1993). Proteins: Structures and Molecular Properties (2nd ed.). W H Freeman and Company. pp. 78–86. ISBN 0-7167-2317-4.
2. P H Hirel; M J Schmitter; P Dessen; G Fayat; S Blanquet (1989). "Extent of N-terminal methionine excision from Escherichia coli proteins is governed by the side-chain length of the penultimate amino acid". Proc Natl Acad Sci U S A. 86 (21): 8247–51. doi:10.1073/pnas.86.21.8247. PMC 298257 . PMID 2682640.
3. Hanson, M.A., Marzluf, G.A., 1975. Control of the synthesis of a single enzyme by multiple regulatory circuits in Neurospora crassa. Proc. Natl. Acad. Sci. U.S.A. 72, 1240–1244.
4. Sims, G. K., and M. M. Wander. 2002. Proteolytic activity under nitrogen or sulfur limitation. Appl. Soil Ecol. 568:1-5.
5. Thomas E Creighton (1993). "Chapter 10 - Degradation". Proteins: Structures and Molecular Properties (2nd ed.). W H Freeman and Company. pp. 463–473. ISBN 0-7167-2317-4.
6. Voet & Voet (1995). Biochemistry (2nd ed.). John Wiley & Sons. pp. 1010–1014. ISBN 0-471-58651-X.
7. Tompa, P.; Prilusky, J.; Silman, I.; Sussman, J. L. (2008-05-01). "Structural disorder serves as a weak signal for intracellular protein degradation". Proteins. 71 (2): 903–909. doi:10.1002/prot.21773. ISSN 1097-0134. PMID 18004785.
8. Inobe, Tomonao; Matouschek, Andreas (2014-02-01). "Paradigms of protein degradation by the proteasome". Current Opinion in Structural Biology. 24: 156–164. doi:10.1016/j.sbi.2014.02.002. ISSN 1879-033X. PMC 4010099 . PMID 24632559.
9. van der Lee, Robin; Lang, Benjamin; Kruse, Kai; Gsponer, Jörg; Sánchez de Groot, Natalia; Huynen, Martijn A.; Matouschek, Andreas; Fuxreiter, Monika; Babu, M. Madan (25 September 2014). "Intrinsically Disordered Segments Affect Protein Half-Life in the Cell and during Evolution". Cell Reports. 8 (6): 1832–1844. doi:10.1016/j.celrep.2014.07.055. ISSN 2211-1247. PMC 4358326 . PMID 25220455.
10. Silk DB (1974). "Progress report. Peptide absorption in man". Gut. 15 (6): 494–501. doi:10.1136/gut.15.6.494. PMC 1413009 . PMID 4604970.
11. Michael S. Brown; Joseph L. Goldstein (May 1997). "The SREBP Pathway: Regulation of Cholesterol Metabolism by Proteolysis of a Membrane-Bound Transcription Factor". Cell. 89 (3): 331–340. doi:10.1016/S0092-8674(00)80213-5. PMID 9150132.
12. Shaun R. Coughlin (2000). "Thrombin signalling and protease-activated receptors". Nature. 407 (6801): 258–264. doi:10.1038/35025229. PMID 11001069.
13. Glotzer M, Murray AW, Kirschner MW (1991). "Cyclin is degraded by the ubiquitin pathway". Nature. 349 (6305): 132–8. doi:10.1038/349132a0. PMID 1846030.

14. Kathleen M. Sakamoto (2002). "Ubiquitin-dependent proteolysis: its role in human diseases and the design of therapeutic strategies"(PDF). Molecular Genetics and Metabolism. 77 (1–2): 44–56. doi:10.1016/S1096-7192(02)00146-4. PMID 12359129.
15. De Strooper B. (2010). "Proteases and proteolysis in Alzheimer disease: a multifactorial view on the disease process". Physiological Reviews. 90 (2): 465–94. doi:10.1152/physrev.00023.2009. PMID 20393191
16. Abboud RT1, Vimalanathan S (2008). "Pathogenesis of COPD. Part I. The role of protease-antiprotease imbalance in emphysema". International Journal of Tuberculosis and Lung Diseases. 12 (4): 361–7. PMID 18371259.
17. Daniel. Kahne; W. Clark Still (1988). "Hydrolysis of a peptide bond in neutral water". J. Am. Chem. Soc. 110 (22): 7529–7534. doi:10.1021/ja00230a041.
18. Radzicka, Anna; Wolfenden, Richard (January 1996). "Rates of Uncatalyzed Peptide Bond Hydrolysis in Neutral Solution and the Transition State Affinities of Proteases". Journal of the American Chemical Society. 118 (26): 6105–6109. doi:10.1021/ja954077c.
19. Bernard Testa, Joachim M. Mayer (1 July 2003). Hydrolysis in Drug and Prodrug Metabolism. Wiley VCH. pp. 270–288. ISBN 978-3906390253.
20. Thomas E Creighton (1993). Proteins: Structures and Molecular Properties (2nd ed.). W H Freeman and Company. p. 6. ISBN 0-7167-2317-4.
21. "Ribonuclease A". Protein Data Bank.
22. Bryan John Smith (2002). "Chapter 71-75". In John M. Walker. The Protein Protocols Handbook (2 ed.). Humana Press. pp. 485–510. doi:10.1385/1592591698. ISBN 978-0-89603-940-7.
23. White RH (1984). "Hydrolytic stability of biomolecules at high temperatures and its implication for life at 250 degrees C". Nature. 310 (5976): 430–2. doi:10.1038/310430a0. PMID 6462230.
24. Ramesh K. Sharmaa; W.Geoffrey Chana; Jeffrey I. Seemanb; Mohammad R. Hajaligola (January 2003). "Formation of low molecular weight heterocycles and polycyclic aromatic compounds (PACs) in the pyrolysis of α-amino acids". Journal of Analytical and Applied Pyrolysis. 66 (1–2,): 97–121. doi:10.1016/S0165-2370(02)00108-0.
25. Fabbri D, Adamiano A, Torri C (2010). "GC-MS determination of polycyclic aromatic hydrocarbons evolved from pyrolysis of biomass". Anal Bioanal Chem. 397 (1): 309–17. doi:10.1007/s00216-010-3563-5. PMID 20213167.
26. White JL, Conner BT, Perfetti TA, Bombick BR, Avalos JT, Fowler KW, Smith CJ, Doolittle DJ (May 2001). "Effect of pyrolysis temperature on the mutagenicity of tobacco smoke condensate". Food Chem Toxicol. 39 (5): 499–505. doi:10.1016/s0278-6915(00)00155-1. PMID 11313117.
27. "Chemicals in Meat Cooked at High Temperatures and Cancer Risk". National Cancer Institute.

28. Hilz H, Wiegers U, Adamietz P (1975). "Stimulation of Proteinase K action by denaturing agents: application to the isolation of nucleic acids and the degradation of 'masked' proteins". European Journal of Biochemistry. 56 (1): 103–108. doi:10.1111/j.1432-1033.1975.tb02211.x. PMID 1236799.

29. Klenow H, Henningsen I (1970). "Selective Elimination of the Exonuclease Activity of the Deoxyribonucleic Acid Polymerase from Escherichia coli B by Limited Proteolysis". Proc. Natl. Acad. Sci. USA. 65 (1): 168–175. doi:10.1073/pnas.65.1.168. PMC 286206 . PMID 4905667.

30. Minde DP; Maurice, Madelon M.; Rüdiger, Stefan G. D. (2012). Uversky, Vladimir N, ed. "Determining biophysical protein stability in lysates by a fast proteolysis assay, FASTpp". PLoS ONE. 7 (10): e46147. doi:10.1371/journal.pone.0046147. PMC 3463568 . PMID 23056252.

31. Wernimont, A; Edwards, A (2009). Song, Haiwei, ed. "In situ proteolysis to generate crystals for structure determination: An update". PLoS ONE. 4 (4): e5094. doi:10.1371/journal.pone.0005094. PMC 2661377 . PMID 19352432.

32. Kohei Oda (2012). "New families of carboxyl peptidases: serine-carboxyl peptidases and glutamic peptidases". Journal of Biochemistry. 151 (1): 13–25. doi:10.1093/jb/mvr129. PMID 22016395.

33. Hayes WK. 2005. Research on Biological Roles and Variation of Snake Venoms. Loma Linda University

CHAPTER 7

Quantitative Proteomics

Chapter Contents

Quantitative proteomics is a powerful approach used for both discovery and targeted proteomic analyses to understand global proteomic dynamics in a cell, tissue or organism. Most quantitative proteomic analyses entail the isotopic labeling of proteins or peptides in the experimental groups, which can then be differentiated by mass spectrometry. Relative quantitation methods (SILAC, ICAT, ICPL and isobaric tags) are used to compare protein or peptide abundance between samples, while spiking unlabeled samples with known concentrations of isotopically labeled synthetic peptides can yield absolute quantitation of target peptides (via SRM). Label-free strategies are also available for both relative and absolute quantitation. Although these strategies are more complex than mere protein identification, quantitative proteomics is critical for our understanding global protein expression and modifications underlying the molecular mechanisms of biological processes and disease states.

INTRODUCTION

Quantitative proteomics is an analytical chemistry technique for determining the amount of proteins in a sample. Rather than just providing lists of proteins identified in a certain sample, quantitative proteomics yields information about differences between samples.

For example, this approach can be used to compare samples from healthy and diseased patients. The methods for protein identification are identical to those used in general (i.e. qualitative) proteomics, but include quantification as an additional dimension. Quantitative proteomics is mainly performed by two-dimensional gel electrophoresis (2-DE) or mass spectrometry (MS). In contrast to 2-DE, which requires MS for the downstream protein identification, MS technology can identify and quantify the changes.

TECHNOLOGIES

Mass spectrometry (MS) and two-dimensional gel electrophoresis (2-DE) represent the main technologies for quantitative proteomics with advantages and disadvantages. 2-DE provides information about the protein quantity, charge, and mass of the intact protein. It has limitations for the analysis of proteins larger than 150 kDa or smaller than 5kDa and low solubility proteins. Quantitative MS has higher sensitivity but does not provide information about the intact protein data.

Classical 2-DE based on post-electrophoretic dye staining has limitations: at least three technical replicates are required to verify the reproducibility. Difference gel electrophoresis (DIGE) uses fluorescence-based labeling of the proteins prior to separation has increased the precision of quantification as well as the sensitivity in the protein detection. Therefore, DIGE represents the current main approach for the 2-DE based study of proteomes.

For quantitative MS, a commonly applied approach is isotope-coded affinity tags (ICAT), which uses two reagents with heavy and light isotopes, respectively, and a biotin affinity tag to modify cysteine containing peptides. This technology has been used to label whole *Saccharomyces cerevisiae* cells, and, in conjunction with mass spectrometry, helped lay the foundation of quantitative proteomics.

DISCOVERY AND TARGETED PROTEOMICS

Strategies to improve the sensitivity and scope of proteomic analysis often require large sample quantities and multi-dimensional fractionation, which sacrifices throughput. Alternatively, efforts to improve the sensitivity and throughput of protein quantification limit the number of peptides that can be monitored per MS run. For this reason, proteomics research is typically divided into two categories: discovery and targeted proteomics. Discovery proteomics optimizes protein identification by spending more time and effort per sample and reducing the number of samples analyzed. In contrast, targeted proteomics strategies limit the number of features that will be monitored and then optimize the chromatography, instrument tuning and acquisition methods to achieve the highest sensitivity and throughput for hundreds or thousands of samples.

RELATIVE AND ABSOLUTE QUANTIFICATION

Mass spectrometry is not inherently quantitative because of differences in the ionization efficiency and/or detectability of the many peptides in a given sample, which has sparked the development of methods to determine relative and absolute abundance of proteins in samples. The intensity of a peak in a mass spectrum is not a good indicator of the amount of the analyte in the sample, although differences in peak intensity of the *same* analyte between multiple samples accurately reflect relative differences in its abundance.

Label-free quantification

One approach for relative quantification is to separately analyze samples by MS and compare the spectra to determine peptide abundance in one sample relative to another, as in Label-free quantification strategies.

Stable Isotope Labels

An approach for relative quantification that is more costly and time-consuming, though less sensitive to experimental bias than label-free quantification, entails labeling the samples with stable isotope labels that allow the mass spectrometer to distinguish between identical proteins in separate samples. One type of label, isotopic tags, consist of stable isotopes incorporated into protein crosslinkers that causes a known mass shift of the labeled protein or peptide in the mass spectrum. Differentially labeled samples are combined and analyzed together, and the differences in the peak intensities of the isotope pairs accurately reflect difference in the abundance of the corresponding proteins.

Absolute proteomic quantification using isotopic peptides entails spiking known concentrations of synthetic, heavy isotopologues of target peptides into an experimental sample and then performing LC-MS/MS. As with relative quantification using isotopic labels, peptides of equal chemistry co-elute and are analyzed by MS simultaneously. Unlike relative quantification, though, the abundance of the target peptide in the experimental sample is compared to that of the heavy peptide and back-calculated to the initial concentration of the standard using a pre-determined standard curve to yield the absolute quantification of the target peptide.

Relative quantification methods include isotope-coded affinity tags (ICAT), isobaric labeling (tandem mass tags (TMT) and isobaric tags for relative and absolute quantification (iTRAQ)), label-free quantification Metal-coded tags (MeCAT), N-terminal labelling, stable isotope labeling with amino acids in cell culture (SILAC), and Terminal amine isotopic labeling of substrates (TAILS).

Absolute quantification is performed using selected reaction monitoring (SRM).

MeCAT can be used in combination with element mass spectrometry ICP-MS allowing first-time absolute quantification of the metal bound by MeCAT reagent to a protein or biomolecule. Thus it is possible to determine the absolute amount of protein down to attomol range using external calibration by metal standard solution. It is compatible to protein separation by 2D electrophoresis and chromatography in multiplex experiments. Protein identification and relative quantification can be performed by MALDI-MS/MS and ESI-MS/MS.

Mass spectrometers have a limited capacity to detect low-abundance peptides in samples with a high dynamic range. The limited duty cycle of mass spectrometers also restricts the collision rate, resulting in an undersampling Sample preparation protocols represent sources of experimental bias.

Quantitative Proteomics

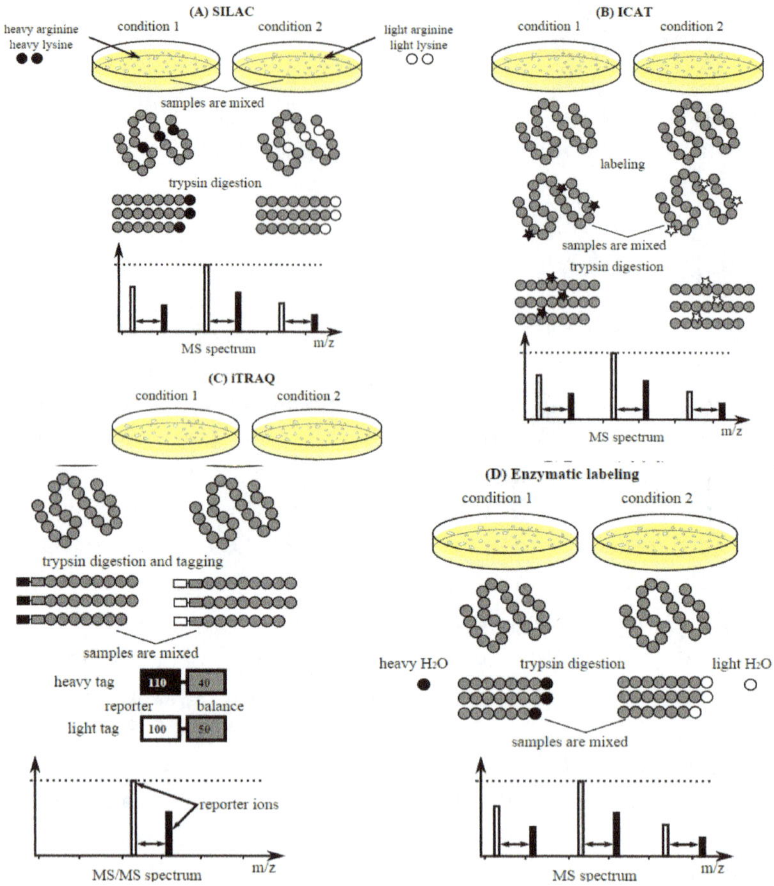

Quantitative Mass Spectrometry.

Mass spectrometry (MS) is commonly regarded as an instrumental technique for separation of electrically charged species in the gas phase (for general information, see for example). The charged species (ions) are produced in the ion source. In some cases, the ion source also assists the transfer of solid-phase or liquid-phase analytes into the gas phase. The gas-phase ions subsequently are transferred into the mass analyser. The mass analyser sorts the ions—in space or time—according to the mass-to-charge ratios (m/z). The separated ions are detected by an ion detector in the space or time domain. Electric signals, produced by the ion detector, are subsequently processed to produce mass spectra. In fact, mass spectra can be viewed as histograms, which provide information on the number of ions at different m/z values. The detected ions may correspond to the original molecules, their fragments or other species formed during the ionization process. MS enables direct identification of molecules based on the mass-to-charge ratio as well as fragmentation patterns. Thus, it fulfils the role of a qualitative analytical technique with high selectivity.

Technologies

Mass spectrometry (MS) and two-dimensional gel electrophoresis (2-DE) represent the main technologies for quantitative proteomics with advantages and disadvantages. 2-DE provides information about the protein quantity, charge, and mass of the intact protein. It has limitations for the analysis of proteins larger than 150 kDa or smaller than 5kDa and low solubility proteins. Quantitative MS has higher sensitivity but does not provide information about the intact protein data.

Classical 2-DE based on post-electrophoretic dye staining has limitations: at least three technical replicates are required to verify the reproducibility. Difference gel electrophoresis (DIGE) uses fluorescence-based labeling of the proteins prior to separation has increased the precision of quantification as well as the sensitivity in the protein detection. Therefore, DIGE represents the current main approach for the 2-DE based study of proteomes.

For quantitative MS, a commonly applied approach is isotope-coded affinity tags (ICAT), which uses two reagents with heavy and light isotopes, respectively, and a biotin affinity tag to modify cysteine containing peptides. This technology has been used to label whole *Saccharomyces cerevisiae* cells, and, in conjunction with mass spectrometry, helped lay the foundation of quantitative proteomics.

Discovery and Targeted Proteomics

Strategies to improve the sensitivity and scope of proteomic analysis often require large sample quantities and multi-dimensional fractionation, which sacrifices throughput. Alternatively, efforts to improve the sensitivity and throughput of protein quantification limit the number of peptides that can be monitored per MS run. For this reason, proteomics research is typically divided into two categories: discovery and targeted proteomics. Discovery proteomics optimizes protein identification by spending more time and effort per sample and reducing the number of samples analyzed. In contrast, targeted proteomics strategies limit the number of features that will be monitored and then optimize the chromatography, instrument tuning and acquisition methods to achieve the highest sensitivity and throughput for hundreds or thousands of samples.

Relative and Absolute Quantification

Mass spectrometry is not inherently quantitative because of differences in the ionization efficiency and/or detectability of the many peptides in a given sample, which has sparked the development of methods to determine relative and absolute abundance of proteins in samples. The intensity of a peak in a mass spectrum is not a good indicator of the amount of the analyte in the sample, although differences in peak intensity of the *same* analyte between multiple samples accurately reflect relative differences in its abundance.

Label-free Quantification

One approach for relative quantification is to separately analyze samples by MS and compare the spectra to determine peptide abundance in one sample relative to another, as in Label-free quantification strategies.

Stable isotope Labels

An approach for relative quantification that is more costly and time-consuming, though less sensitive to experimental bias than label-free quantification, entails labeling the samples with stable isotope labels that allow the mass spectrometer to distinguish between identical proteins in separate samples. One type of label, isotopic tags, consist of stable isotopes incorporated into protein crosslinkers that causes a known mass shift of the labeled protein or peptide in the mass spectrum. Differentially labeled samples are combined and analyzed together, and the differences in the peak intensities of the isotope pairs accurately reflect difference in the abundance of the corresponding proteins.

Absolute proteomic quantification using isotopic peptides entails spiking known concentrations of synthetic, heavy isotopologues of target peptides into an experimental sample and then performing LC-MS/MS. As with relative quantification using isotopic labels, peptides of equal chemistry co-elute and are analyzed by MS simultaneously. Unlike relative quantification, though, the abundance of the target peptide in the experimental sample is compared to that of the heavy peptide and back-calculated to the initial concentration of the standard using a pre-determined standard curve to yield the absolute quantification of the target peptide.

Relative quantification methods include isotope-coded affinity tags (ICAT), isobaric labeling (tandem mass tags (TMT) and isobaric tags for relative and absolute quantification (iTRAQ)), label-free quantification Metal-coded tags (MeCAT), N-terminal labelling, stable isotope labeling with amino acids in cell culture (SILAC), and Terminal amine isotopic labeling of substrates (TAILS).

Absolute quantification is performed using selected reaction monitoring (SRM).

MeCAT can be used in combination with element mass spectrometry ICP-MS allowing first-time absolute quantification of the metal bound by MeCAT reagent to a protein or biomolecule. Thus it is possible to determine the absolute amount of protein down to attomol range using external calibration by metal standard solution. It is compatible to protein separation by 2D electrophoresis and chromatography in multiplex experiments. Protein identification and relative quantification can be performed by MALDI-MS/MS and ESI-MS/MS.

Mass spectrometers have a limited capacity to detect low-abundance peptides in samples with a high dynamic range. The limited duty cycle of mass spectrometers also restricts the collision rate, resulting in an undersampling Sample preparation protocols represent sources of experimental bias.

MASS SPECTROMETRY

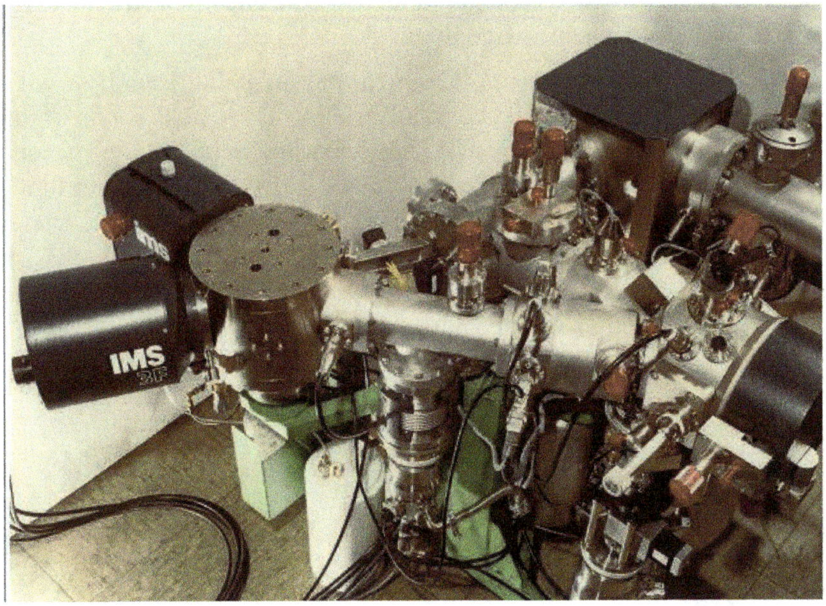

SIMS mass spectrometer, model IMS 3f.

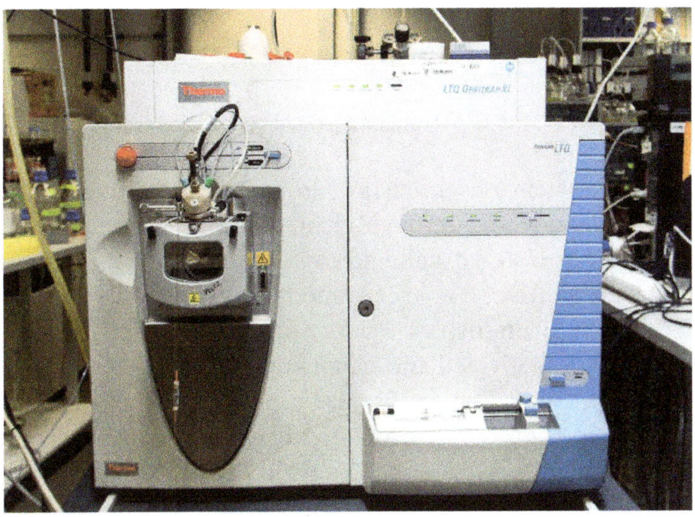

Orbitrap mass spectrometer.

Mass spectrometry (**MS**) is an analytical technique that ionizes chemical species and sorts the ions based on their mass to charge ratio. In simpler terms, a mass spectrum measures the masses within a sample. Mass spectrometry is used in many different fields and is applied to pure samples as well as complex mixtures.

A mass spectrum is a plot of the ion signal as a function of the mass-to-charge ratio. These spectra are used to determine the elemental or isotopic signature of a sample, the masses of particles and of molecules, and to elucidate the chemical structures of molecules, such as peptides and other chemical compounds.

In a typical MS procedure, a sample, which may be solid, liquid, or gas, is ionized, for example by bombarding it with electrons. This may cause some of the sample›s molecules to break into charged fragments. These ions are then separated according to their mass-to-charge ratio, typically by accelerating them and subjecting them to an electric or magnetic field: ions of the same mass-to-charge ratio will undergo the same amount of deflection. The ions are detected by a mechanism capable of detecting charged particles, such as an electron multiplier. Results are displayed as spectra of the relative abundance of detected ions as a function of the mass-to-charge ratio. The atoms or molecules in the sample can be identified by correlating known masses to the identified masses or through a characteristic fragmentation pattern.

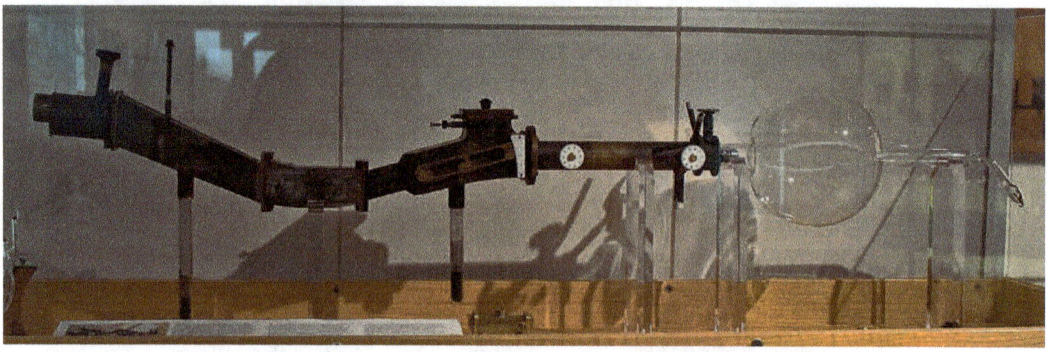

Replica of J.J. Thompson's third mass spectrometer.

In 1886, Eugen Goldstein observed rays in gas discharges under low pressure that traveled away from the anode and through channels in a perforated cathode, opposite to the direction of negatively charged cathode rays (which travel from cathode to anode). Goldstein called these positively charged anode rays "Kanalstrahlen "; the standard translation of this term into English is "canal rays ". Wilhelm Wien found that strong electric or magnetic fields deflected the canal rays and, in 1899, constructed a device with parallel electric and magnetic fields that separated the positive rays according to their charge-to-mass ratio (*Q/m*). Wien found that the charge-to-mass ratio depended on the nature of the gas in the discharge tube. English scientist J.J. Thomson later improved on the work of Wien by reducing the pressure to create the mass spectrograph.

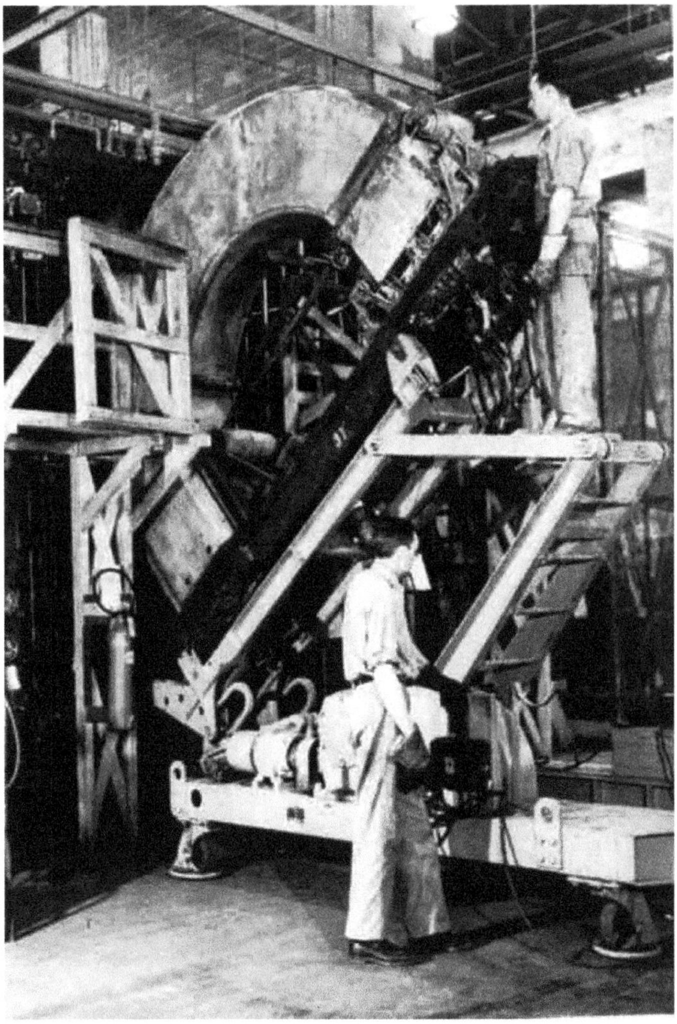

Calutron mass spectrometers were used in the Manhattan Project for uranium enrichment.

The word *spectrograph* had become part of the international scientific vocabulary by 1884.Early *spectrometry* devices that measured the mass-to-charge ratio of ions were called *mass spectrographs* which consisted of instruments that recorded a spectrum of mass values on a photographic plate. A *mass spectroscope* is similar to a *mass spectrograph* except that the beam of ions is directed onto a phosphor screen.A mass spectroscope configuration was used in early instruments when it was desired that the effects of adjustments be quickly observed. Once the instrument was properly adjusted, a photographic plate was inserted and exposed. The term mass spectroscope continued to be used even though the direct illumination of a phosphor screen was replaced by indirect measurements with an oscilloscope. The use of the term *mass spectroscopy* is now discouraged due to the possibility of confusion with light spectroscopy.Mass spectrometry is often abbreviated as *mass-spec* or simply as *MS*.

Modern techniques of mass spectrometry were devised by Arthur Jeffrey Dempster and F.W. Aston in 1918 and 1919 respectively.

Sector mass spectrometers known as calutrons were used for separating the isotopes of uranium developed by Ernest O. Lawrence during the Manhattan Project. Calutron mass spectrometers were used for uranium enrichment at the Oak Ridge, Tennessee Y-12 plant established during World War II.

In 1989, half of the Nobel Prize in Physics was awarded to Hans Dehmelt and Wolfgang Paul for the development of the ion trap technique in the 1950s and 1960s.

In 2002, the Nobel Prize in Chemistry was awarded to John Bennett Fenn for the development of electrospray ionization (ESI) and Koichi Tanaka for the development of soft laser desorption (SLD) and their application to the ionization of biological macromolecules, especially proteins.

Parts of a Mass Spectrometer

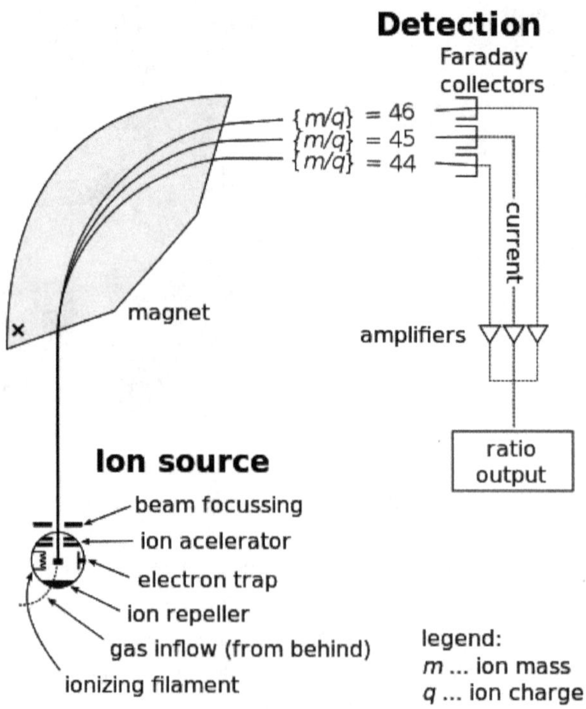

Schematics of a simple mass spectrometer with sector type mass analyzer. This one is for the measurement of carbon dioxide isotope ratios (IRMS) as in the carbon-13 urea breath test

A mass spectrometer consists of three components: an ion source, a mass analyzer, and a detector. The *ionizer* converts a portion of the sample into ions. There is a wide variety of ionization techniques, depending on the phase (solid, liquid, gas) of the sample and the efficiency of various ionization mechanisms for the unknown species.

An extraction system removes ions from the sample, which are then targeted through the mass analyzer and onto the *detector*. The differences in masses of the fragments allows the mass analyzer to sort the ions by their mass-to-charge ratio. The detector measures the value of an indicator quantity and thus provides data for calculating the abundances of each ion present. Some detectors also give spatial information, e.g., a multichannel plate.

Theoretical example

The following example describes the operation of a spectrometer mass analyzer, which is of the sector type. (Other analyzer types are treated below.) Consider a sample of sodium chloride (table salt). In the ion source, the sample is vaporized (turned into gas) and ionized (transformed into electrically charged particles) into sodium (Na^+) and chloride (Cl^-) ions. Sodium atoms and ions are monoisotopic, with a mass of about 23 u. Chloride atoms and ions come in two isotopes with masses of approximately 35 u (at a natural abundance of about 75 percent) and approximately 37 u (at a natural abundance of about 25 percent). The analyzer part of the spectrometer contains electric and magnetic fields, which exert forces on ions traveling through these fields. The speed of a charged particle may be increased or decreased while passing through the electric field, and its direction may be altered by the magnetic field. The magnitude of the deflection of the moving ion's trajectory depends on its mass-to-charge ratio. Lighter ions get deflected by the magnetic force more than heavier ions (based on Newton›s second law of motion, $F = ma$). The streams of sorted ions pass from the analyzer to the detector, which records the relative abundance of each ion type. This information is used to determine the chemical element composition of the original sample (i.e. that both sodium and chlorine are present in the sample) and the isotopic composition of its constituents (the ratio of ^{35}Cl to ^{37}Cl).

Creating Ions

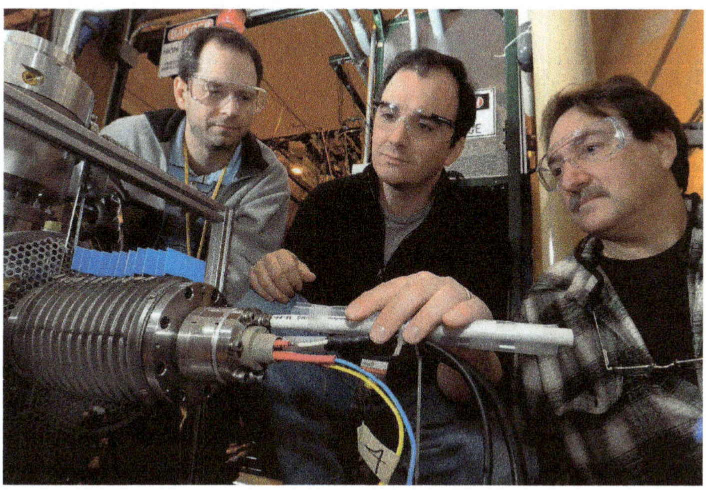

Surface ionization source at the Argonne National Laboratory linear accelerator.

The ion source is the part of the mass spectrometer that ionizes the material under analysis (the analyte). The ions are then transported by magnetic or electric fields to the mass analyzer.

Techniques for ionization have been key to determining what types of samples can be analyzed by mass spectrometry. Electron ionization and chemical ionization are used for gases and vapors. In chemical ionization sources, the analyte is ionized by chemical ion-molecule reactions during collisions in the source. Two techniques often used with liquid and solid biological samples include electrospray ionization (invented by John Fenn) and matrix-assisted laser desorption/ionization (MALDI, initially developed as a similar technique "Soft Laser Desorption (SLD) « by K. Tanaka for which a Nobel Prize was awarded and as MALDI by M. Karas and F. Hillenkamp).

Hard Ionization and Soft Ionization

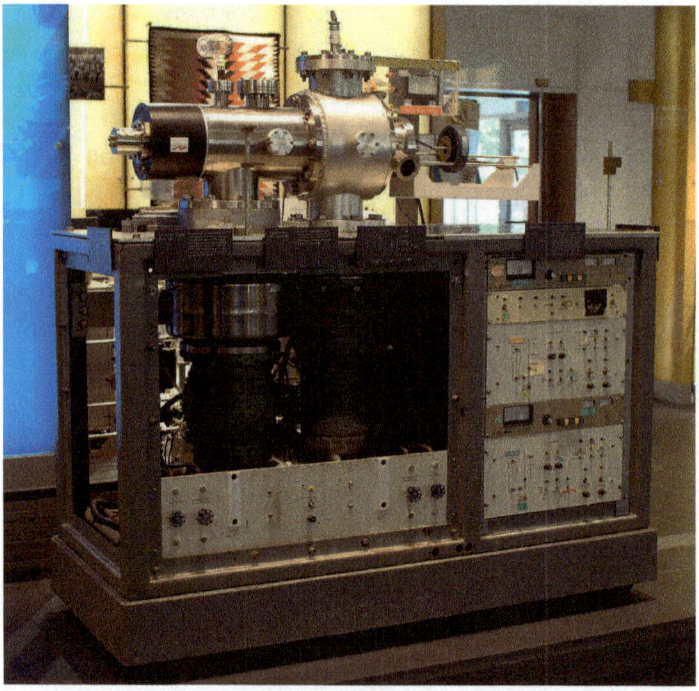

Quadrupole mass spectrometer and electrospray ion source used for Fenn's early work.

In mass spectrometry, ionization refers to the production of gas phase ions suitable for resolution in the mass analyser or mass filter. Ionization occurs in the ion source. There are several ion sources available; each has advantages and disadvantages for particular applications. For example, electron ionization (EI) gives a high degree of fragmentation, yielding highly detailed mass spectra which when skilfully analysed can provide important information for structural elucidation/characterisation and facilitate identification of unknown compounds by comparison to mass spectral libraries obtained under identical operating conditions. However, EI is not suitable for coupling to HPLC, i.e. LC-MS, since at atmospheric pressure, the filaments used to generate electrons burn out rapidly. Thus EI is coupled predominantly with GC, i.e. GC-MS, where the entire system is under high vacuum.

Hard ionization techniques are processes which impart high quantities of residual energy in the subject molecule invoking large degrees of fragmentation (i.e. the systematic rupturing of bonds acts to remove the excess energy, restoring stability to the resulting ion). Resultant ions tend to have *m/z* lower than the molecular mass (other than in the case of proton transfer and not including isotope peaks). The most common example of hard ionization is electron ionization (EI).

Soft ionization refers to the processes which impart little residual energy onto the subject molecule and as such result in little fragmentation. Examples include fast atom bombardment (FAB), chemical ionization (CI), atmospheric-pressure chemical ionization (APCI), electrospray ionization (ESI), and matrix-assisted laser desorption/ionization (MALDI)

Inductively Coupled Plasma

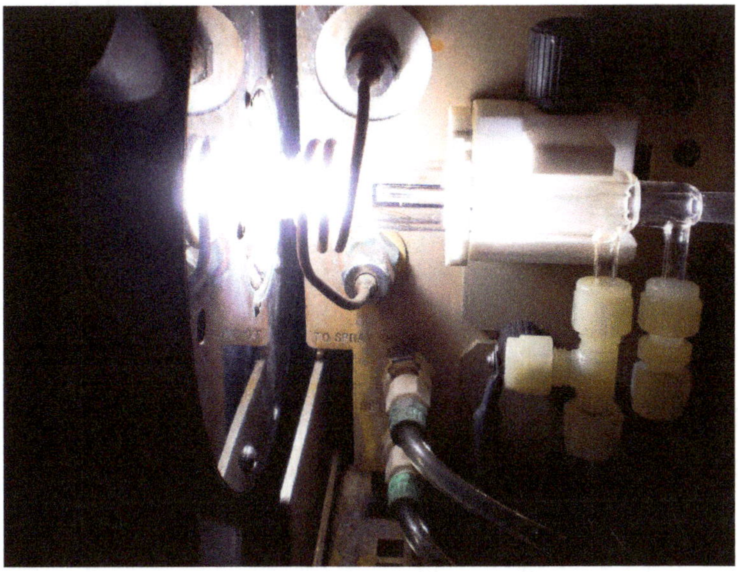

Inductively coupled plasma ion source.

Inductively coupled plasma (ICP) sources are used primarily for cation analysis of a wide array of sample types. In this source, a plasma that is electrically neutral overall, but that has had a substantial fraction of its atoms ionized by high temperature, is used to atomize introduced sample molecules and to further strip the outer electrons from those atoms. The plasma is usually generated from argon gas, since the first ionization energy of argon atoms is higher than the first of any other elements except He, O, F and Ne, but lower than the second ionization energy of all except the most electropositive metals.

The heating is achieved by a radio-frequency current passed through a coil surrounding the plasma.

Other Ionization Techniques

Others include photoionization, glow discharge, field desorption (FD), fast atom bombardment (FAB), thermospray, desorption/ionization on silicon (DIOS), Direct Analysis in Real Time (DART), atmospheric pressure chemical ionization (APCI), secondary ion mass spectrometry (SIMS), spark ionization and thermal ionization (TIMS).

Mass selection

Mass analyzers separate the ions according to their mass-to-charge ratio. The following two laws govern the dynamics of charged particles in electric and magnetic fields in vacuum:

$\mathbf{F} = Q(\mathbf{E} + \mathbf{v} \times \mathbf{B})$ (Lorentz force law);

$\mathbf{F} = m\mathbf{a}$ (Newton's second law of motion in non-relativistic case, i.e. valid only at ion velocity much lower than the speed of light).

Here **F** is the force applied to the ion, *m* is the mass of the ion, **a** is the acceleration, *Q* is the ion charge, **E** is the electric field, and **v** × **B** is the vector cross product of the ion velocity and the magnetic field

Equating the above expressions for the force applied to the ion yields:

$$(m/Q)\mathbf{a} = \mathbf{E} + \mathbf{v} \times \mathbf{B}.$$

This differential equation is the classic equation of motion for charged particles. Together with the particle›s initial conditions, it completely determines the particle›s motion in space and time in terms of *m/Q*. Thus mass spectrometers could be thought of as "mass-to-charge spectrometers". When presenting data, it is common to use the (officially) dimensionless *m/z*, where z is the number of elementary charges (*e*) on the ion (z=Q/e). This quantity, although it is informally called the mass-to-charge ratio, more accurately speaking represents the ratio of the mass number and the charge number, *z*.

There are many types of mass analyzers, using either static or dynamic fields, and magnetic or electric fields, but all operate according to the above differential equation. Each analyzer type has its strengths and weaknesses. Many mass spectrometers use two or more mass analyzers for tandem mass spectrometry (MS/MS). In addition to the more common mass analyzers listed below, there are others designed for special situations.

There are several important analyser characteristics. The mass resolving power is the measure of the ability to distinguish two peaks of slightly different *m/z*. The mass accuracy is the ratio of the *m/z* measurement error to the true m/z. Mass accuracy is usually measured in ppm or milli mass units. The mass range is the range of *m/z* amenable to analysis by a given analyzer. The linear dynamic range is the range over which ion signal is linear with analyte concentration. Speed refers to the time frame of the experiment and ultimately is used to determine the number of spectra per unit time that can be generated.

Sector Instruments

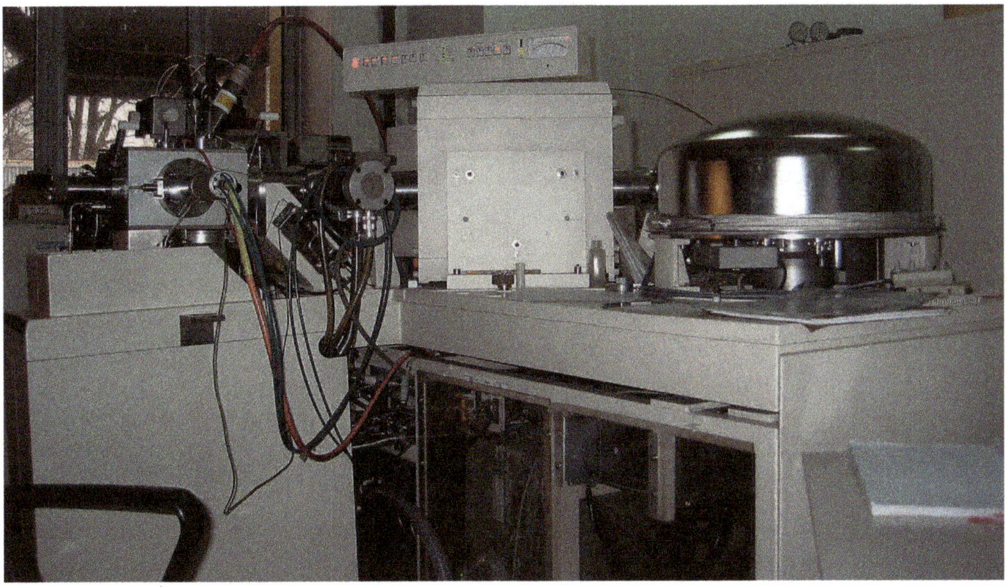

ThermoQuest AvantGarde sector mass spectrometer

A sector field mass analyzer uses an electric and/or magnetic field to affect the path and/or velocity of the charged particles in some way. As shown above, sector instruments bend the trajectories of the ions as they pass through the mass analyzer, according to their mass-to-charge ratios, deflecting the more charged and faster-moving, lighter ions more. The analyzer can be used to select a narrow range of m/z or to scan through a range of m/z to catalog the ions present.

Time-of-flight

The time-of-flight (TOF) analyzer uses an electric field to accelerate the ions through the same potential, and then measures the time they take to reach the detector. If the particles all have the same charge, the kinetic energies will be identical, and their velocities will depend only on their masses. Ions with a lower mass will reach the detector first.

Quadrupole Mass Filter

Quadrupole mass analyzers use oscillating electrical fields to selectively stabilize or destabilize the paths of ions passing through a radio frequency (RF) quadrupole field created between 4 parallel rods. Only the ions in a certain range of mass/charge ratio are passed through the system at any time, but changes to the potentials on the rods allow a wide range of m/z values to be swept rapidly, either continuously or in a succession of discrete hops. A quadrupole mass analyzer acts as a mass-selective filter and is closely related to the quadrupole ion trap, particularly the linear quadrupole ion trap except that it is designed to pass the untrapped ions rather than collect the trapped ones, and is for that reason referred to as a transmission quadrupole. A magnetically enhanced quadrupole mass analyzer includes the addition of a magnetic field, either applied axially or transversely. This novel type of instrument leads to an additional performance enhancement in terms of resolution and/or sensitivity depending upon the magnitude and orientation of the applied magnetic field. A common variation of the transmission quadrupole is the triple quadrupole mass spectrometer. The "triple quad" has three consecutive quadrupole stages, the first acting as a mass filter to transmit a particular incoming ion to the second quadrupole, a collision chamber, wherein that ion can be broken into fragments. The third quadrupole also acts as a mass filter, to transmit a particular fragment ion to the detector. If a quadrupole is made to rapidly and repetitively cycle through a range of mass filter settings, full spectra can be reported. Likewise, a triple quad can be made to perform various scan types characteristic of tandem mass spectrometry.

Ion Traps

Three-Dimensional Quadrupole Ion Trap

The quadrupole ion trap works on the same physical principles as the quadrupole mass analyzer, but the ions are trapped and sequentially ejected. Ions are trapped in a mainly quadrupole RF field, in a space defined by a ring electrode (usually connected to the main RF potential) between two endcap electrodes (typically connected to DC or auxiliary AC potentials). The sample is ionized either internally (e.g. with an electron or laser beam), or externally, in which case the ions are often introduced through an aperture in an endcap electrode.

There are many mass/charge separation and isolation methods but the most commonly used is the mass instability mode in which the RF potential is ramped so that the orbit of ions with a mass $a > b$ are stable while ions with mass b become unstable and are ejected on the z-axis onto a detector. There are also non-destructive analysis methods.

Ions may also be ejected by the resonance excitation method, whereby a supplemental oscillatory excitation voltage is applied to the endcap electrodes, and the trapping voltage amplitude and/or excitation voltage frequency is varied to bring ions into a resonance condition in order of their mass/charge ratio.

Cylindrical Ion Trap

The cylindrical ion trap mass spectrometer (CIT) is a derivative of the quadrupole ion trap where the electrodes are formed from flat rings rather than hyperbolic shaped electrodes. The architecture lends itself well to miniaturization because as the size of a trap is reduced, the shape of the electric field near the center of the trap, the region where the ions are trapped, forms a shape similar to that of a hyperbolic trap.

Linear Quadrupole Ion Trap

A linear quadrupole ion trap is similar to a quadrupole ion trap, but it traps ions in a two dimensional quadrupole field, instead of a three-dimensional quadrupole field as in a 3D quadrupole ion trap. Thermo Fisher›s LTQ (“linear trap quadrupole “) is an example of the linear ion trap.

A toroidal ion trap can be visualized as a linear quadrupole curved around and connected at the ends or as a cross section of a 3D ion trap rotated on edge to form the toroid, donut shaped trap. The trap can store large volumes of ions by distributing them throughout the ring-like trap structure. This toroidal shaped trap is a configuration that allows the increased miniaturization of an ion trap mass analyzer. Additionally all ions are stored in the same trapping field and ejected together simplifying detection that can be complicated with array configurations due to variations in detector alignment and machining of the arrays.

As with the toroidal trap, linear traps and 3D quadrupole ion traps are the most commonly miniaturized mass analyzers due to their high sensitivity, tolerance for mTorr pressure, and capabilities for single analyzer tandem mass spectrometry (e.g. product ion scans).

Orbitrap

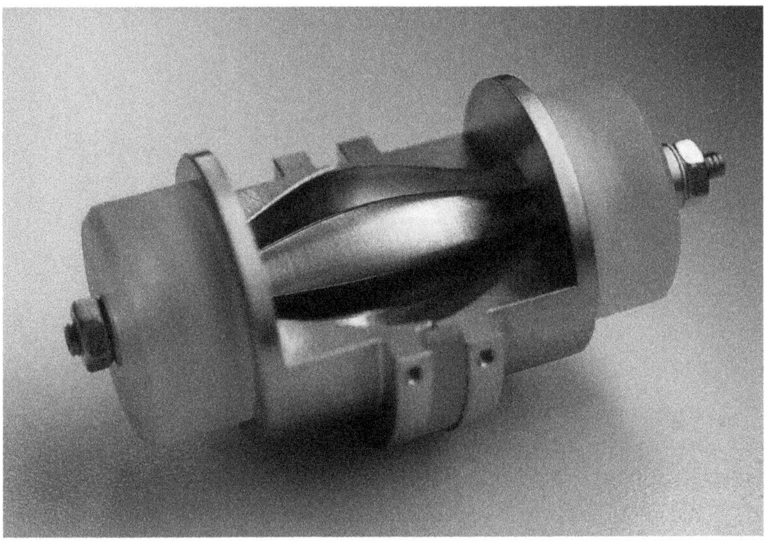

Orbitrap Mass Analyzer.

Orbitrap instruments are similar to Fourier transform ion cyclotron resonance mass spectrometers (see text below). Ions are electrostatically trapped in an orbit around a central, spindle shaped electrode. The electrode confines the ions so that they both orbit around the central electrode and oscillate back and forth along the central electrode's long axis. This oscillation generates an image current in the detector plates which is recorded by the instrument. The frequencies of these image currents depend on the mass to charge ratios of the ions. Mass spectra are obtained by Fourier transformation of the recorded image currents.

Orbitraps have a high mass accuracy, high sensitivity and a good dynamic range.

Fourier transform ion Cyclotron Resonance

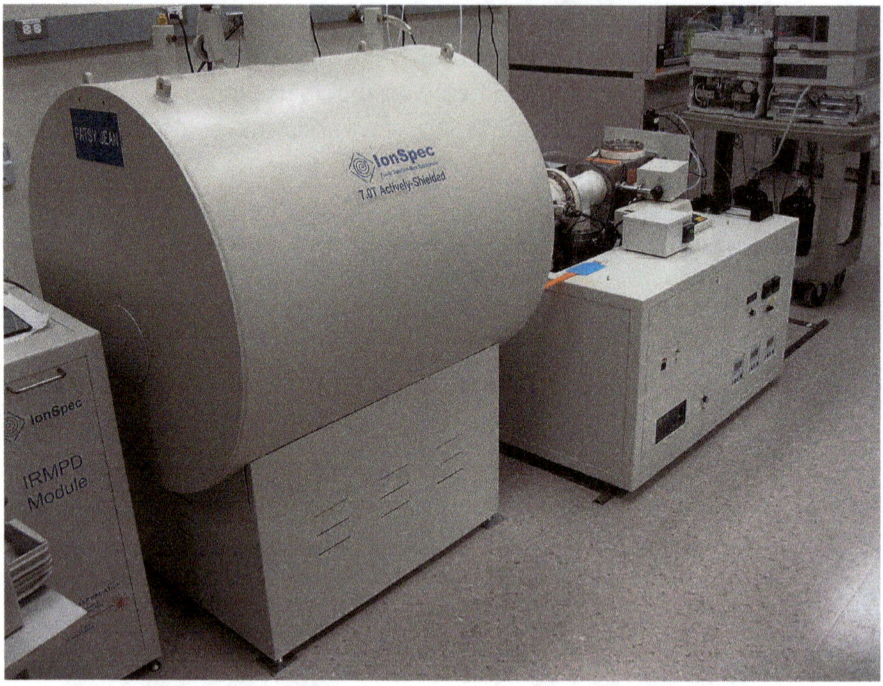

Fourier transform ion cyclotron resonance mass spectrometer.

Fourier transform mass spectrometry (FTMS), or more precisely Fourier transform ion cyclotron resonance MS, measures mass by detecting the image current produced by ions cyclotroning in the presence of a magnetic field. Instead of measuring the deflection of ions with a detector such as an electron multiplier, the ions are injected into a Penning trap (a static electric/magnetic ion trap) where they effectively form part of a circuit. Detectors at fixed positions in space measure the electrical signal of ions which pass near them over time, producing a periodic signal. Since the frequency of an ion›s cycling is determined by its mass to charge ratio, this can be deconvoluted by performing a Fourier transform on the signal. FTMS has the advantage of high sensitivity (since each ion is "counted" more than once) and much higher resolution and thus precision.

Ion cyclotron resonance (ICR) is an older mass analysis technique similar to FTMS except that ions are detected with a traditional detector. Ions trapped in a Penning trap are excited by an RF electric field until they impact the wall of the trap, where the detector is located. Ions of different mass are resolved according to impact time.

Detectors

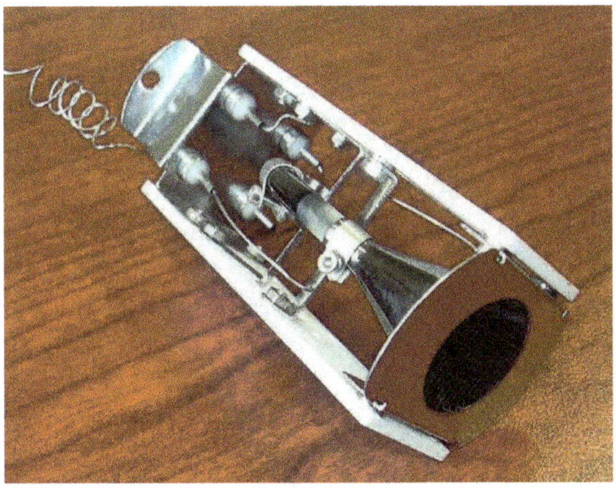

A continuous dynode particle multiplier detector.

The final element of the mass spectrometer is the detector. The detector records either the charge induced or the current produced when an ion passes by or hits a surface. In a scanning instrument, the signal produced in the detector during the course of the scan versus where the instrument is in the scan (at what *m/Q*) will produce a mass spectrum, a record of ions as a function of *m/Q*.

Typically, some type of electron multiplier is used, though other detectors including Faraday cups and ion-to-photon detectors are also used. Because the number of ions leaving the mass analyzer at a particular instant is typically quite small, considerable amplification is often necessary to get a signal. Microchannel plate detectors are commonly used in modern commercial instruments. In FTMS and Orbitraps, the detector consists of a pair of metal surfaces within the mass analyzer/ion trap region which the ions only pass near as they oscillate. No direct current is produced, only a weak AC image current is produced in a circuit between the electrodes. Other inductive detectors have also been used.

Tandem Mass Spectrometry

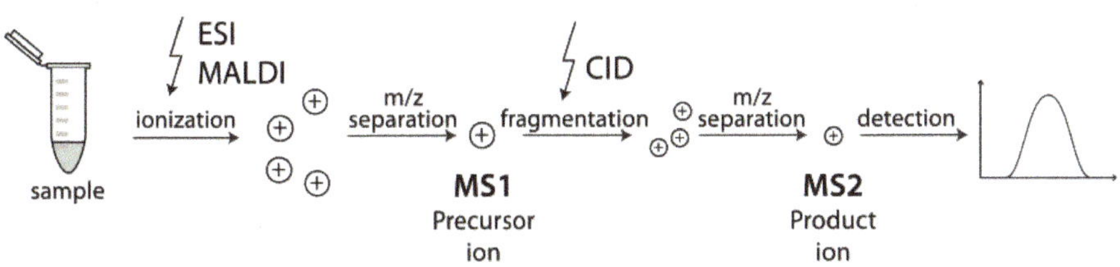

Tandem mass spectrometry for biological molecules using ESI or MALDI.

A tandem mass spectrometer is one capable of multiple rounds of mass spectrometry, usually separated by some form of molecule fragmentation. For example, one mass analyzer can isolate one peptide from many entering a mass spectrometer. A second mass analyzer then stabilizes the peptide ions while they collide with a gas, causing them to fragment by collision-induced dissociation (CID). A third mass analyzer then sorts the fragments produced from the peptides. Tandem MS can also be done in a single mass analyzer over time, as in a quadrupole ion trap. There are various methods for fragmenting molecules for tandem MS, including collision-induced dissociation (CID), electron capture dissociation (ECD), electron transfer dissociation (ETD), infrared multiphoton dissociation (IRMPD), blackbody infrared radiative dissociation (BIRD), electron-detachment dissociation (EDD) and surface-induced dissociation (SID). An important application using tandem mass spectrometry is in protein identification.

Tandem mass spectrometry enables a variety of experimental sequences. Many commercial mass spectrometers are designed to expedite the execution of such routine sequences as selected reaction monitoring (SRM) and precursor ion scanning. In SRM, the first analyzer allows only a single mass through and the second analyzer monitors for multiple user-defined fragment ions. SRM is most often used with scanning instruments where the second mass analysis event is duty cycle limited. These experiments are used to increase specificity of detection of known molecules, notably in pharmacokinetic studies. Precursor ion scanning refers to monitoring for a specific loss from the precursor ion. The first and second mass analyzers scan across the spectrum as partitioned by a user-defined *m/z* value. This experiment is used to detect specific motifs within unknown molecules.

Another type of tandem mass spectrometry used for radiocarbon dating is accelerator mass spectrometry (AMS), which uses very high voltages, usually in the mega-volt range, to accelerate negative ions into a type of tandem mass spectrometer.

Common Mass Spectrometer Configurations and Techniques

When a specific configuration of source, analyzer, and detector becomes conventional in practice, often a compound acronym arises to designate it, and the compound acronym may be better known among nonspectrometrists than the component acronyms. The epitome of this is MALDI-TOF, which simply refers to combining a matrix-assisted laser desorption/ionization source with a time-of-flight mass analyzer. The MALDI-TOF moniker is more widely recognized by the non-mass spectrometrists than MALDI or TOF individually. Other examples include inductively coupled plasma-mass spectrometry (ICP-MS), accelerator mass spectrometry (AMS), thermal ionization-mass spectrometry (TIMS) and spark source mass spectrometry (SSMS). Sometimes the use of the generic "MS " actually connotes a very specific mass analyzer and detection system, as is the case with AMS, which is always sector based.

Certain applications of mass spectrometry have developed monikers that although strictly speaking would seem to refer to a broad application, in practice have come instead to connote a specific or a limited number of instrument configurations. An example of this is isotope ratio mass spectrometry (IRMS), which refers in practice to the use of a limited number of sector based mass analyzers; this name is used to refer to both the application and the instrument used for the application.

Separation Techniques Combined with Mass Spectrometry

An important enhancement to the mass resolving and mass determining capabilities of mass spectrometry is using it in tandem with chromatographic and other separation techniques.

Gas Chromatography

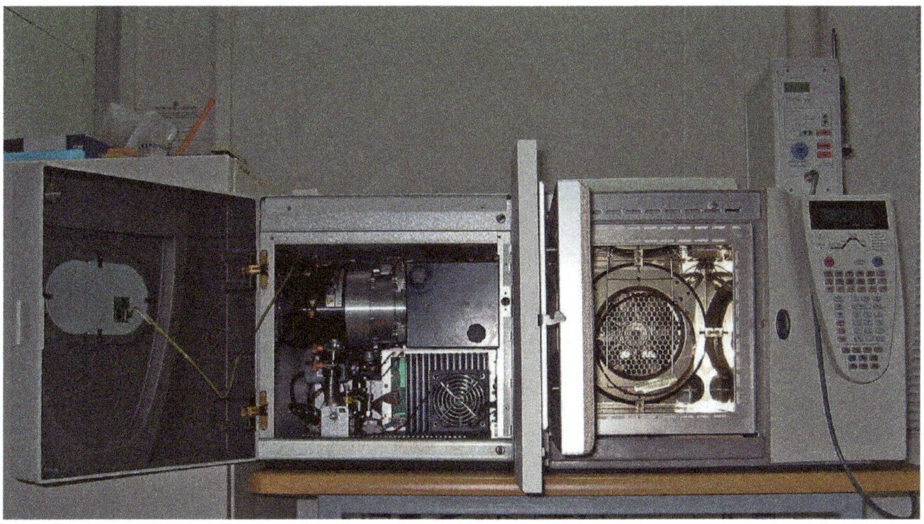

A gas chromatograph (right) directly coupled to a mass spectrometer (left).

A common combination is gas chromatography-mass spectrometry (GC/MS or GC-MS). In this technique, a gas chromatograph is used to separate different compounds. This stream of separated compounds is fed online into the ion source, a metallic filament to which voltage is applied. This filament emits electrons which ionize the compounds. The ions can then further fragment, yielding predictable patterns. Intact ions and fragments pass into the mass spectrometer's analyzer and are eventually detected.

Liquid Chromatography

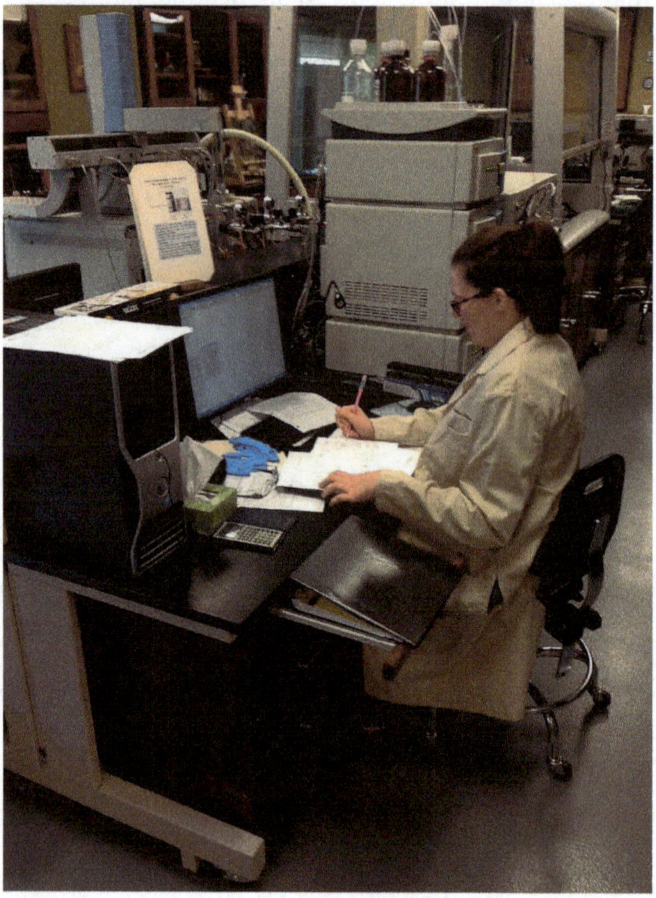

Indianapolis Museum of Art conservation scientist performing liquid chromatography–mass spectrometry.

Similar to gas chromatography MS (GC/MS), liquid chromatography-mass spectrometry (LC/MS or LC-MS) separates compounds chromatographically before they are introduced to the ion source and mass spectrometer. It differs from GC/MS in that the mobile phase is liquid, usually a mixture of water and organic solvents, instead of gas. Most commonly, an electrospray ionization source is used in LC/MS. Other popular and commercially available LC/MS ion sources are atmospheric pressure chemical ionization and atmospheric pressure photoionization. There are also some newly developed ionization techniques like laser spray.

Capillary Electrophoresis–Mass Spectrometry

Capillary electrophoresis–mass spectrometry (CE-MS) is a technique that combines the liquid separation process of capillary electrophoresis with mass spectrometry. CE-MS is typically coupled to electrospray ionization.

Ion Mobility

Ion mobility spectrometry-mass spectrometry (IMS/MS or IMMS) is a technique where ions are first separated by drift time through some neutral gas under an applied electrical potential gradient before being introduced into a mass spectrometer. Drift time is a measure of the radius relative to the charge of the ion. The duty cycle of IMS (the time over which the experiment takes place) is longer than most mass spectrometric techniques, such that the mass spectrometer can sample along the course of the IMS separation. This produces data about the IMS separation and the mass-to-charge ratio of the ions in a manner similar to LC/MS.

The duty cycle of IMS is short relative to liquid chromatography or gas chromatography separations and can thus be coupled to such techniques, producing triple modalities such as LC/IMS/MS.

Data and Analysis

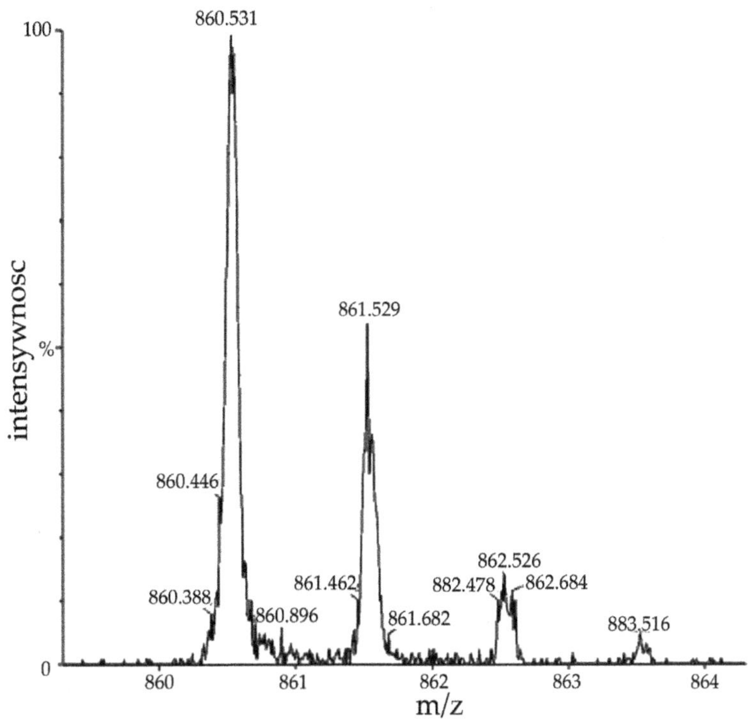

Mass spectrum of a peptide showing the isotopic distribution.

Data Representations

Mass spectrometry produces various types of data. The most common data representation is the mass spectrum.

Certain types of mass spectrometry data are best represented as a mass chromatogram. Types of chromatograms include selected ion monitoring (SIM), total ion current (TIC), and selected reaction monitoring (SRM), among many others.

Other types of mass spectrometry data are well represented as a three-dimensional contour map. In this form, the mass-to-charge, *m/z* is on the *x*-axis, intensity the *y*-axis, and an additional experimental parameter, such as time, is recorded on the *z*-axis.

Data Analysis

Mass spectrometry data analysis is specific to the type of experiment producing the data. General subdivisions of data are fundamental to understanding any data.

Many mass spectrometers work in either *negative ion mode* or *positive ion mode*. It is very important to know whether the observed ions are negatively or positively charged. This is often important in determining the neutral mass but it also indicates something about the nature of the molecules.

Different types of ion source result in different arrays of fragments produced from the original molecules. An electron ionization source produces many fragments and mostly single-charged (1-) radicals (odd number of electrons), whereas an electrospray source usually produces non-radical quasimolecular ions that are frequently multiply charged. Tandem mass spectrometry purposely produces fragment ions post-source and can drastically change the sort of data achieved by an experiment.

Knowledge of the origin of a sample can provide insight into the component molecules of the sample and their fragmentations. A sample from a synthesis/manufacturing process will probably contain impurities chemically related to the target component. A crudely prepared biological sample will probably contain a certain amount of salt, which may form adducts with the analyte molecules in certain analyses.

Results can also depend heavily on sample preparation and how it was run/introduced. An important example is the issue of which matrix is used for MALDI spotting, since much of the energetics of the desorption/ionization event is controlled by the matrix rather than the laser power. Sometimes samples are spiked with sodium or another ion-carrying species to produce adducts rather than a protonated species.

Mass spectrometry can measure molar mass, molecular structure, and sample purity. Each of these questions requires a different experimental procedure; therefore, adequate definition of the experimental goal is a prerequisite for collecting the proper data and successfully interpreting it.

Interpretation of Mass Spectra

Since the precise structure or peptide sequence of a molecule is deciphered through the set of fragment masses, the interpretation of mass spectra requires combined use of various techniques. Usually the first strategy for identifying an unknown compound is to compare its experimental mass spectrum against a library of mass spectra. If no matches result from the search, then manual interpretation or software assisted interpretation of mass spectra must be performed. Computer simulation of ionization and fragmentation processes occurring in mass spectrometer is the primary tool for assigning structure or peptide sequence to a molecule. An *a priori* structural information is fragmented *in silico* and the resulting pattern is compared with observed spectrum. Such simulation is often supported by a fragmentation library that contains published patterns of known decomposition reactions. Software taking advantage of this idea has been developed for both small molecules and proteins.

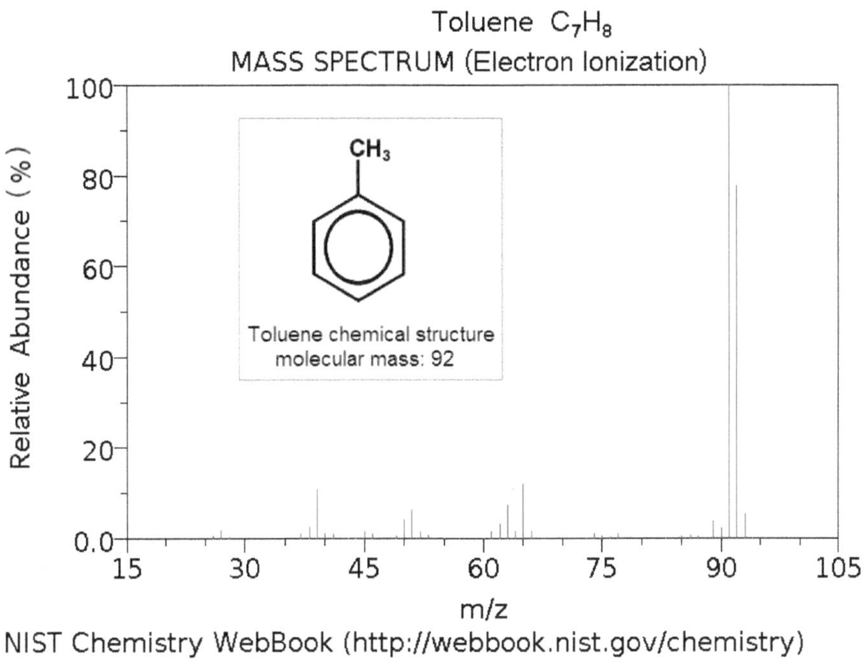

Toluene electron ionization mass spectrum

Analysis of mass spectra can also be spectra with accurate mass. A mass-to-charge ratio value (*m/z*) with only integer precision can represent an immense number of theoretically possible ion structures; however, more precise mass figures significantly reduce the number of candidate molecular formulas. A computer algorithm called formula generator calculates all molecular formulas that theoretically fit a given mass with specified tolerance.

A recent technique for structure elucidation in mass spectrometry, called precursor ion fingerprinting, identifies individual pieces of structural information by conducting a search of the tandem spectra of the molecule under investigation against a library of the product-ion spectra of structurally characterized precursor ions.

Applications

Mass spectrometry has both qualitative and quantitative uses. These include identifying unknown compounds, determining the isotopic composition of elements in a molecule, and determining the structure of a compound by observing its fragmentation. Other uses include quantifying the amount of a compound in a sample or studying the fundamentals of gas phase ion chemistry (the chemistry of ions and neutrals in a vacuum). MS is now in very common use in analytical laboratories that study physical, chemical, or biological properties of a great variety of compounds.

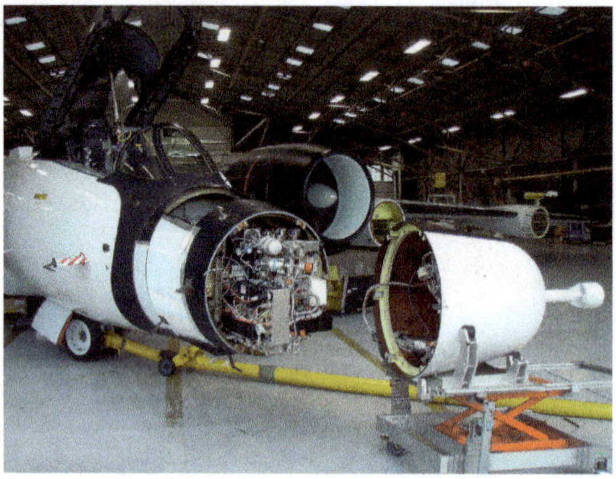

NOAA Particle Analysis by Laser Mass Spectrometry aerosol mass spectrometer aboard a NASA WB-57 high-altitude research aircraft.

As an analytical technique it possesses distinct advantages such as: Increased sensitivity over most other analytical techniques because the analyzer, as a mass-charge filter, reduces background interference, Excellent specificity from characteristic fragmentation patterns to identify unknowns or confirm the presence of suspected compounds, Information about molecular weight, Information about the isotopic abundance of elements, Temporally resolved chemical data.

A few of the disadvantages of the method is that often fails to distinguish between optical and geometrical isomers and the positions of substituent in o-, m- and p- positions in an aromatic ring. Also, its scope is limited in identifying hydrocarbons that produce similar fragmented ions.

Isotope ratio MS: Isotope Dating and Tracing

Mass spectrometry is also used to determine the isotopic composition of elements within a sample. Differences in mass among isotopes of an element are very small, and the less abundant isotopes of an element are typically very rare, so a very sensitive instrument is required. These instruments, sometimes referred to as isotope ratio mass spectrometers (IR-MS), usually use a single magnet to bend a beam of ionized particles towards a series of Faraday cups which convert particle impacts to electric current. A fast on-line analysis of deuterium content of water can be done using flowing afterglow mass spectrometry, FA-MS. Probably the most sensitive and accurate mass spectrometer for this purpose is the accelerator mass spectrometer (AMS). This is because it provides ultimate sensitivity, capable of measuring individual atoms and measuring nuclides with a dynamic range of $\sim 10^{15}$ relative to the major stable isotope.Isotope ratios are important markers of a variety of processes. Some isotope ratios are used to determine the age of materials for example as in carbon dating. Labeling with stable isotopes is also used for protein quantification. (see protein characterization below)

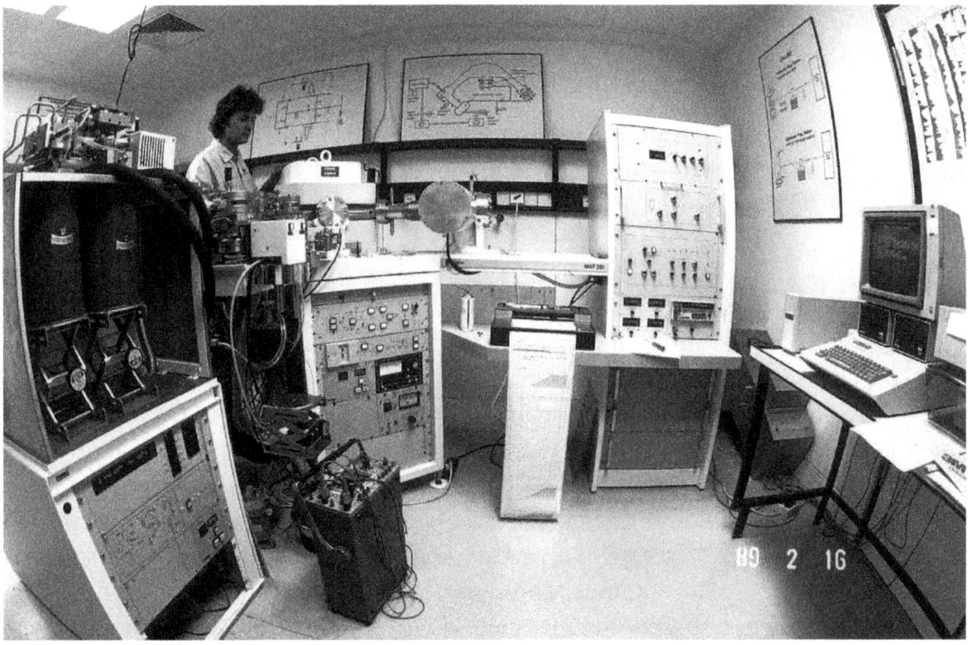

Mass spectrometer to determine the $^{16}O/^{18}O$ and $^{12}C/^{13}C$ isotope ratio on biogenous carbonate.

Trace Gas Analysis

Several techniques use ions created in a dedicated ion source injected into a flow tube or a drift tube: selected ion flow tube (SIFT-MS), and proton transfer reaction (PTR-MS), are variants of chemical ionization dedicated for trace gas analysis of air, breath or liquid headspace using well defined reaction time allowing calculations of analyte concentrations from the known reaction kinetics without the need for internal standard or calibration.

Atom Probe

An atom probe is an instrument that combines time-of-flight mass spectrometry and field-evaporation microscopy to map the location of individual atoms.

Pharmacokinetics

Pharmacokinetics is often studied using mass spectrometry because of the complex nature of the matrix (often blood or urine) and the need for high sensitivity to observe low dose and long time point data. The most common instrumentation used in this application is LC-MS with a triple quadrupole mass spectrometer. Tandem mass spectrometry is usually employed for added specificity. Standard curves and internal standards are used for quantitation of usually a single pharmaceutical in the samples. The samples represent different time points as a pharmaceutical is administered and then metabolized or cleared from the body. Blank or t=0 samples taken before administration are important in determining background and ensuring data integrity with such complex sample matrices. Much attention is paid to the linearity of the standard curve; however it is not uncommon to use curve fitting with more complex functions such as quadratics since the response of most mass spectrometers is less than linear across large concentration ranges.

There is currently considerable interest in the use of very high sensitivity mass spectrometry for microdosing studies, which are seen as a promising alternative to animal experimentation.

Protein Characterization

Mass spectrometry is an important method for the characterization and sequencing of proteins. The two primary methods for ionization of whole proteins are electrospray ionization (ESI) and matrix-assisted laser desorption/ionization (MALDI). In keeping with the performance and mass range of available mass spectrometers, two approaches are used for characterizing proteins. In the first, intact proteins are ionized by either of the two techniques described above, and then introduced to a mass analyzer. This approach is referred to as "top-down " strategy of protein analysis. The top-down approach however is largely limited to low-throughput single-protein studies. In the second, proteins are enzymatically digested into smaller peptides using proteases such as trypsin or pepsin, either in solution or in gel after electrophoretic separation. Other proteolytic agents are also used. The collection of peptide products are then introduced to the mass analyzer. When the characteristic pattern of peptides is used for the identification of the protein the method is called peptide mass fingerprinting (PMF), if the identification is performed using the sequence data determined in tandem MS analysis it is called de novo peptide sequencing. These procedures of protein analysis are also referred to as the "bottom-up " approach. A third approach however is beginning to be used, this intermediate "middle-down " approach involves analyzing proteolytic peptide larger than the typical tryptic peptide.

Glycan Analysis

Mass spectrometry (MS), with its low sample requirement and high sensitivity, has been predominantly used in glycobiology for characterization and elucidation of glycan structures. Mass spectrometry provides a complementary method to HPLC for the analysis of glycans. Intact glycans may be detected directly as singly charged ions by matrix-assisted laser desorption/ionization mass spectrometry (MALDI-MS) or, following permethylation or peracetylation, by fast atom bombardment mass spectrometry (FAB-MS). Electrospray ionization mass spectrometry (ESI-MS) also gives good signals for the smaller glycans. Various free and commercial software are now available which interpret MS data and aid in Glycan structure characterization.

Space Exploration

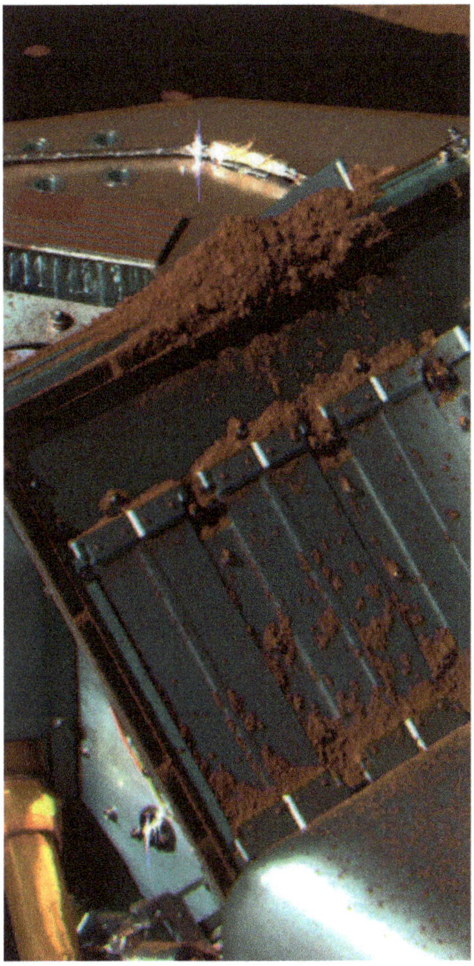

NASA's Phoenix Mars Lander analyzing a soil sample from the "Rosy Red" trench with the TEGA mass spectrometer.

As a standard method for analysis, mass spectrometers have reached other planets and moons. Two were taken to Mars by the Viking program. In early 2005 the Cassini–Huygens mission delivered a specialized GC-MS instrument aboard the Huygens probe through the atmosphere of Titan, the largest moon of the planet Saturn. This instrument analyzed atmospheric samples along its descent trajectory and was able to vaporize and analyze samples of Titan›s frozen, hydrocarbon covered surface once the probe had landed. These measurements compare the abundance of isotope(s) of each particle comparatively to earth›s natural abundance. Also on board the Cassini–Huygens spacecraft is an ion and neutral mass spectrometer which has been taking measurements of Titan›s atmospheric composition as well as the composition of Enceladus› plumes. A Thermal and Evolved Gas Analyzer mass spectrometer was carried by the Mars Phoenix Lander launched in 2007.

Mass spectrometers are also widely used in space missions to measure the composition of plasmas. For example, the Cassini spacecraft carries the Cassini Plasma Spectrometer (CAPS),which measures the mass of ions in Saturn›s magnetosphere.

Respired Gas Monitor

Mass spectrometers were used in hospitals for respiratory gas analysis beginning around 1975 through the end of the century.

Found mostly in the operating room, they were a part of a complex system, in which respired gas samples from patients undergoing anesthesia were drawn into the instrument through a valve mechanism designed to sequentially connect up to 32 rooms to the mass spectrometer. A computer directed all operations of the system. The data collected from the mass spectrometer was delivered to the individual rooms for the anesthesiologist to use.

The uniqueness of this magnetic sector mass spectrometer may have been the fact that a plane of detectors, each purposely positioned to collect all of the ion species expected to be in the samples, allowed the instrument to simultaneously report all of the gases respired by the patient. Although the mass range was limited to slightly over 120 u, fragmentation of some of the heavier molecules negated the need for a higher detection limit.

Preparative Mass Spectrometry

The primary function of mass spectrometry is as a tool for chemical analyses based on detection and quantification of ions according to their mass-to-charge ratio. However, mass spectrometry also shows promise for material synthesis. Ion soft landing is characterized by deposition of intact species on surfaces at low kinetic energies which precludes the fragmentation of the incident species. The soft landing technique was first reported in 1977 for the reaction of low energy sulfur containing ions on a lead surface.

LABEL-FREE QUANTIFICATION

Label-free quantification is a method in mass spectrometry that aims to determine the relative amount of proteins in two or more biological samples. Unlike other methods for protein quantification, label-free quantification does not use a stable isotope containing compound to chemically bind to and thus label the protein.

Implementation

Label-free quantification may be based on precursor signal intensity or on spectral counting. The first method is useful when applied to high precision mass spectra, such as those obtained using the new generation of time-of-flight (ToF), fourier transform ion cyclotron resonance (FTICR), or Orbitrap mass analyzers. The high-resolution power facilitates the extraction of peptide signals on the MS^1 level and thus uncouples the quantification from the identification process. In contrast, spectral counting simply counts the number of spectra identified for a given peptide in different biological samples and then integrates the results for all measured peptides of the protein(s) that are quantified.

The computational framework of label free approach includes detecting peptides, matching the corresponding peptides across multiple LC-MS data, selecting discriminatory peptides.

Intact protein expression spectrometry (IPEx) is a label-free quantification approach in mass spectrometry under development by the analytical chemistry group at the United States Food and Drug Administration Center for Food Safety and Applied Nutrition and elsewhere. Intact proteins are analyzed by an LCMS instrument, usually a quadrupole time-of-flight in profile mode, and the full protein profile is determined and quantified using data reduction software. Early results are very encouraging. In one study, two groups of treatment replicates from mammalian samples (different organisms with similar treatment histories, but not technical replicates) show dozens of low CV protein biomarkers, suggesting that IPEx is a viable technology for studying protein expression.

Detecting Peptides

Typically, peptide signals are detected at the MS1 level and distinguished from chemical noise through their characteristic isotopic pattern. These patterns are then tracked across the retention time dimension and used to reconstruct a chromatographic elution profile of the mono-isotopic peptide mass. The total ion current of the peptide signal is then integrated and used as a quantitative measurement of the original peptide concentration. For each detected peptide, all isotopic peaks are first found and the charge state is then assigned.

Label-free quantification may be based on precursor signal intensity and has problems due to the identity of the peptide precursor ion that is being measured which, in high-throughput studies, could easily be a completely different peptide happening to display a similar m/z ratio and elutes at the same time or overlapping with other peptides. Spectral counting has problems due to the fact that the peptides are identified, thus making it necessary to run an additional MS/MS scan which takes time and therefore reduces the resolution of the experiment.

Matching Corresponding Peptides

In contrast to differential labelling, every biological specimen needs to be measured separately in a label-free experiment. The extracted peptide signals are then mapped across few or multiple LC-MS measurements using their coordinates on the mass-to-charge and retention-time dimensions. Data from high mass precision instruments greatly facilitate this process and increase the certainty of matching correct peptide signals across runs.

Clearly, differential processing of biological samples makes it necessary to have a standard which can be used to adjust the results. Peptides that are not expected to change in their expression levels in different biological samples may be used for this purpose. However, not all peptides ionize well and therefore the choice of candidates should be done after an initial study which should only characterize the protein content of the biological samples that will be investigated.

Selecting Discriminatory Peptides

Finally, sophisticated normalization methods are used to remove systematic artefacts in the peptide intensity values between LC-MS measurements. Then, discriminatory peptides are identified by selecting the peptides whose normalized intensities are different (e.g., p-value < 0.05) among multiple groups of samples.

In addition, newer hybrid mass spectrometers like LTQ OrbiTrap offer the possibility to acquire MS/MS peptide identifications in parallel to the high mass precision measurement of peptides on the MS1 level. This raises the computational challenge for the processing and integration of these two sources of information and has led to the development of novel promising quantification strategies.

STABLE ISOTOPE LABELING BY AMINO ACIDS IN CELL CULTURE

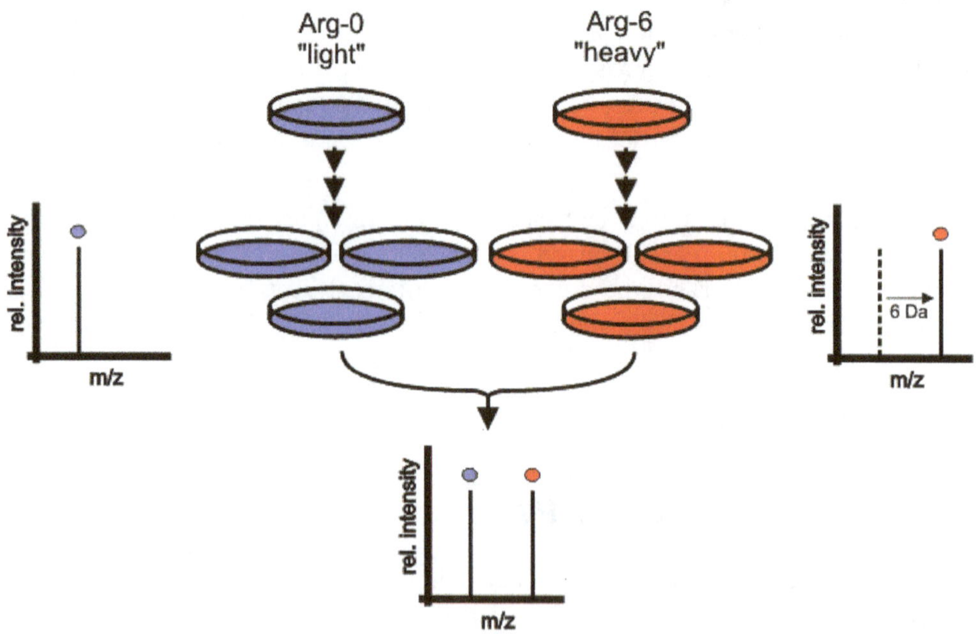

The principle of SILAC. Cells are differentially labeled by growing them in light medium with normal arginine (Arg-0, blue color) or medium with heavy arginine (Arg-6, red color). Metabolic incorporation of the amino acids into the proteins results in a mass shift of the corresponding peptides. This mass shift can be detected by a mass spectrometer as indicated by the depicted mass spectra. When both samples are combined, the ratio of peak intensities in the mass spectrum reflects the relative protein abundance. In this example, the labeled protein has the same abundance in both samples (ratio 1).

SILAC (Stable Isotope Labeling by/with Amino acids in Cell culture) is a technique based on mass spectrometry that detects differences in protein abundance among samples using non-radioactive isotopic labeling. It is a popular method for quantitative proteomics.

Procedure

Two populations of cells are cultivated in cell culture. One of the cell populations is fed with growth medium containing normal amino acids. In contrast, the second population is fed with growth medium containing amino acids labeled with stable (non-radioactive) heavy isotopes. For example, the medium can contain arginine labeled with six carbon-13 atoms (^{13}C) instead of the normal carbon-12 (^{12}C). When the cells are growing in this medium, they incorporate the heavy arginine into all of their proteins. Thereafter, all peptides containing a single arginine are 6 Da heavier than their normal counterparts. Alternatively, uniform labeling with ^{13}C or ^{15}N can be used. The trick is that the proteins from both cell populations can be combined and analyzed together by mass spectrometry. Pairs of chemically identical peptides of different stable-isotope composition can be differentiated in a mass spectrometer owing to their mass difference. The ratio of peak intensities in the mass spectrum for such peptide pairs reflects the abundance ratio for the two proteins.

Applications

A SILAC approach involving incorporation of tyrosine labeled with nine carbon-13 atoms (^{13}C) instead of the normal carbon-12 (^{12}C) has been utilized to study tyrosine kinase substrates in signaling pathways. SILAC has emerged as a very powerful method to study cell signaling, post translation modifications such as phosphorylation, protein–protein interaction and regulation of gene expression. In addition, SILAC has become an important method in secretomics, the global study of secreted proteins and secretory pathways. It can be used to distinguish between proteins secreted by cells in culture and serum contaminants. Standardized protocols of SILAC for various application have also been published.

While SILAC had been mostly used in studying eukaryotic cells and cell cultures, it had been recently employed in bacteria and its multicellular biofilm in antibiotic tolerance, to differentiate tolerance and sensitive subpopulations.

Pulsed SILAC

Pulsed SILAC (pSILAC) is a variation of the SILAC method where the labelled amino acids are added to the growth medium for only a short period of time. This allows monitoring differences in *de novo* protein production rather than raw concentration.

It had also been used to study biofilm tolerance to antibiotics to differentiate tolerant and sensitive subpopulations

ISOBARIC LABELING

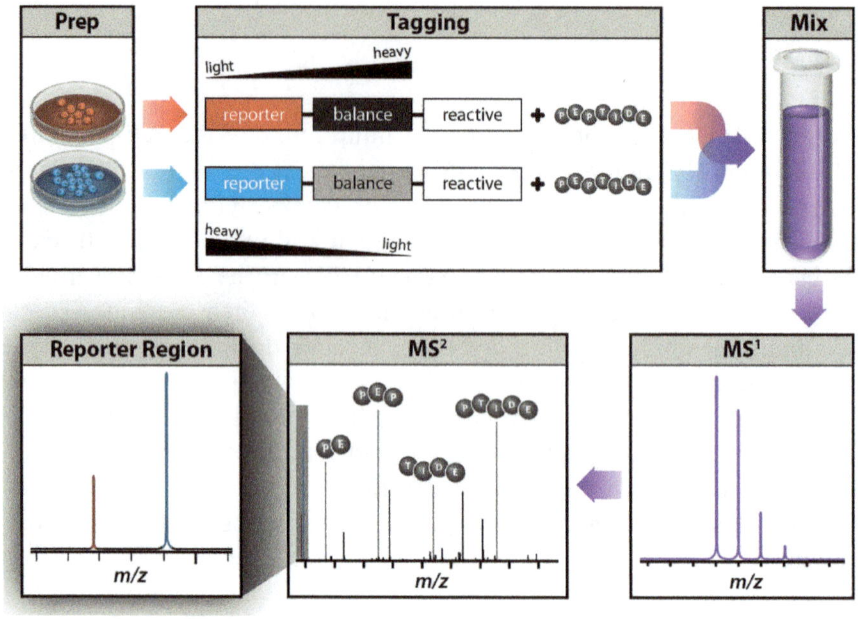

A schematic of isobaric labeling. Proteins are extracted from different conditions or cell types, digested into peptides, and labeled with isobaric stable isotope tags. These tags consist of reporter, balance, and reactive regions. Lighter reporter regions are paired with heavier balance regions, such that the entire tag attached to the peptide adds the same mass shift. Therefore, after mixing, in MS^1, the peptides appear as a single precursor. However, when fragmented during MS^2, in addition to the normal fragment ions, the reporter regions dissociate to produce ion signals which provide quantitative information regarding the relative amount of the peptide in the samples.

Isobaric labeling is a mass spectrometry strategy used in quantitative proteomics. Peptides or proteins are labeled with various chemical groups that are (at least nominally) isobaric, or the same in mass, but which fragment during tandem mass spectrometry to yield reporter ions of different mass. In a typical bottom-up proteomics workflow, proteins are enzymatically digested by a protease to produce peptides, which are then labeled with different isobaric tags. The samples are mixed in equal ratios. During a liquid chromatography-mass spectrometry analysis, the peptides are fragmented to produce sequence-specific product ions, which help to determine the peptide sequence, as well as the reporter tags, whose abundances reflect the relative ratio of the peptide in the samples that were combined.

Availability

There are two types of isobaric tags commercially available: tandem mass tags (TMT) and isobaric tags for relative and absolute quantitation (iTRAQ). TMT is available in duplex and 6-plex forms, while iTRAQ is available in 4-plex and 8-plex forms.

ISOBARIC TAG FOR RELATIVE AND ABSOLUTE QUANTITATION

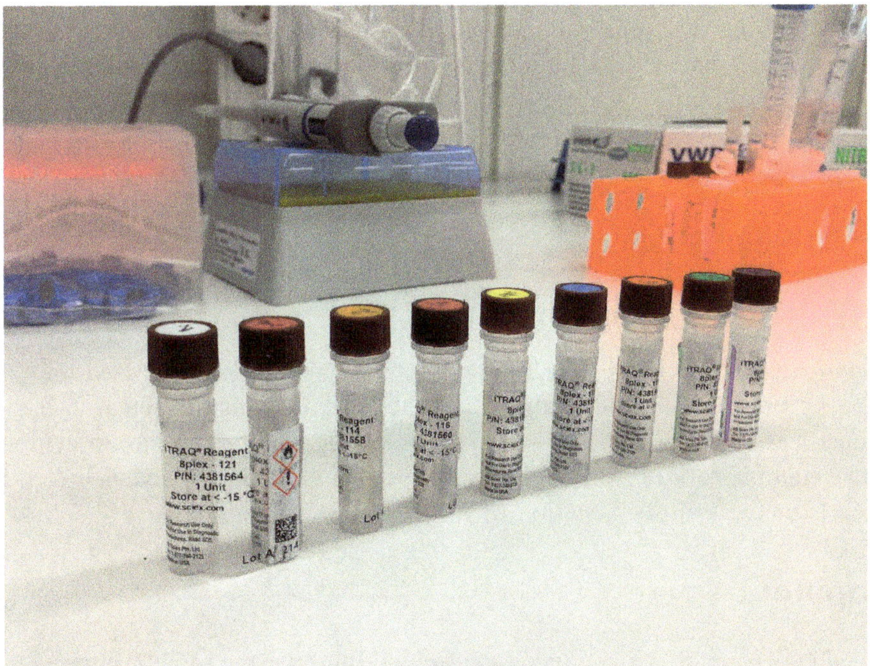

8plex iTRAQ kit.

Isobaric tags for relative and absolute quantitation (**iTRAQ**) is an isobaric labeling method used in quantitative proteomics by tandem mass spectrometry to determine the amount of proteins from different sources in a single experiment. It uses stable isotope labeled molecules that can be covalent bonded to the N-terminus and side chain amines of proteins.

Procedure

The ITRAQ method is based on the covalent labeling of the N-terminus and side chain amines of peptides from protein digestions with tags of varying mass. There are currently two mainly used reagents: 4-plex and 8-plex, which can be used to label all peptides from different samples/treatments. These samples are then pooled and usually fractionated by liquid chromatography and analyzed by tandem mass spectrometry (MS/MS). A database search is then performed using the fragmentation data to identify the labeled peptides and hence the corresponding proteins. The fragmentation of the attached tag generates a low molecular mass reporter ion that can be used to relatively quantify the peptides and the proteins from which they originated.

Data Evaluation

At the peptide level, the signals of the reporter ions of each MS/MS spectrum allow for calculating the relative abundance (ratio) of the peptide(s) identified by this spectrum. The abundance of the reporter ions may consist of more than one single signal in the MS/MS data and the signals have to be integrated in some way from the histogram spectrum.

At the protein level, the combined ratios a proteins' peptides represent the relative quantification of that protein.

The MS/MS spectra can be analyzed using software that is freely available: i-Tracker and jTraqX

ISOTOPE-CODED AFFINITY TAG

An **Isotope-coded affinity tag (ICAT)** is an isotopic labeling method used for quantitative proteomics by mass spectrometry that uses chemical labeling reagents. These chemical probes consist of three elements: a reactive group for labeling an amino acid side chain (e.g., iodoacetamide to modify cysteine residues), an isotopically coded linker, and a tag (e.g., biotin) for the affinity isolation of labeled proteins/peptides.

Development

The original tags were developed using deuterium, but later the same group redesigned the tags using 13C instead to circumvent issues of peak separation during liquid chromatography due to the deuterium interacting with the stationary phase of the column.

Quantitative Proteomics

For the quantitative comparison of two proteomes, one sample is labeled with the isotopically light (d0) probe and the other with the isotopically heavy (d8) version. To minimize error, both samples are then combined, digested with a protease (i.e., trypsin), and subjected to avidin affinity chromatography to isolate peptides labeled with isotope-coded tagging reagents. These peptides are then analyzed by liquid chromatography-mass spectrometry (LC-MS). The ratios of signal intensities of differentially mass-tagged peptide pairs are quantified to determine the relative levels of proteins in the two samples.

METAL-CODED AFFINITY TAG

Metal-coded affinity tag is a method used for quantitative proteomics by mass spectrometry that uses a metal chelate complex 1,4,7,10-tetraazacyclododecane-1,4,7,10-tetraacetate (DOTA) coupled to different lanthanide ions. The metal complexes attach to the cysteine residues of proteins in a sample.

Proteomic analysis

For bottom-up proteomics, the proteins can be separated by two-dimensional gel electrophoresis and analyzed by matrix-assisted laser desorption/ionization (MALDI) or electrospray ionization mass spectrometry for relative quantification or by inductively coupled plasma mass spectrometry for absolute quantification. For top-down proteomics, the undigested labeled proteins are analyzed.

SHOTGUN PROTEOMICS

Shotgun proteomics refers to the use of bottom-up proteomics techniques in identifying proteins in complex mixtures using a combination of high performance liquid chromatography combined with mass spectrometry. The name is derived from shotgun sequencing of DNA which is itself named after the rapidly expanding, quasi-random firing pattern of a shotgun. The most common method of shotgun proteomics starts with the proteins in the mixture being digested and the resulting peptides are separated by liquid chromatography. Tandem mass spectrometry is then used to identify the peptides.

Targeted proteomics using SRM and Data-independent acquisition methods are often considered alternatives to shotgun proteomics in the field of bottom-up proteomics. While shotgun proteomics uses data-dependent selection of precursor ions to generate fragment ion scans, the aforementioned methods use a deterministic method for acquisition of fragment ion scans.

Shotgun proteomics arose from the difficulties of using previous technologies to separate complex mixtures. In 1975, two-dimensional polyacrylamide gel electrophoresis (2D-PAGE) was described by O'Farrell and Klose with the ability to resolve complex protein mixtures. The development of matrix-assisted laser desorption ionization (MALDI), electrospray ionization (ESI), and database searching continued to grow the field of proteomics. However these methods still had difficulty identifying and separating low-abundance proteins, aberrant proteins, and membrane proteins. Shotgun proteomics emerged as a method that could resolve even these proteins.

Advantages

Shotgun proteomics allows global protein identification as well as the ability to systematically profile dynamic proteomes. It also avoids the modest separation efficiency and poor mass spectral sensitivity associated with intact protein analysis.

Disadvantages

The dynamic exclusion filtering that is often used in shotgun proteomics maximizes the number of identified proteins at the expense of random sampling. This problem may be exacerbated by the undersampling inherent in shotgun proteomics.

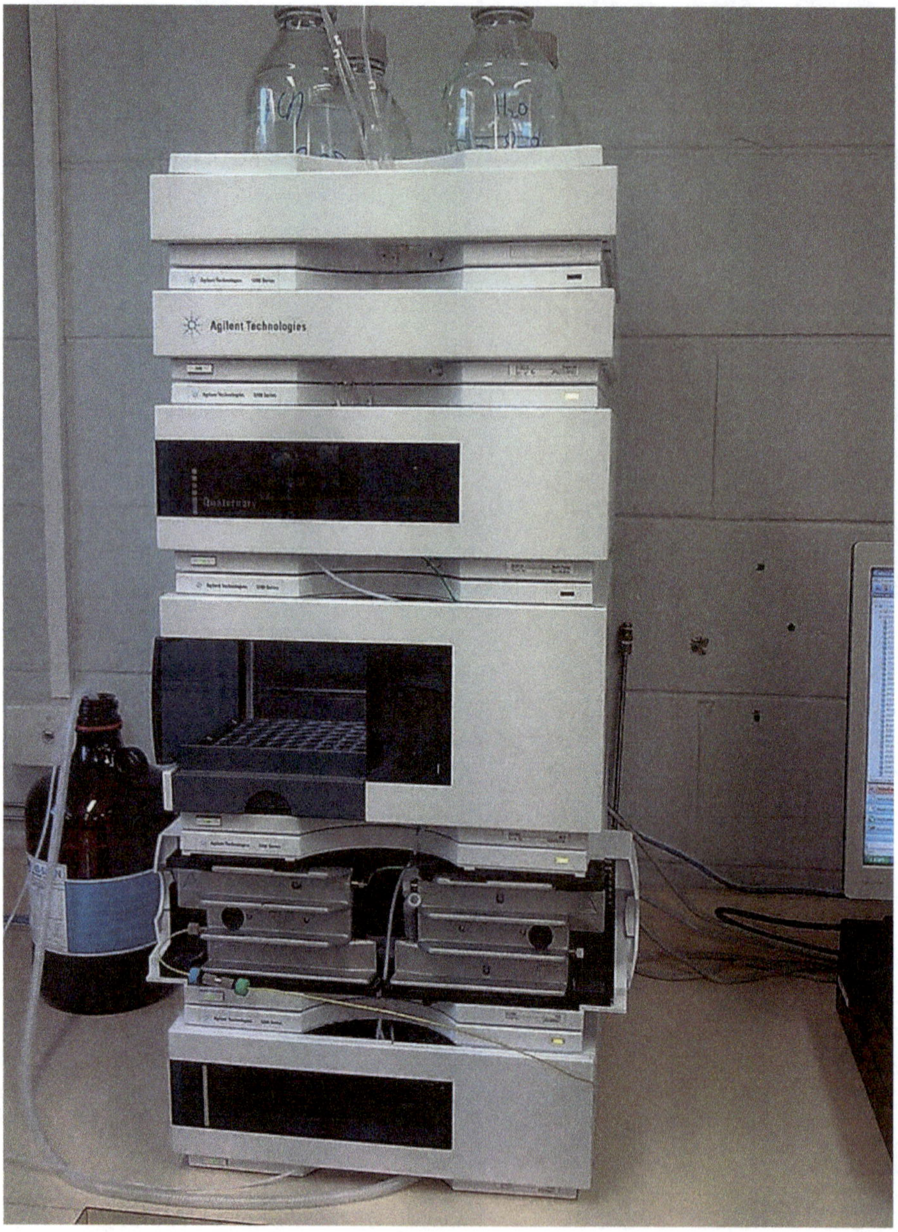

Agilent 1200 HPLC.

Workflow

Cells containing the protein complement desired are grown. Proteins are then extracted from the mixture and digested with a protease to produce a peptide mixture. The peptide mixture is then loaded directly onto a microcapillary column and the peptides are separated by hydrophobicity and charge. As the peptides elute from the column, they are ionized and separated by m/z in the first stage of tandem mass spectrometry. The selected ions undergo collision-induced dissociation or other process to induce fragmentation. The charged fragments are separated in the second stage of tandem mass spectrometry.

The "fingerprint " of each peptide›s fragmentation mass spectrum is used to identify the protein from which they derive by searching against a sequence database with commercially available software (e.g. SEQUEST or MASCOT). Examples of sequence databases are the Genpept database or the PIR database. After the database search, each peptide-spectrum match (PSM) needs to be evaluated for validity. This analysis allows researchers to profile various biological systems.

Issues with Peptide Identification

Peptides that are degenerate (shared by two or more proteins in the database) may make it difficult to identify the protein to which they belong. Additionally, some proteome samples of vertebrates have a large number of paralogs. Finally, alternative splicing in higher eukaryotes can result in many identical protein subsequences.

Practical Applications

With the human genome sequenced, the next step is the verification and functional annotation of all predicted genes and their protein products. Shotgun proteomics can be used for functional classification or comparative analysis of these protein products. It can be used in projects ranging from large-scale whole proteome to focusing on a single protein family. It can be done in research labs or commercially.

Large-scale analysis

One example of this is a study by Washburn, Wolters, & Yates in which they used shotgun proteomics on the proteome of a Saccharomyces cerevisiae strain grown to mid-log phase. They were able to detect and identify 1,484 proteins as well as identify proteins rarely seen in proteome analysis, including low-abundance proteins like transcription factors and protein kinases. They were also able to identify 131 proteins with three or more predicted transmembrane domains.

Protein Family

Vaisar et al. uses shotgun proteomics to implicate protease inhibition and complement activation in the antiinflammatory properties of high-density lipoprotein. In a study by Lee et al., higher expression level of hnRNP A2/B1 and Hsp90 were observed in human hepatoma HepG2 cells than in wild type cells. This led to a search for reported functional roles mediated in concert by both these multifunctional cellular chaperones.

SELECTED REACTION MONITORING

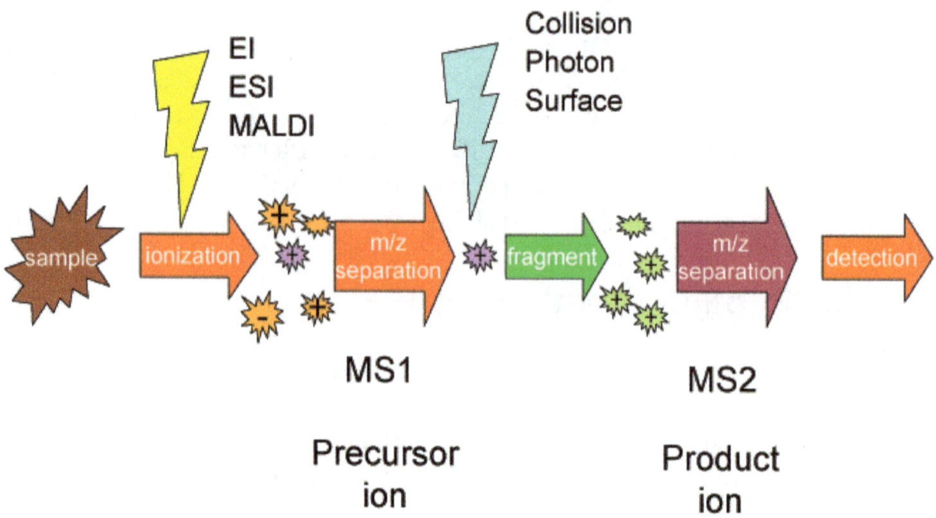

In selected reaction monitoring, the mass selection stage MS1 selects precursor ions that undergo fragmentation followed by product ion selection in the MS2 stage. Additional stages of selection and fragmentation can be performed.

Selected reaction monitoring (SRM) is a method used in tandem mass spectrometry in which an ion of a particular mass is selected in the first stage of a tandem mass spectrometer and an ion product of a fragmentation reaction of the precursor ion is selected in the second mass spectrometer stage for detection.

Variants

A general case of SRM can be represented by

$$ABCD^+ \rightarrow AB + CD^+$$

where the precursor ion $ABCD^+$ is selected by the first stage of mass spectrometry (MS1), dissociates into molecule AB and product ion CD^+, and the latter is selected by the second stage of mass spectrometry (MS2) and detected. The precursor and product ion pair is called a SRM "transition." **Consecutive reaction monitoring (CRM)** is the serial application of three or more stages of mass spectrometry to SRM, represented in a simple case by

$$ABCD^+ \rightarrow AB + CD^+ \rightarrow C + D^+$$

where $ABCD^+$ is selected by MS1, dissociates into molecule AB and ion CD^+. The ion is selected in the second mass spectrometry stage MS2 then undergoes further fragmentation to form ion D^+ which is selected in the third mass spectrometry stage MS3 and detected. **Multiple reaction monitoring (MRM)** is the application of selected reaction monitoring to multiple product ions from one or more precursor ions, for example

$$ABCD^+ \rightarrow AB + CD^+$$

$$ABCD^+ \rightarrow AB^+ + CD$$

where $ABCD^+$ is selected by MS1 and dissociates by two pathways, forming either AB^+ or CD^+. The ions are selected sequentially by MS2 and detected. **Parallel reaction monitoring (PRM)** is the application of SRM with parallel detection of all transitions in a single analysis using a high resolution mass spectrometer.

Proteomics

SRM can be used for targeted quantitative proteomics by mass spectrometry. Following ionization in, for example, an electrospray source, a peptide precursor is first isolated to obtain a substantial ion population of mostly the intended species. This population is then fragmented to yield product ions whose signal abundances are indicative of the abundance of the peptide in the sample. This experiment can be performed on triple quadrupole mass spectrometers, where mass-resolving Q_1 isolates the precursor, q_2 acts as a collision cell, and mass-resolving Q_3 is cycled through the product ions which are detected upon exiting the last quadrupole by an electron multiplier. A precursor/product pair is often referred to as a *transition*. Much work goes into ensuring that transitions are selected that have maximum specificity.

Using isotopic labeling with heavy-labeled (e.g., D, ^{13}C, or ^{15}N) peptides to a complex matrix as concentration standards, SRM can be used to construct a calibration curve that can provide the absolute quantification (i.e., copy number per cell) of the native, light peptide, and by extension, its parent protein.

SRM has been used to identify the proteins encoded by wild-type and mutant genes (mutant proteins) and quantify their absolute copy numbers in tumors and biological fluids, thus answering the basic questions about the absolute copy number of proteins in a single cell, which will be essential in digital modelling of mammalian cells and human body, and the relative levels of genetically abnormal proteins in tumors, and proving useful for diagnostic applications. SRM has also been used as a method of triggering full product ion scans of peptides to either a) confirm the specificity of the SRM transition, or b) detect specific post-translational modifications which are below the limit of detection of standard MS analyses.

DATA-INDEPENDENT ACQUISITION

In mass spectrometry, **data-independent acquisition (DIA)** is a method of molecular structure determination in which all ions within a selected *m/z* range are fragmented and analyzed in a second stage of tandem mass spectrometry. Tandem mass spectra are acquired either by fragmenting all ions that enter the mass spectrometer at a given time (called broadband DIA) or by sequentially isolating and fragmenting ranges of *m/z* . DIA is an alternative to data-dependent acquisition where a fixed number of precursor ions are selected and analyzed by tandem mass spectrometry.

Broadband

One of the first DIA approaches was a nozzle-skimmer dissociation method called shotgun collision-induced dissociation (CID). Fragmentation can be in the ion source of the mass spectrometer by increasing the nozzle-skimmer voltage in electrospray ionization.

MS^E is a broadband DIA technique that uses alternating low-energy CID and high-energy CID. The low-energy CID is used to acquire precursor ion mass spectra whereas the high-energy CID is used to obtain product ion information by tandem mass spectrometry.

Data Analysis

Data analysis is generally challenging for DIA methods as the resulting fragment ion spectra are highly multiplexed. In DIA spectra therefore the direct relation between a precursor ion and its fragment ions is lost since the fragment ions in DIA spectra may potentially result from multiple precursor ions (any precursor ion present in the m/z range from which the DIA spectrum was derived).

One approach to DIA data analysis attempts to use database-based search engines used in data-dependent acquisition to search the produced multiplexed spectra. This approach can be improved by assigning individual fragment ion to precursor ions observed in precursor ion scans, using the elution profile of the fragment ions and the precursor ions, and then searching the resulting "pseudo-spectra".

A second approach to DIA data analysis is based on a targeted analysis, also known as SWATH-MS (Sequential Windowed Acquisition of All Theoretical Fragment Ion Mass Spectra). This approach uses targeted extraction of fragment ion traces directly for identification and quantification without an explicit attempt to de-multiplex the DIA fragment ion spectra.

REFERENCES

1. Jürgen Cox and Matthias Mann (July 2011). "Quantitative, High-Resolution Proteomics for Data-Driven Systems Biology". Annual Review of Biochemistry. 80: 273–299. doi:10.1146/annurev-biochem-061308-093216. PMID 21548781. – via Annual Reviews (subscription required)
2. Nelson P. Barrera and Carol V. Robinson (July 2011). "Advances in the Mass Spectrometry of Membrane Proteins: From Individual Proteins to Intact Complexes". Annual Review of Biochemistry. 80: 247–71. doi:10.1146/annurev-biochem-062309-093307. PMID 21548785. – via Annual Reviews (subscription required)
3. Karas, M.; Bachmann, D.; Hillenkamp, F. (1985). "Influence of the Wavelength in High-Irradiance Ultraviolet Laser Desorption Mass Spectrometry of Organic Molecules". Analytical Chemistry. 57 (14): 2935–9. doi:10.1021/ac00291a042.
4. Karas, M.; Bachmann, D.; Bahr, U.; Hillenkamp, F. (1987). "Matrix-Assisted Ultraviolet Laser Desorption of Non-Volatile Compounds". International Journal of Mass Spectrometry and Ion Processes. 78: 53–68. Bibcode:1987IJMSI..78...53K.

doi:10.1016/0168-1176(87)87041-6.

5. Dole M, Mack LL, Hines RL, Mobley RC, Ferguson LD, Alice MB (1968). "Molecular Beams of Macroions". Journal of Chemical Physics. 49 (5): 2240–2249. Bibcode:1968JChPh..49.2240D. doi:10.1063/1.1670391.
6. Birendra N. Pramanik; A.K. Ganguly; Michael L. Gross (28 February 2002). Applied Electrospray Mass Spectrometry: Practical Spectroscopy Series. CRC Press. pp. 4–. ISBN 978-0-8247-4419-9.
7. "Press Release: The Nobel Prize in Chemistry 2002". The Nobel Foundation. 2002-10-09. Retrieved 2011-04-02.
8. s Chait, Brian T. (2011). "Mass Spectrometry in the Postgenomic Era". 80: 239–46. doi:10.1146/annurev-biochem-110810-095744. PMID 21675917. – via Annual Reviews (subscription required)
9. Trauger, A. Sunia and W. Webb and G. Siuzdak (2002). "Peptide and protein analysis with mass spectrometry". Spectroscopy. 16 (1): 15–28. doi:10.1155/2002/320152.
10. W. Wells, G. Wang & S. J. Baek (2006). "Comparative Study of Three Proteomic Quantitative Methods, DIGE, cICAT, and iTRAQ, Using 2D Gel- or LC–MALDI TOF/TOF". Journal of Proteome Research. 5 (3): 651–658. doi:10.1021/pr050405o.
11. Issaq, J. Haleem & T. D. Veenstra (2008). "Two-dimensional polyacrylamide gel electrophoresis (2D-PAGE): advances and perspectives". BioTechniques. 46 (5): 697–700. doi:10.2144/000112823.
12. Bret, Cooper and J. Feng and W. Garrett (2010). "Relative, Label-free Protein Quantitation: Spectral Counting Error Statistics from Nine Replicate MudPIT Samples". Spectroscopy. 21 (9): 1534–1546. doi:10.1016/j.jasms.2010.05.001.
13. Augustin, Scalbert and L. Brennan and O. Fiehn (2009). "Mass-spectrometry-based metabolomics: limitations and recommendations for future progress with particular focus on nutrition research". NCBI. 5 (4): 435–458. doi:10.1007/s11306-009-0168-0.
14. P. Hernandez, M. Müller & R. D. Appel (2006). "Automated protein identification by tandem mass spectrometry: Issues and strategies". Mass Spectrometry Reviews. 25 (2): 235–254. doi:10.1002/mas.20068. PMID 16284939.
15. Snijders AP, de Vos MG, Wright PC (2005). "Novel approach for peptide quantitation and sequencing based on 15N and 13C metabolic labeling". J. Proteome Res. 4 (2): 578–85. doi:10.1021/pr0497733. PMID 15822937.
16. M. Miyagi & K. C. S. Rao (2007). "Proteolytic 18O-labeling strategies for quantitative proteomics". Mass Spectrometry Reviews. 26 (1): 121–136. doi:10.1002/mas.20116. PMID 17086517.
17. Haqqani AS, Kelly JF, Stanimirovic DB (2008). "Quantitative protein profiling by mass spectrometry using label-free proteomics". Methods Mol. Biol. 439: 241–56. doi:10.1007/978-1-59745-188-8_17. PMID 18370108.
18. Z. Zhang; D. L. Smith (1994). "Probing noncovalent structural features of

proteins by mass spectrometry". Mass Spectrometry Reviews. 13 (5–6): 411–429. doi:10.1002/mas.1280130503.

19. T. E. Wales & J. R. Engen (2006). "Hydrogen exchange mass spectrometry for the analysis of protein dynamics". Mass Spectrometry Reviews. 25 (1): 158–170. doi:10.1002/mas.20064. PMID 16208684.
20. R.E Iacob & J. R. Engen (2012). "Hydrogen Exchange Mass Spectrometry: Are We Out of the Quicksand?". Mass Spectrometry Reviews. 23 (6): 1003–1010. doi:10.1007/s13361-012-0377-z. PMID 22476891.
21. B. B. Stocks & L. Konermann (2009). "Structural Characterization of Short-Lived Protein Unfolding Intermediates by Laser-Induced Oxidative Labeling and Mass Spectrometry". Anal. Chem. 81 (1): 20–27. doi:10.1021/ac801888h.
22. Gupta N.; Tanner S.; Jaitly N.; Adkins J.N.; Lipton M.; Edwards R.; Romine M.; Osterman A.; Bafna V.; Smith R.D.; et al. (2007). "Whole proteome analysis of post-translational modifications: Applications of mass-spectrometry for proteogenomic annotation". Genome Res. 17: 1362–1377. doi:10.1101/gr.6427907. PMC 1950905 . PMID 17690205.
23. Gupta N.; Benhamida J.; Bhargava V.; Goodman D.; Kain E.; Kerman I.; Nguyen N.; Ollikainen N.; Rodriguez J.; Wang J.; et al. (2008). "Comparative proteogenomics: Combining mass spectrometry and comparative genomics to analyze multiple genomes". Genome Res. 18: 1133–1142. doi:10.1101/gr.074344.107. PMC 2493402 . PMID 18426904.
24. Sparkman, O. David (2000). Mass spectrometry desk reference. Pittsburgh: Global View Pub. ISBN 0-9660813-2-3.
25. "Definition of spectrograph." Merriam Webster. Accessed 13 June 2008.
26. Downard, Kevin (2004). "Mass Spectrometry - A Foundation Course". Royal Society of Chemistry. doi:10.1039/9781847551306. ISBN 978-0-85404-609-6.
27. Squires, Gordon (1998). "Francis Aston and the mass spectrograph". Dalton Transactions (23): 3893–3900. doi:10.1039/a804629h.
28. KM Downard (2007). "Francis William Aston – the man behind the mass spectrograph". European Journal of Mass Spectrometry. 13 (3): 177–190. doi:10.1255/ejms.878. PMID 17881785.
29. Thomson, J.J. (1913). Rays Of Positive Electricity and Their Application to Chemical Analysis. London: Longman's Green and Company.
30. Siri, William (1947). "Mass spectroscope for analysis in the low-mass range". Review of Scientific Instruments. 18 (8): 540–545. Bibcode:1947RScI...18..540S. doi:10.1063/1.1740998.
31. Price, Phil (1991). "Standard definitions of terms relating to mass spectrometry. A report from the Committee on Measurements and Standards of the American Society for Mass Spectrometry". Journal of the American Society for Mass Spectrometry. 2 (4): 336–348. doi:10.1016/1044-0305(91)80025-3. PMID 24242353.
32. Parkins, William E. (2005). "The uranium bomb, the calutron, and the space-

charge problem". Physics Today. 58 (5): 45–51. Bibcode:2005PhT....58e..45P. doi:10.1063/1.1995747. ISSN 0031-9228.

33. "The Nobel Prize in Chemistry 2002: Information for the Public". The Nobel Foundation. 9 October 2002. Retrieved 2007-08-29.
34. Fenn, J. B.; Mann, M.; Meng, C. K.; Wong, S. F.; Whitehouse, C. M. (1989). "Electrospray ionization for mass spectrometry of large biomolecules". Science. 246 (4926): 64–71. Bibcode:1989Sci...246...64F. doi:10.1126/science.2675315. PMID 2675315.
35. Tanaka, K.; Waki, H.; Ido, Y.; Akita, S.; Yoshida, Y.; Yoshida, T. (1988). "Protein and Polymer Analyses up to m/z 100 000 by Laser Ionization Time-of flight Mass Spectrometry". Rapid Commun Mass Spectrom. 2 (20): 151–3. doi:10.1002/rcm.1290020802.
36. Karas, M.; Bachman, D.; Bahr, U.; Hillenkamp, F. (1987). "Matrix-Assisted Ultraviolet Laser Desorption of Non-Volatile Compounds". Int J Mass Spectrom Ion Proc. 78: 53–68. Bibcode:1987IJMSI..78...53K. doi:10.1016/0168-1176(87)87041-6.
37. Bruins, A. P. (1991). "Mass spectrometry with ion sources operating at atmospheric pressure". Mass Spectrometry Reviews. 10 (1): 53–77. doi:10.1002/mas.1280100104.
38. Cottrell, John S & Greathead, Roger J (1986). "Extending the Mass Range of a Sector Mass Spectrometer". Mass Spectrometry Reviews. 5 (3): 215–247. doi:10.1002/mas.1280050302.
39. In the event that the ions do not start at identical kinetic energies, some ions may lag behind higher kinetic energy ions decreasing resolution. Reflectron geometries are commonly employed to correct this problem. Wollnik, H. (1993). "Time-of-flight mass analyzers". Mass Spectrometry Reviews. 12 (2): 89–114. doi:10.1002/mas.1280120202.
40. Syed S; Maher S; Taylor S (2013). "Quadrupole mass filter operation under the influence of magnetic field". Journal of Mass Spectrometry. 48 (12): 1325–1339. doi:10.1002/jms.3293.
41. Maher S; Syed S; Hughes D; Gibson J; Taylor S (2013). "Mapping the stability diagram of a quadrupole mass spectrometer with a static transverse magnetic field applied". Journal of the American Society for Mass Spectrometry. 24 (8): 1307–1314. Bibcode:2013JASMS..24.1307M. doi:10.1007/s13361-013-0654-5.
42. Paul, W.; Steinwedel, H. (1953). "Ein neues Massenspektrometer ohne Magnetfeld". Zeitschrift für Naturforschung A. 8 (7): 448–450. Bibcode:1953ZNatA...8..448P. doi:10.1515/zna-1953-0710.
43. March, R. E. (2000). "Quadrupole ion trap mass spectrometry: a view at the turn of the century". International Journal of Mass Spectrometry. 200 (1–3): 285–312. Bibcode:2000IJMSp.200..285M. doi:10.1016/S1387-3806(00)00345-6.
44. Schwartz, Jae C.; Senko, Michael W.; Syka, John E. P. (2002). "A two-dimensional quadrupole ion trap mass spectrometer". Journal of the American Society for Mass Spectrometry. 13 (6): 659–669. doi:10.1016/S1044-0305(02)00384-7.

PMID 12056566.

45. Lammert SA, Rockwood AA, Wang M, Lee ML, Lee ED, Tolley SE, Oliphant JR, Jones JL, Waite RW (2006). "Miniature Toroidal Radio Frequency Ion Trap Mass Analyzer". Journal of the American Society for Mass Spectrometry. 17 (7): 916–922. doi:10.1016/j.jasms.2006.02.009. PMID 16697659.
46. Snyder, Dalton; Pulliam, Christopher; Ouyang, Zheng; Cooks, R. Graham (2016). "Miniature and fieldable mass spectrometers: Recent advances". Anal. Chem. 88: 2–29. doi:10.1021/acs.analchem.5b03070.
47. Hu, Qizhi; Noll, Robert J.; Li, Hongyan; Makarov, Alexander; Hardman, Mark; Graham Cooks, R. (2005). "The Orbitrap: a new mass spectrometer". Journal of Mass Spectrometry. 40 (4): 430–443. doi:10.1002/jms.856. PMID 15838939.
48. Comisarow, M. B. & Marshall, A. G. (1974). "Fourier transform ion cyclotron resonance spectroscopy". Chemical Physics Letters. 25 (2): 282–283. Bibcode:1974CPL....25..282C. doi:10.1016/0009-2614(74)89137-2.
49. Marshall, A. G.; Hendrickson, C. L.; Jackson, G. S. (1998). "Fourier transform ion cyclotron resonance mass spectrometry: a primer". Mass Spectrometry Reviews. 17 (1): 1–34. doi:10.1002/(SICI)1098-2787(1998)17:1<1::AID-MAS1>3.0.CO;2-K. PMID 9768511.
50. Dubois, F.; Knochenmuss, R.; Zenobi, R.; Brunelle, A.; Deprun, C.; Le Beyec, Y. (1999). "A comparison between ion-to-photon and microchannel plate detectors". Rapid Communications in Mass Spectrometry. 13 (9): 786–791. doi:10.1002/(SICI)1097-0231(19990515)13:9<786::AID-RCM566>3.0.CO;2-3.
51. Park, Melvin A.; Callahan, John H.; Vertes, Akos (1994). "An inductive detector for time-of-flight mass spectrometry". Rapid Communications in Mass Spectrometry. 8 (4): 317–322. doi:10.1002/rcm.1290080407.
52. Boyd, Robert K. (1994). "Linked-scan techniques for MS/MS using tandem-in-space instruments". Mass Spectrometry Reviews. 13 (5–6): 359–410. doi:10.1002/mas.1280130502.
53. Eiceman, G.A. (2000). Gas Chromatography. In R.A. Meyers (Ed.), Encyclopedia of Analytical Chemistry: Applications, Theory, and Instrumentation, pp. 10627. Chichester: Wiley. ISBN 0-471-97670-9
54. Loo JA, Udseth HR, Smith RD (June 1989). "Peptide and protein analysis by electrospray ionization-mass spectrometry and capillary electrophoresis-mass spectrometry". Anal. Biochem. 179 (2): 404–12. doi:10.1016/0003-2697(89)90153-X. PMID 2774189.
55. Maxwell EJ, Chen DD (October 2008). "Twenty years of interface development for capillary electrophoresis-electrospray ionization-mass spectrometry". Anal. Chim. Acta. 627 (1): 25–33. doi:10.1016/j.aca.2008.06.034. PMID 18790125.
56. Verbeck GF, Ruotolo BT, Sawyer HA, Gillig KJ, Russell DH (2002). "A fundamental introduction to ion mobility mass spectrometry applied to the analysis of biomolecules". J Biomol Tech. 13 (2): 56–61. PMC 2279851 . PMID 19498967.

57. Matz, Laura M.; Asbury, G. Reid; Hill, Herbert H. (2002). "Two-dimensional separations with electrospray ionization ambient pressure high-resolution ion mobility spectrometry/quadrupole mass spectrometry". Rapid Communications in Mass Spectrometry. 16 (7): 670–675. doi:10.1002/rcm.623. PMID 11921245.

58. Sowell, Renã A.; Koeniger, Stormy L.; Valentine, Stephen J.; Moon, Myeong Hee; Clemmer, David E. (2004). "Nanoflow LC/IMS-MS and LC/IMS-CID/MS of Protein Mixtures". Journal of the American Society for Mass Spectrometry. 15 (9): 1341–1353. doi:10.1016/j.jasms.2004.06.014. PMID 15337515.

59. Tureček, František; McLafferty, Fred W. (1993). Interpretation of mass spectra. Sausalito: University Science Books. ISBN 0-935702-25-3.

60. Mistrik, R. (2004). A New Concept for the Interpretation of Mass Spectra Based on a Combination of a Fragmentation Mechanism Database and a Computer Expert System. in Ashcroft, A.E., Brenton, G., Monaghan,J.J. (Eds.), Advances in Mass Spectrometry, Elsevier, Amsterdam, vol. 16, pp. 821

61. Sheldon, Michelle T.; Mistrik, Robert; Croley, Timothy R. (2009). "Determination of ion structures in structurally related compounds using precursor ion fingerprinting". Journal of the American Society for Mass Spectrometry. 20 (3): 370–376. doi:10.1016/j.jasms.2008.10.017. PMID 19041260.

62. Maher S, Jjunju FP, Taylor S (2015). "100 years of mass spectrometry: Perspectives and future trends". Rev. Mod. Phys. 87 (1): 113–135. Bibcode:2015RvMP...87..113M. doi:10.1103/RevModPhys.87.113.

63. Hsieh, Yunsheng; Korfmacher, WA (2006). "Systems for Drug Metabolism and Pharmacokinetic Screening, Y. Hsieh and W.A. Korfmacher, Current Drug Metabolism". Current Drug Metabolism. 7 (5): 479–489. doi:10.2174/138920006777697963. PMID 16787157.

64. Covey, T.R.; Lee, E.D.; Henion, J.D. (1986). "Mass Spectrometry for the Determination of Drugs in Biological Samples". Anal. Chem. 58 (12): 2453–2460. doi:10.1021/ac00125a022. PMID 3789400.

65. Covey, Tom R.; Crowther, Jonathan B.; Dewey, Elizabeth A.; Henion, Jack D. (1985). "Mass Spectrometry Determination of Drugs and Their Metabolites in Biological Fluids". Anal. Chem. 57 (2): 474–81. doi:10.1021/ac50001a036. PMID 3977076.

66. Chait, Brian T. (2011). "Mass Spectrometry in the Postgenomic Era". 80: 239–46. doi:10.1146/annurev-biochem-110810-095744. PMID 21675917. – via Annual Reviews (subscription required)

67. Apte A, Meitei NS (2009). "Bioinformatics in Glycomics: Glycan Characterization with Mass Spectrometric Data Using SimGlycan". Methods in molecular biology. Methods in Molecular Biology. 600: 269–281. doi:10.1007/978-1-60761-454-8_19. ISBN 978-1-60761-453-1. PMID 19882135.

68. Harvey, D.; Dwek, R.A.; Rudd, P.M. (2000). "Determining the Structure of Glycan Moieties by Mass Spectrometry". Current Protocols in Protein Science. Chapter 12: 12.7–12.7.15. doi:10.1002/0471140864.ps1207s43. ISBN 0-471-14086-4. PMID 18429296.

69. Blow, Nathan (2009). "Glycobiology: A spoonful of sugar". Nature. 457 (7229): 617–620. Bibcode:2009Natur.457..617B. doi:10.1038/457617a. PMID 19177129.

70. Petrie, S. & Bohme, D. K. (2007). "Ions in space". Mass Spectrometry Reviews. 26 (2): 258–280. doi:10.1002/mas.20114. PMID 17111346.

71. Hoffman, J; Chaney, R; Hammack, H (2008). "Phoenix Mars Mission—The Thermal Evolved Gas Analyzer". Journal of the American Society for Mass Spectrometry. 19 (10): 1377–83. doi:10.1016/j.jasms.2008.07.015. PMID 18715800.

72. "Cassini Plasma Spectrometer". Southwest Research Institute. Retrieved 2008-01-04.

73. Riker JB, Haberman B (1976). "Expired gas monitoring by mass spectrometry in a respiratory intensive care unit". Crit. Care Med. 4 (5): 223–9. doi:10.1097/00003246-197609000-00002. PMID 975846.

74. Gothard, J.W.W.; Busst, C.M.; Branthwaite, M.A.; Davies, N.J.H.; Denison, D.M. (1980). "Applications of respiratory mass spectrometry to intensive care". Anaesthesia. 35 (9): 890–895. doi:10.1111/j.1365-2044.1980.tb03950.x. PMID 6778243.

75. Verbeck G, Hoffmann W, Walton B (2012). "Soft-landing preparative mass spectrometry". Analyst. 137 (19): 4393–4407. Bibcode:2012Ana...137.4393V. doi:10.1039/C2AN35550G.

76. Franchetti V, Solka BH, Baitinger WE, Amy JW, Cooks RG (1977). "Soft landing of ions as a means of surface modification". Mass Spectrom. Ion Phys. 23 (1): 29–35. Bibcode:1977IJMSI..23...29F. doi:10.1016/0020-7381(77)80004-1.

CHAPTER 8

Post-translational Modification of Proteins

Chapter Contents

Protein post-translational modification (PTM) increases the functional diversity of the proteome by the covalent addition of functional groups or proteins, proteolytic cleavage of regulatory subunits or degradation of entire proteins. These modifications include phosphorylation, glycosylation, ubiquitination, nitrosylation, methylation, acetylation, lipidation and proteolysis and influence almost all aspects of normal cell biology and pathogenesis. Therefore, identifying and understanding PTMs is critical in the study of cell biology and disease treatment and prevention.

INTRODUCTION

Post-translational modification (PTM) refers to the covalent and generally enzymatic modification of proteins during or after protein biosynthesis. Proteins are synthesized by ribosomes translating mRNA into polypeptide chains, which may then undergo PTM to form the mature protein product. PTMs are important components in cell signaling.

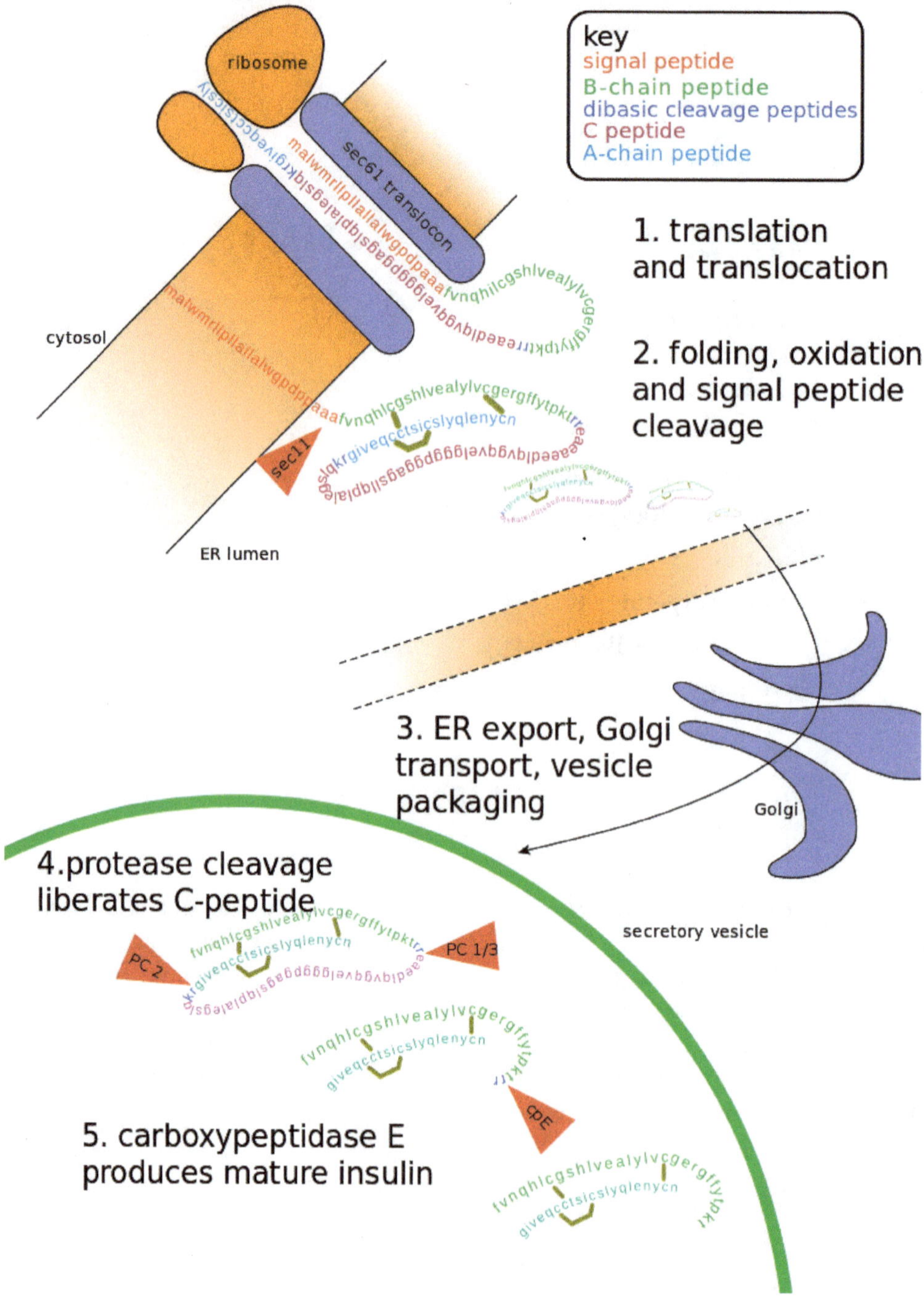

Post-translational modification of insulin. At the top, the ribosome translates a mRNA sequence into a protein, insulin, and passes the protein through the endoplasmic reticulum, where it is cut, folded and held in shape by disulfide (-S-S-) bonds. Then the protein passes through the golgi apparatus, where it is packaged into a vesicle. In the vesicle, more parts are cut off, and it turns into mature insulin.

Post-translational modifications can occur on the amino acid side chains or at the protein's C- or N- termini.They can extend the chemical repertoire of the 20 standard amino acids by introducing new functional groups such as phosphate, acetate, amide groups, or methyl groups. Phosphorylation is a very common mechanism for regulating the activity of enzymes and is the most common post-translational modification. Many eukaryotic proteins also have carbohydrate molecules attached to them in a process called glycosylation, which can promote protein folding and improve stability as well as serving regulatory functions. Attachment of lipid molecules, known as lipidation, often targets a protein or part of a protein attached to the cell membrane.

Other forms of post-translational modification consist of cleaving peptide bonds, as in processing a propeptide to a mature form or removing the initiator methionine residue. The formation of disulfide bonds from cysteine residues may also be referred to as a post-translational modification. For instance, the peptide hormoneinsulin is cut twice after disulfide bonds are formed, and a propeptide is removed from the middle of the chain; the resulting protein consists of two polypeptide chains connected by disulfide bonds.

Some types of post-translational modification are consequences of oxidative stress. Carbonylation is one example that targets the modified protein for degradation and can result in the formation of protein aggregates. Specific amino acid modifications can be used as biomarkers indicating oxidative damage.

Sites that often undergo post-translational modification are those that have a functional group that can serve as a nucleophile in the reaction: the hydroxyl groups of serine, threonine, and tyrosine; the amine forms of lysine, arginine, and histidine; the thiolate anion of cysteine; the carboxylates of aspartate and glutamate; and the N- and C-termini. In addition, although the amides of asparagine and glutamine are weak nucleophiles, both can serve as attachment points for glycans. Rarer modifications can occur at oxidized methionines and at some methylenes in side chains.

Post-translational modification of proteins can be experimentally detected by a variety of techniques, including mass spectrometry, Eastern blotting, and Western blotting.

PTMs Involving Addition of Functional Groups

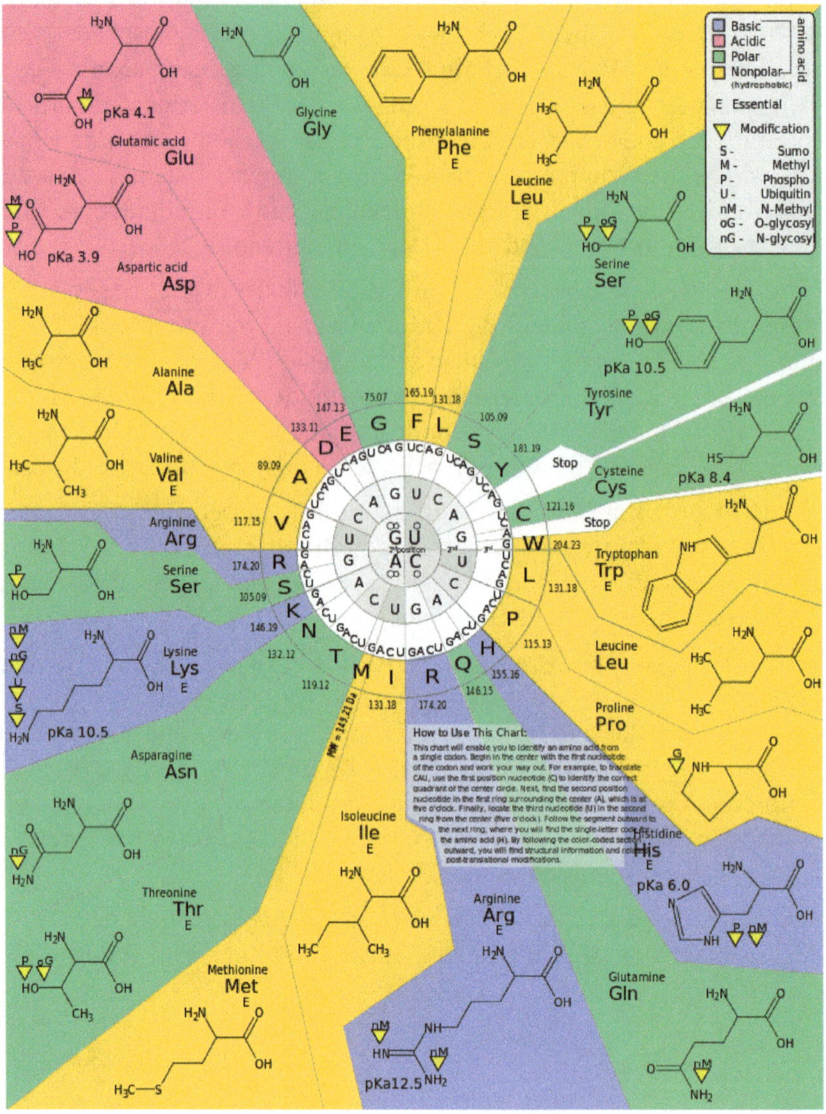

The genetic code diagram showing the amino acid residues as target of modification.

Addition by an enzyme *in vivo*

Hydrophobic groups for membrane localization

- myristoylation, attachment of myristate, a C_{14} saturated acid
- palmitoylation, attachment of palmitate, a C_{16} saturated acid
- isoprenylation or prenylation, the addition of an isoprenoid group (e.g. farnesol and geranylgeraniol)

  - farnesylation
  - geranylgeranylation
- glypiation, glycosylphosphatidylinositol (GPI) anchor formation via an amide bond to C-terminal tail

Cofactors for Enhanced Enzymatic Activity

- lipoylation, attachment of a lipoate (C_8) functional group
- flavin moiety (FMN or FAD) may be covalently attached
- heme C attachment via thioether bonds with cysteins
- phosphopantetheinylation, the addition of a 4›-phosphopantetheinyl moiety from coenzyme A, as in fatty acid, polyketide, non-ribosomal peptide and leucine biosynthesis
- retinylidene Schiff base formation

Modifications of Translation Factors

- diphthamide formation (on a histidine found in eEF2)
- ethanolamine phosphoglycerol attachment (on glutamate found in eEF1α)
- hypusine formation (on conserved lysine of eIF5A (eukaryotic) and aIF5A (archaeal))

Smaller Chemical Groups

- acylation, e.g. *O*-acylation (esters), *N*-acylation (amides), *S*-acylation (thioesters)
  - acetylation, the addition of an acetyl group, either at the N-terminus of the protein or at lysine residues. *See also histone acetylation*. The reverse is called deacetylation.
  - formylation
- alkylation, the addition of an alkyl group, e.g. methyl, ethyl
  - methylation the addition of a methyl group, usually at lysine or arginine residues. The reverse is called demethylation.
- amide bond formation
- amidation at C-terminus
- amino acid addition
- arginylation, a tRNA-mediation addition
- polyglutamylation, covalent linkage of glutamic acid residues to the N-terminus of tubulin and some other proteins. (See tubulin polyglutamylase)
- polyglycylation, covalent linkage of one to more than 40 glycine residues to the tubulin C-terminal tail

- butyrylation
- gamma-carboxylation dependent on Vitamin K
- glycosylation, the addition of a glycosyl group to either arginine, asparagine, cysteine, hydroxylysine, serine, threonine, tyrosine, or tryptophan resulting in a glycoprotein. Distinct from glycation, which is regarded as a nonenzymatic attachment of sugars.
- polysialylation, addition of polysialic acid, PSA, to NCAM
- malonylation
- hydroxylation: addition of an oxygen atom to the side-chain of Pro or Lys residues.
- iodination (e.g. of thyroglobulin)
- nucleotide addition such as ADP-ribosylation
- phosphate ester (*O*-linked) or phosphoramidate (*N*-linked) formation
- phosphorylation, the addition of a phosphate group, usually to serine, threonine, and tyrosine (*O*-linked), or histidine (*N*-linked)
- adenylylation, the addition of an adenylyl moiety, usually to tyrosine (*O*-linked), or histidine and lysine (*N*-linked)
- propionylation
- pyroglutamate formation
- *S*-glutathionylation
- *S*-nitrosylation
- *S*-sulfenylation (*aka* *S*-sulphenylation), reversible covalent attachment of hydroxide to the thiol group of cysteine residues
- succinylation addition of a succinyl group to lysine
- sulfation, the addition of a sulfate group to a tyrosine.

Non-enzymatic additions *in vivo*

- glycation, the addition of a sugar molecule to a protein without the controlling action of an enzyme.
- carbamylation the addition of Isocyanic acid to an N-terminus of either lysine, histidine, taurine, arginine, or cysteine.
- carbonylation the addition of carbon monoxide to other organic/inorganic compounds.

Non-enzymatic additions *in vitro*

- biotinylation: covalent attachment of a biotin moiety using a biotinylation reagent, typically for the purpose of labeling a protein.

- oxidation: addition of one or more Oxygen atoms to a susceptible side-chain, principally of Met, Trp, His or Cys residues. Formation of disulfide bonds between Cys residues.
- pegylation: covalent attachment of polyethylene glycol (PEG) using a pegylation reagent, typically to the N-terminus or the side-chains of Lys residues. Pegylation is used to improve the efficacy of protein pharmaceuticals.

OTHER PROTEINS OR PEPTIDES

- ISGylation, the covalent linkage to the ISG15 protein (Interferon-Stimulated Gene 15)
- SUMOylation, the covalent linkage to the SUMO protein (Small Ubiquitin-related MOdifier)
- ubiquitination, the covalent linkage to the protein ubiquitin.
- Neddylation, the covalent linkage to Nedd
- Pupylation, the covalent linkage to the Prokaryotic ubiquitin-like protein

CHEMICAL MODIFICATION OF AMINO ACIDS

- citrullination, or **deimination**, the conversion of arginine to citrulline
- deamidation, the conversion of glutamine to glutamic acid or asparagine to aspartic acid
- eliminylation, the conversion to an alkene by beta-elimination of phosphothreonine and phosphoserine, or dehydration of threonine and serine, as well as by decarboxylation of cysteine
- carbamylation of the N-terminus (an α-amine) and the side-chain amino groups of lysine and, usually to a lesser extent, arginine

STRUCTURAL CHANGES

- disulfide bridges, the covalent linkage of two cysteine amino acids
- proteolytic cleavage, cleavage of a protein at a peptide bond
- racemization
    - of proline by prolyl isomerase
    - of serine by protein-serine epimerase
    - of alanine in dermorphin, a frog opioid peptide
    - of methionine in deltorphin, also a frog opioid peptide
- protein splicing, self-catalytic removal of inteins analogous to mRNA processing

STATISTICS

In 2011, statistics of each post-translational modification experimentally and putatively detected have been compiled using proteome-wide information from the Swiss-Prot database. The 10 most common experimentally found modifications were as follows:

Frequency	Modification
58383	Phosphorylation
6751	Acetylation
5526	N-linked glycosylation
2844	Amidation
1619	Hydroxylation
1523	Methylation
1133	O-linked glycosylation
878	Ubiquitylation
826	Pyrrolidone Carboxylic Acid
504	Sulfation

More details can be found at http://selene.princeton.edu/PTMCuration/.

PROTEIN TARGETING

Protein targeting or **protein sorting** is the biological mechanism by which proteins are transported to the appropriate destinations in the cell or outside of it. Proteins can be targeted to the inner space of an organelle, different intracellular membranes, plasma membrane, or to exterior of the cell via secretion. This delivery process is carried out based on information contained in the protein itself. Correct sorting is crucial for the cell; errors can lead to diseases.

Targeting signals

Targeting signals are the pieces of information that enable the cellular transport machinery to correctly position a protein inside or outside the cell. This information is contained in the polypeptide chain or in the folded protein. The continuous stretch of amino acid residues in the chain that enables targeting are called signal peptides or targeting peptides. There are two types of targeting peptides, the presequences and the internal targeting peptides. The presequences of the targeting peptide are often found at the N-terminal extension and is composed of between 6-136 basic and hydrophobic amino acids. In case of peroxisomes the targeting sequence is on the C-terminal extension mostly. Other signals, known as signal patches, are composed of parts which are separate in the primary sequence. They become functional when folding brings them together on the protein surface. In addition, protein modifications like glycosylations can induce targeting.

Protein Translocation

In 1970, Günter Blobel conducted experiments on the translocation of proteins across membranes. He was awarded the 1999 Nobel prize for his findings. He discovered that many proteins have a signal sequence, that is, a short amino acid sequence at one end that functions like a postal code for the target organelle. The translation of mRNA into protein by a ribosome takes place within the cytosol. If the synthesized proteins "belong " in a different organelle, they can be transported there in either of two ways depending on the protein: Co-translational translocation (translocation during the process of translation), and Post-translational translocation (translocation after the process of translation is complete).

Co-translational Translocation

Most proteins that are secretory, membrane-bound, or reside in the endoplasmic reticulum (ER), golgi or endosomes use the co-translational translocation pathway. This process begins with the N-terminal signal peptide of the protein being recognized by a signal recognition particle (SRP) *while the protein is still being synthesized on the ribosome*. The synthesis pauses while the ribosome-protein complex is transferred to an SRP receptor on the ER in eukaryotes, and the plasma membrane in prokaryotes. There, the nascent protein is inserted into the translocon, a membrane-bound protein conducting channel composed of the Sec61 translocation complex in eukaryotes, and the homologous SecYEG complex in prokaryotes. In secretory proteins and type I transmembrane proteins, the signal sequence is immediately cleaved from the nascent polypeptide once it has been translocated into the membrane of the ER (eukaryotes) or plasma membrane (prokaryotes) by signal peptidase. The signal sequence of type II membrane proteins and some polytopic membrane proteins are not cleaved off and therefore are referred to as signal anchor sequences. Within the ER, the protein is first covered by a chaperone protein to protect it from the high concentration of other proteins in the ER, giving it time to fold correctly. Once folded, the protein is modified as needed (for example, by glycosylation), then transported to the Golgi for further processing and goes to its target organelles or is retained in the ER by various ER retention mechanisms.

The amino acid chain of transmembrane proteins, which often are transmembrane receptors, passes through a membrane one or several times. They are inserted into the membrane by translocation, until the process is interrupted by a stop-transfer sequence, also called a membrane anchor sequence. These complex membrane proteins are at the moment mostly understood using the same model of targeting that has been developed for secretory proteins. However, many complex multi-transmembrane proteins contain structural aspects that do not fit the model. Seven transmembrane G-protein coupled receptors (which represent about 5% of the genes in humans) mostly do not have an amino-terminal signal sequence. In contrast to secretory proteins, the first transmembrane domain acts as the first signal sequence, which targets them to the ER membrane. This also results in the translocation of the amino terminus of the protein into the ER membrane lumen. This would seem to break the rule of "co-translational " translocation which has always held for mammalian proteins targeted to the ER. This has been demonstrated with opsin with in vitro experiments. A great deal of the mechanics of transmembrane topology and folding remains to be elucidated.

Post-translational Translocation

Even though most secretory proteins are co-translationally translocated, some are translated in the cytosol and later transported to the ER/plasma membrane by a post-translational system. In prokaryotes this requires certain cofactors such as SecA and SecB. This pathway is poorly understood in eukaryotes, but is facilitated by Sec62 and Sec63, two membrane-bound proteins.

In addition, proteins targeted to other destinations, such as mitochondria, chloroplasts, or peroxisomes, use specialized post-translational pathways. Also, proteins targeted for the nucleus are translocated post-translation. They pass through the nuclear envelope via nuclear pores.

Sorting of Proteins to Mitochondria

Most mitochondrial proteins are synthesized as cytosolic precursors containing uptake peptide signals. Cytosolic chaperones deliver preproteins to channel linked receptors in the mitochondrial membrane. The preprotein with presequence targeted for the mitochondria is bound by receptors and the General Import Pore (GIP) (Receptors and GIP are collectively known as Translocase of Outer Membrane or TOM) at the outer membrane. The preprotein is translocated through TOM as hairpin loops. The preprotein is transported through the intermembrane space by small TIMs (which also acts as molecular chaperones) to the TIM23 or 22 (Translocase of Inner Membrane) at the inner membrane. Within the matrix the targeting sequence is cleaved off by mtHsp70.

Three mitochondrial outer membrane receptors are known: TOM20, TOM22 and TOM70

TOM70: Binds to internal targeting peptides and acts as a docking point for cytosolic chaperones.

TOM20: Binds presequencesTOM22: Binds both presequences and internal targeting peptides

The TOM channel (TOM40) is a cation specific high conductance channel with a molecular weight of 410 kDa and a pore diameter of 21Å.

The presequence translocase23 (TIM23) is localized to the mitochondrial inner membrane and acts a pore forming protein which binds precursor proteins with its N-terminus. TIM23 acts a translocator for preproteins for the mitochondrial matrix, the inner mitochondrial membrane as well as for the intermembrane space. TIM50 is bound to TIM23 at the inner mitochondrial side and found to bind presequences. TIM44 is bound on the matrix side and found binding to mtHsp70.

The presequence translocase22 (TIM22) binds preproteins exclusively bound for the inner mitochondrial membrane.

Mitochondrial matrix targeting sequences are rich in positively charged amino acids and hydroxylated ones.

Proteins are targeted to submitochondrial compartments by multiple signals and several pathways.

Targeting to the outer membrane, intermembrane space, and inner membrane often requires another signal sequence in addition to the matrix targeting sequence.

Sorting of Proteins to Chloroplasts

The preprotein for chloroplasts may contain a stromal import sequence or a stromal and thylakoid targeting sequence. The majority of preproteins are translocated through the Toc and Tic complexes located within the chloroplast envelope. In the stroma the stromal import sequence is cleaved off and folded as well as intra-chloroplast sorting to thylakoids continues. Proteins targeted to the envelope of chloroplasts usually lack cleavable sorting sequence.

Sorting of proteins to both chloroplasts and mitochondria

Many proteins are needed in both mitochondria and chloroplasts. In general the targeting peptide is of intermediate character to the two specific ones. The targeting peptides of these proteins have a high content of basic and hydrophobic amino acids, a low content of negatively charged amino acids. They have a lower content of alanine and a higher content of leucine and phenylalanine. The dual targeted proteins have a more hydrophobic targeting peptide than both mitochondrial and chloroplastic ones.

Sorting of Proteins to Peroxisomes

All peroxisomal proteins are encoded by nuclear genes.

To date there are two types of known Peroxisome Targeting Signals (PTS):

Peroxisome targeting signal 1 (PTS1): a C-terminal tripeptide with a consensus sequence (S/A/C)-(K/R/H)-(L/A). The most common PTS1 is serine-lysine-leucine (SKL). Most peroxisomal matrix proteins possess a PTS1 type signal.

Peroxisome targeting signal 2 (PTS2): a nonapeptide located near the N-terminus with a consensus sequence (R/K)-(L/V/I)-XXXXX-(H/Q)-(L/A/F) (where X can be any amino acid).

There are also proteins that possess neither of these signals. Their transport may be based on a so-called "piggy-back" mechanism: such proteins associate with PTS1-possessing matrix proteins and are translocated into the peroxisomal matrix together with them.

Diseases

Peroxisomal protein transport is defective in the following genetic diseases:

- Zellweger syndrome.
- Adrenoleukodystrophy (ALD).
- Refsum disease

Protein Targeting in Bacteria and Archaea

As discussed above (see protein translocation), most prokaryotic membrane-bound and secretory proteins are targeted to the plasma membrane by either a co-translation pathway that uses bacterial SRP or a post-translation pathway that requires SecA and SecB. At the plasma membrane, these two pathways deliver proteins to the SecYEG translocon for translocation. Bacteria may have a single plasma membrane (Gram-positive bacteria), or an inner membrane plus an outer membrane separated by the periplasm (Gram-negative bacteria). Besides the plasma membrane the majority of prokaryotes lack membrane-bound organelles as found in eukaryotes, but they may assemble proteins onto various types of inclusions such as gas vesicles and storage granules.

GRAM-NEGATIVE BACTERIA

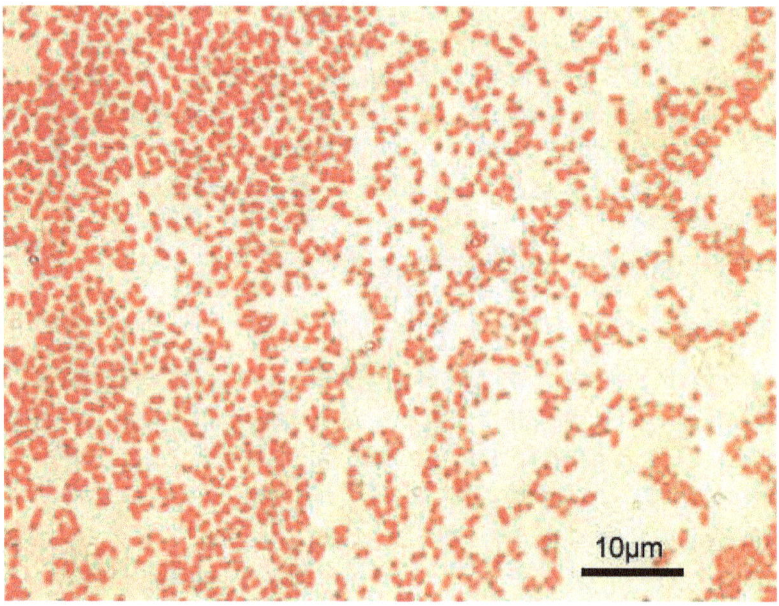

Microscopic image of gram-negative *Pseudomonas aeruginosa* bacteria (pink-red rods).

Gram-negative bacteria are a group of bacteria that do not retain the crystal violet stain used in the Gram staining method of bacterial differentiation. They are characterized by their cell envelopes, which are composed of a thin peptidoglycan cell wall sandwiched between an inner cytoplasmic cell membrane and a bacterial outer membrane.

Gram-negative bacteria are spread worldwide, in virtually all environments that support life. The gram-negative bacteria include the model organism *Escherichia coli*, as well as many pathogenic bacteria, such as *Pseudomonas aeruginosa*, *Neisseria gonorrhoeae*, Chlamydia trachomatis, and *Yersinia pestis*. Several classes of antibiotics target gram-negative bacteria specifically, including aminoglycosides and carbapenems.

Characteristics

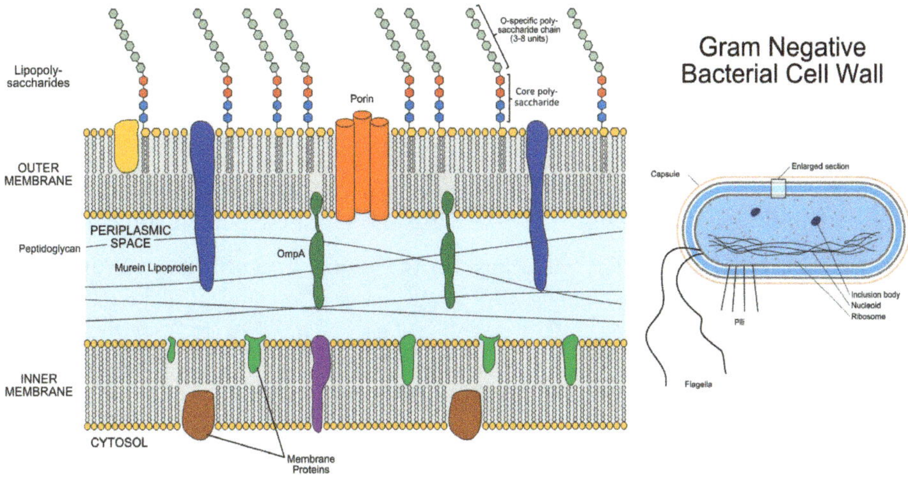

Gram-negative cell wall structure.

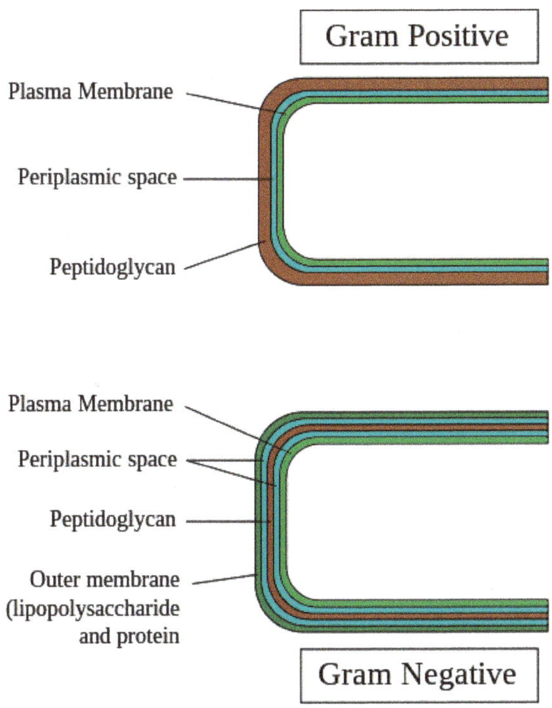

Gram-positive and -negative bacteria are differentiated chiefly by their cell wall structure.

Gram-negative bacteria display these characteristics:

- An inner cell membrane is present (cytoplasmic)

- A thin peptidoglycan layer is present (This is much thicker in gram-positive bacteria)
- Has outer membrane containing lipopolysaccharides (LPS, which consists of lipid A, core polysaccharide, and O antigen) in its outer leaflet and phospholipids in the inner leaflet
- Porins exist in the outer membrane, which act like pores for particular molecules
- Between the outer membrane and the cytoplasmic membrane there is a space filled with a concentrated gel-like substance called periplasm
- The S-layer is directly attached to the outer membrane rather than to the peptidoglycan
- If present, flagella have four supporting rings instead of two
- Teichoic acids or lipoteichoic acids are absent
- Lipoproteins are attached to the polysaccharide backbone
- Some contain Braun›s lipoprotein, which serves as a link between the outer membrane and the peptidoglycan chain by a covalent bond
- Most, with very few exceptions, do not form spores

Classification

Along with cell shape, Gram staining is a rapid diagnostic tool and once was used to group species at the subdivision of Bacteria. Historically, the kingdom Monera was divided into four divisions based on Gram staining: Firmacutes (+), Gracillicutes (−), Mollicutes (0) and Mendocutes (var.). Since 1987, the monophyly of the gram-negative bacteria has been disproven with molecular studies. However some authors, such as Cavalier-Smith still treat them as a monophyletic taxon (though not a clade; his definition of monophyly requires a single common ancestor but does not require holophyly, the property that all descendents be encompassed by the taxon) and refer to the group as subkingdom "Negibacteria ".

Taxonomy

Bacteria are traditionally divided into the two groups: gram-positive and gram-negative, based on their Gram stain retention. These groups are often thought of as lineages, with gram-negative bacteria more closely-related to one another than to gram-positive bacteria. While this is often true, the classification system breaks down in some cases. A given bacteria's Gram stain result, bacterial membrane organization, and lineage groupings do not always match up. As such, the Gram stain cannot be reliably used to assess familial relationships of bacteria. That said, Gram staining does often give reliable information about the composition of the cell membrane, distinguishing between the presence or absence of an outer lipid membrane.

Of these two structurally distinct groups of prokaryotic organisms, monoderm prokaryotes are indicated to be ancestral. Based upon a number of different observations including that the gram-positive bacteria are the major reactors to antibiotics and that gram-negative bacteria are, in general, resistant to them, it has been proposed that the outer cell membrane in gram-negative bacteria (diderms) evolved as a protective mechanism against antibiotic selection pressure. Some bacteria such as Deinococcus, which stain gram-positive due to the presence of a thick peptidoglycan layer, but also possess an outer cell membrane are suggested as intermediates in the transition between monoderm (gram-positive) and diderm (gram-negative) bacteria. The diderm bacteria can also be further differentiated between simple diderms lacking lipopolysaccharide; the archetypical diderm bacteria, in which the outer cell membrane contains lipopolysaccharide; and the diderm bacteria, in which the outer cell membrane is made up of mycolic acid (e. g. Mycobacterium).

In addition, a number of bacterial taxa (viz. Negativicutes, Fusobacteria, Synergistetes, and Elusimicrobia) that are either part of the phylum Firmicutes or branches in its proximity are also found to possess a diderm cell structure. However, a conserved signature indel (CSI) in the HSP60 (GroEL) protein distinguishes all traditional phyla of gram-negative bacteria (e.g., Proteobacteria, Aquificae, Chlamydiae, Bacteroidetes, Chlorobi, Cyanobacteria, Fibrobacteres, Verrucomicrobia, Planctomycetes, Spirochetes, Acidobacteria) from these other atypical diderm bacteria as well as other phyla of monoderm bacteria (e.g., Actinobacteria, Firmicutes, Thermotogae, Chloroflexi). The presence of this CSI in all sequenced species of conventional lipopolysaccharide-containing gram-negative bacterial phyla provides evidence that these phyla of bacteria form a monophyletic clade and that no loss of the outer membrane from any species from this group has occurred.

Example species

The proteobacteria are a major group of gram-negative bacteria, including *Escherichia coli* (*E. coli*), *Salmonella*, *Shigella*, and other Enterobacteriaceae, *Pseudomonas*, *Moraxella*, *Helicobacter*, *Stenotrophomonas*, *Bdellovibrio*, acetic acid bacteria, *Legionella* etc. Other notable groups of gram-negative bacteria include the cyanobacteria, spirochaetes, green sulfur, and green non-sulfur bacteria.

Medically relevant gram-negative cocci include the four types that cause a sexually transmitted disease (*Neisseria gonorrhoeae*), a meningitis (*Neisseria meningitidis*), and respiratory symptoms (*Moraxella catarrhalis*, *Haemophilus influenzae*).

Medically relevant gram-negative bacilli include a multitude of species. Some of them cause primarily respiratory problems (*Klebsiella pneumoniae*, *Legionella pneumophila*, *Pseudomonas aeruginosa*), primarily urinary problems (*Escherichia coli*, *Proteus mirabilis*, *Enterobacter cloacae*, *Serratia marcescens*), and primarily gastrointestinal problems (*Helicobacter pylori*, *Salmonella enteritidis*, *Salmonella typhi*).

Gram-negative bacteria associated with hospital-acquired infections include *Acinetobacter baumannii*, which cause bacteremia, secondary meningitis, and ventilator-associated pneumonia in hospital intensive-care units.

Bacterial Transformation

Transformation is one of three processes for horizontal gene transfer, in which exogenous genetic material passes from bacterium to another, the other two being conjugation (transfer of genetic material between two bacterial cells in direct contact) and transduction (injection of foreign DNA by a bacteriophage virus into the host bacterium). In transformation, the genetic material passes through the intervening medium, and uptake is completely dependent on the recipient bacterium.

As of 2014 about 80 species of bacteria were known to be capable of transformation, about evenly divided between Gram-positive and Gram-negative bacteria; the number might be an overestimate since several of the reports are supported by single papers. Transformation has been studied in medically important Gram-negative bacteria species such as *Helicobacter pylori*, *Legionella pneumophila*, *Neisseria meningitidis*, *Neisseria gonorrhoeae*, *Haemophilus influenzae* and *Vibrio cholerae*. It has also been studied in gram-negative species found in soil such as *Pseudomonas stutzeri*, *Acinetobacter baylyi*, and gram-negative plant pathogens such as *Ralstonia solanacearum* and *Xylella fastidiosa*.

Medical Treatment

One of the several unique characteristics of gram-negative bacteria is the structure of the bacterial outer membrane. The outer leaflet of this membrane comprises a complex lipopolysaccharide (LPS) whose lipid portion acts as an endotoxin. If gram-negative bacteria enter the circulatory system, the liposaccharide can cause a toxic reaction. This results in fever, an increased respiratory rate, and low blood pressure. This may lead to life-threatening condition of endotoxic shock.

The outer membrane protects the bacteria from several antibiotics, dyes, and detergents that would normally damage either the inner membrane or the cell wall (made of peptidoglycan). The outer membrane provides these bacteria with resistance to lysozyme and penicillin. However, alternative medicinal treatments such as lysozyme with EDTA and the antibiotic ampicillin have been developed to combat the protective outer membrane of some pathogenic gram-negative organisms. Other drugs can also be used, significant ones being chloramphenicol, streptomycin, and nalidixic acid. Chloramphenicol is rarely used in the EU due to the association with drug induced pancytopenia.

The pathogenic capability of gram-negative bacteria is often associated with certain components of their membrane, in particular, the LPS. In humans, the presence of LPS triggers an innate immune response, activating the immune system and producing cytokines (hormonal regulators). Inflammation is a common reaction to cytokine production, which can also produce host toxicity. The innate immune response to LPS, however, is not synonymous with pathogenicity, or the ability to cause disease.

Gram-positive Bacteria

In most gram-positive bacteria, certain proteins are targeted for export across the plasma membrane and subsequent covalent attachment to the bacterial cell wall. A specialized enzyme, sortase, cleaves the target protein at a characteristic recognition site near the protein C-terminus, such as an LPXTG motif (where X can be any amino acid), then transfers the protein onto the cell wall. Several analogous systems are found that likewise feature a signature motif on the extracytoplasmic face, a C-terminal transmembrane domain, and cluster of basic residues on the cytosolic face at the protein's extreme C-terminus.

The PEP-CTERM/exosortase system, found in many Gram-negative bacteria, seems to be related to extracellular polymeric substance production. The PGF-CTERM/archaeosortase A system in archaea is related to S-layer production. The GlyGly-CTERM/rhombosortase system, found in the Shewanella, Vibrio, and a few other genera, seems involved in the release of proteases, nucleases, and other enzymes.

SECRETION

Secretion is the movement of material from one point to another, e.g. secreted chemical substance from a cell or gland. In contrast, excretion, it is the removal of certain substances or waste products from a cell or organism. The classical mechanism of cell secretion is via secretory portals at the cell plasma membrane called porosomes. Porosomes are permanent cup-shaped lipoprotein structure at the cell plasma membrane, where secretory vesicles transiently dock and fuse to release intra-vesicular contents from the cell.

Secretion in bacterial species means the transport or translocation of effector molecules for example: proteins, enzymes or toxins (such as cholera toxin in pathogenic bacteria for example *Vibrio cholerae*) from across the interior (cytoplasm or cytosol) of a bacterial cell to its exterior. Secretion is a very important mechanism in bacterial functioning and operation in their natural surrounding environment for adaptation and survival.

Secretion in Eukaryotic Cells

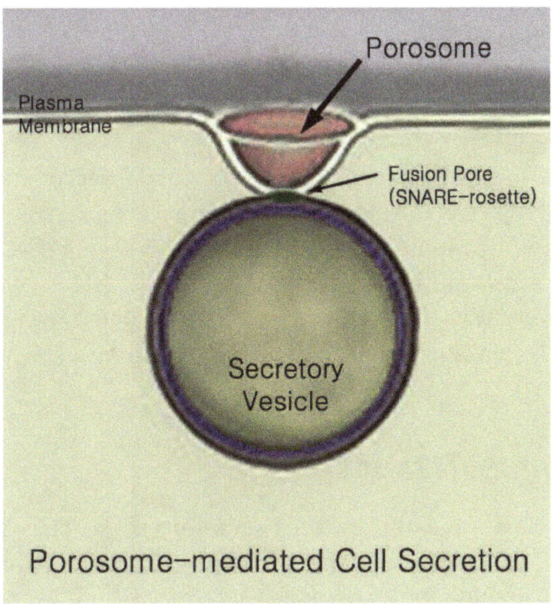

Porosome.

Mechanism

Eukaryotic cells, including human cells, have a highly evolved process of secretion. Proteins targeted for the outside are synthesized by ribosomes docked to the rough endoplasmic reticulum (ER). As they are synthesized, these proteins translocate into the ER lumen, where they are glycosylated and where molecular chaperones aid protein folding. Misfolded proteins are usually identified here and retrotranslocated by ER-associated degradation to the cytosol, where they are degraded by a proteasome. The vesicles containing the properly folded proteins then enter the Golgi apparatus.

In the Golgi apparatus, the glycosylation of the proteins is modified and further posttranslational modifications, including cleavage and functionalization, may occur. The proteins are then moved into secretory vesicles which travel along the cytoskeleton to the edge of the cell. More modification can occur in the secretory vesicles (for example insulin is cleaved from proinsulin in the secretory vesicles).

Eventually, there is vesicle fusion with the cell membrane at a structure called the porosome, in a process called exocytosis, dumping its contents out of the cell›s environment.

Strict biochemical control is maintained over this sequence by usage of a pH gradient: the pH of the cytosol is 7.4, the ER's pH is 7.0, and the cis-golgi has a pH of 6.5. Secretory vesicles have pHs ranging between 5.0 and 6.0; some secretory vesicles evolve into lysosomes, which have a pH of 4.8.

Nonclassical secretion

There are many proteins like FGF1 (aFGF), FGF2 (bFGF), interleukin-1 (IL1) etc. which do not have a signal sequence. They do not use the classical ER-golgi pathway. These are secreted through various nonclassical pathways.

At least four nonclassical (unconventional) protein secretion pathways have been described. They include 1) direct translocation of proteins across the plasma membrane likely through membrane transporters, 2) blebbing, 3) lysosomal secretion, and 4) release via exosomes derived from multivesicular bodies. In addition, proteins can be released from cells by mechanical or physiological wounding and through nonlethal, transient oncotic pores in the plasma membrane induced by washing cells with serum-free media or buffers.

Secretion in Human Tissues

Many human cell types have the ability to be secretory cells. They have a well-developed endoplasmic reticulum and Golgi apparatus to fulfill their function. Tissues in humans that produce secretions include the gastrointestinal tract which secretes digestive enzymes and gastric acid, the lung which secretes surfactants, and sebaceous glands which secrete sebum to lubricate the skin and hair. Meibomian glands in the eyelid secrete sebum to lubricate and protect the eye.

Secretion in Gram Negative Bacteria

Secretion is not unique to eukaryotes alone, it is present in bacteria and archaea as well. ATP binding cassette (ABC) type transporters are common to all the three domains of life. The Sec system constituting the Sec Y-E-G complex (see Type II secretion system (T2SS), below) is another conserved secretion system, homologous to the translocon in the eukaryotic endoplasmic reticulum and the Sec 61 translocon complex of yeast. Some secreted proteins are translocated across the cytoplasmic membrane by the Sec translocon, which requires the presence of an N-terminal signal peptide on the secreted protein. Others are translocated across the cytoplasmic membrane by the twin-arginine translocation pathway (Tat). Gram negative bacteria have two membranes, thus making secretion topologically more complex. There are at least six specialized secretion systems in Gram negative bacteria. Many secreted proteins are particularly important in bacterial pathogenesis.

Type I Secretion System (T1SS or TOSS)

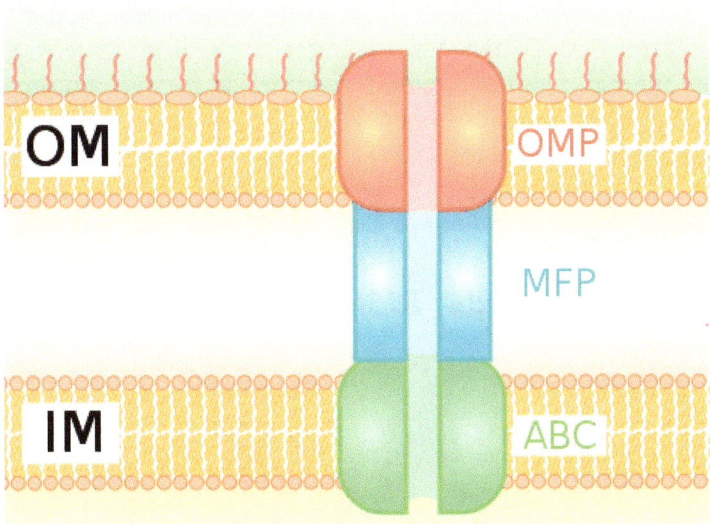

Type I secretion is a chaperone dependent secretion system employing the Hly and Tol gene clusters. The process begins as a leader sequence HlyA is recognized and binds HlyB on the membrane. This signal sequence is extremely specific for the ABC transporter. The HlyAB complex stimulates HlyD which begins to uncoil and reaches the outer membrane where TolC recognizes a terminal molecule or signal on HlyD. HlyD recruits TolC to the inner membrane and HlyA is excreted outside of the outer membrane via a long-tunnel protein channel.

Type I secretion system transports various molecules, from ions, drugs, to proteins of various sizes (20 - 900 kDa). The molecules secreted vary in size from the small *Escherichia coli* peptide colicin V, (10 kDa) to the *Pseudomonas fluorescens* cell adhesion protein LapA of 520 kDa. The best characterized are the RTX toxins and the lipases. Type I secretion is also involved in export of non-proteinaceous substrates like cyclic β-glucans and polysaccharides.

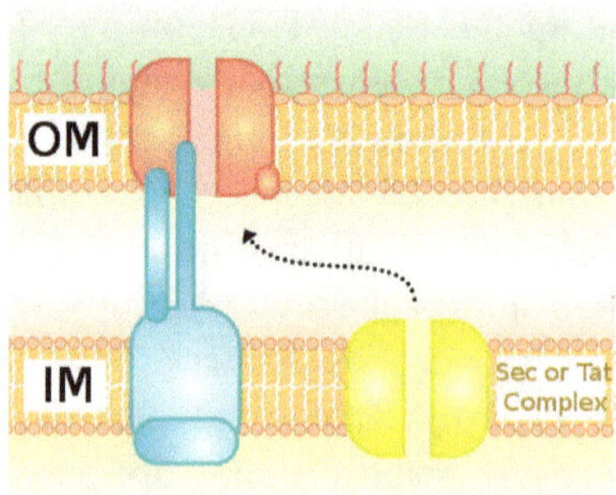

Type II secretion system (T2SS)

Proteins secreted through the type II system, or main terminal branch of the general secretory pathway, depend on the Sec or Tat system for initial transport into the periplasm. Once there, they pass through the outer membrane via a multimeric (12-14 subunits) complex of pore forming secretin proteins. In addition to the secretin protein, 10-15 other inner and outer membrane proteins compose the full secretion apparatus, many with as yet unknown function. Gram-negative type IV pili use a modified version of the type II system for their biogenesis, and in some cases certain proteins are shared between a pilus complex and type II system within a single bacterial species.

Type III Secretion System (T3SS or TTSS)

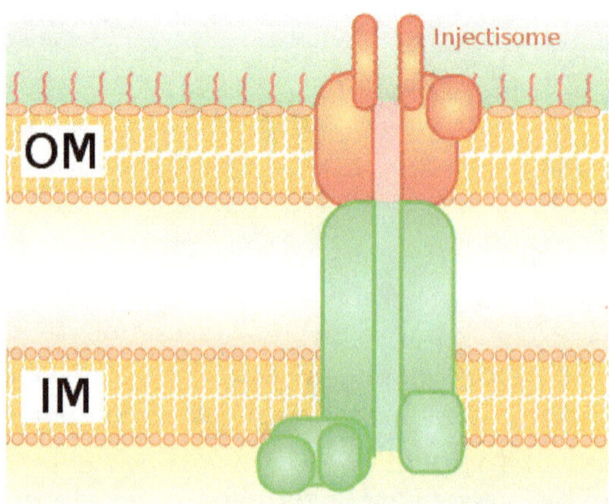

It is homologous to the basal body in bacterial flagella. It is like a molecular syringe through which a bacterium (e.g. certain types of *Salmonella*, *Shigella*, *Yersinia*, *Vibrio*) can inject proteins into eukaryotic cells. The low Ca^{2+}concentration in the cytosol opens the gate that regulates T3SS. One such mechanism to detect low calcium concentration has been illustrated by the lcrV (Low Calcium Response) antigen utilized by *Yersinia pestis*, which is used to detect low calcium concentrations and elicits T3SS attachment. The Hrp system in plant pathogens inject harpins and pathogen effector proteins through similar mechanisms into plants. This secretion system was first discovered in *Yersinia pestis* and showed that toxins could be injected directly from the bacterial cytoplasm into the cytoplasm of its host's cells rather than simply be secreted into the extracellular medium.

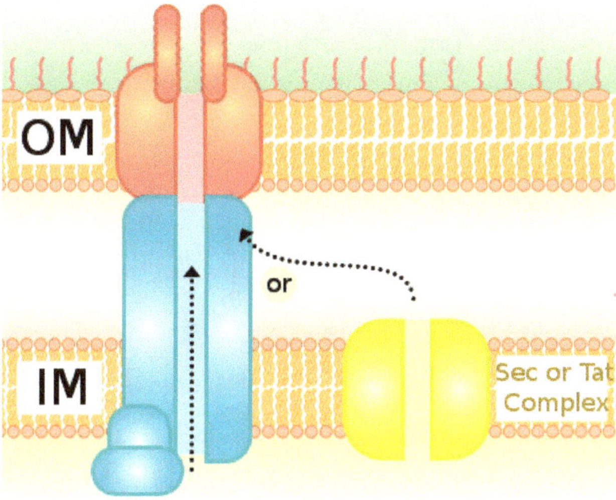

Type IV secretion system (T4SS or TFSS)

It is homologous to conjugation machinery of bacteria. It is capable of transporting both DNA and proteins. It was discovered in *Agrobacterium tumefaciens*, which uses this system to introduce the T-DNA portion of the Ti plasmid into the plant host, which in turn causes the affected area to develop into a crown gall (tumor). *Helicobacter pylori* uses a type IV secretion system to deliver CagA into gastric epithelial cells, which is associated with gastric carcinogenesis. *Bordetella pertussis*, the causative agent of whooping cough, secretes the pertussis toxin partly through the type IV system. *Legionella pneumophila*, the causing agent of legionellosis (Legionnaires' disease) utilizes a type IVB secretion system, known as the icm/dot (**i**ntra**c**ellular **m**ultiplication / **d**efect in **o**rganelle **t**rafficking genes) system, to translocate numerous effector proteins into its eukaryotic host. The prototypic Type IVA secretion system is the VirB complex of *Agrobacterium tumefaciens*.

Protein members of this family are components of the type IV secretion system. They mediate intracellular transfer of macromolecules via a mechanism ancestrally related to that of bacterial conjugation machineries.

Function

In short, Type IV secretion system (T4SS), is the general mechanism by which bacterial cells secrete or take up macromolecules. Their precise mechanism remains unknown. T4SS is encoded on Gram-negative conjugative elements in bacteria.T4SS are cell envelope-spanning complexes or in other words 11-13 core proteins that form a channel through which DNA and proteins can travel from the cytoplasm of the donor cell to the cytoplasm of the recipient cell. Additionally, T4SS also secrete virulence factor proteins directly into host cells as well as taking up DNA from the medium during natural transformation, which shows the versatility of this macromolecular secretion apparatus.

Structure

As shown in the above figure, TraC, in particular consists of a three helix bundle and a loose globular appendage.

Interactions

T4SS has two effector proteins: firstly, ATS-1, which stands for Anaplasma translocated substrate 1, and secondly AnkA, which stands for ankyrin repeat domain-containing protein A. Additionally, T4SS coupling proteins are VirD4, which bind to VirE2.

Type V Secretion System (T5SS)

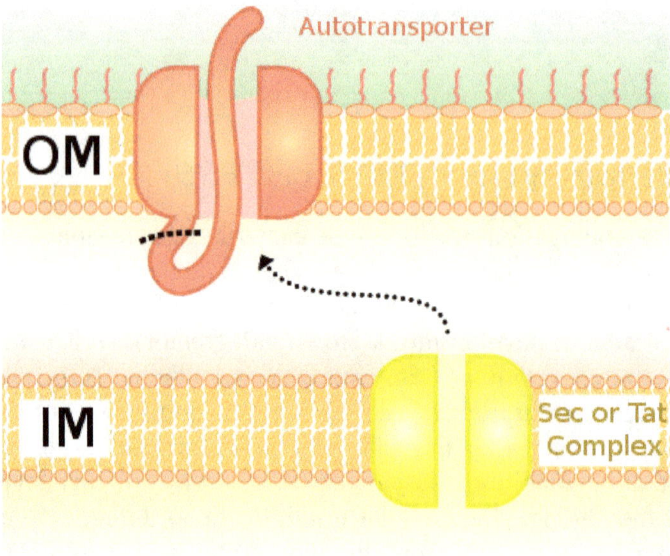

Also called the autotransporter system, type V secretion involves use of the *Sec* system for crossing the inner membrane. Proteins which use this pathway have the capability to form a beta-barrel with their C-terminus which inserts into the outer membrane, allowing the rest of the peptide (the passenger domain) to reach the outside of the cell. Often, autotransporters are cleaved, leaving the beta-barrel domain in the outer membrane and freeing the passenger domain. Some researchers believe remnants of the autotransporters gave rise to the porins which form similar beta-barrel structures. A common example of an autotransporter that uses this secretion system is the Trimeric Autotransporter Adhesins.

Type VI Secretion System (T6SS)

Type VI secretion systems were originally identified in 2006 by the group of John Mekalanos at the Harvard Medical School (Boston, USA) in two bacterial pathogens, *Vibrio cholerae* and *Pseudomonas aeruginosa*. These were identified when mutations in the Hcp and VrgG genes in *Vibrio Cholerae* led to decreased virulence and pathogenicity. Since then, Type VI secretion systems have been found in a quarter of all proteobacterial genomes, including animal, plant, human pathogens, as well as soil, environmental or marine bacteria. While most of the early studies of Type VI secretion focused on its role in the pathogenesis of higher organisms, more recent studies suggested a broader physiological role in defense against simple eukaryotic predators and its role in inter-bacteria interactions. The Type VI secretion system gene clusters contain from 15 to more than 20 genes, two of which, Hcp and VgrG, have been shown to be nearly universally secreted substrates of the system. Structural analysis of these and other proteins in this system bear a striking resemblance to the tail spike of the T4 phage, and the activity of the system is thought to functionally resemble phage infection.

Release of Outer Membrane Vesicles

In addition to the use of the multiprotein complexes listed above, Gram-negative bacteria possess another method for release of material: the formation of bacterial outer membrane vesicles. Portions of the outer membrane pinch off, forming nano-scale spherical structures made of a lipopolysaccharide-rich lipid bilayer enclosing periplasmic materials, and are deployed for membrane vesicle trafficking to manipulate environment or invade at host-pathogen interface. Vesicles from a number of bacterial species have been found to contain virulence factors, some have immunomodulatory effects, and some can directly adhere to and intoxicate host cells. While release of vesicles has been demonstrated as a general response to stress conditions, the process of loading cargo proteins seems to be selective.

Secretion in Gram Positive Bacteria

In some *Staphylococcus* and *Streptococcus* species, the accessory secretory system handles the export of highly repetitive adhesion glycoproteins.

REFERENCES

1. Baron S, Salton MR, Kim KS (1996). "Structure". In Baron S, et al. Baron's Medical Microbiology (4th ed.). Univ of Texas Medical Branch. ISBN 0-9631172-1-1. PMID 21413343.
2. Gibbons, N. E.; Murray, R. G. E. (1978). "Proposals Concerning the Higher Taxa of Bacteria". International Journal of Systematic Bacteriology. 28 (1): 1–6. doi:10.1099/00207713-28-1-1.
3. Woese CR (June 1987). "Bacterial evolution". Microbiol. Rev. 51 (2): 221–71. PMC 373105 . PMID 2439888.

4. Cavalier-Smith, T. (2006). "Rooting the tree of life by transition analyses". Biol. Direct. 1: 19. doi:10.1186/1745-6150-1-19. PMC 1586193 . PMID 16834776.
5. Gupta RS (December 1998). "Protein phylogenies and signature sequences: A reappraisal of evolutionary relationships among archaebacteria, eubacteria, and eukaryotes". Microbiol. Mol. Biol. Rev. 62 (4): 1435–91. PMC 98952 . PMID 9841678.
6. Gupta RS (2000). "The natural evolutionary relationships among prokaryotes". Crit. Rev. Microbiol. 26 (2): 111–31. doi:10.1080/10408410091154219. PMID 10890353.
7. Desvaux M, Hébraud M, Talon R, Henderson IR (April 2009). "Secretion and subcellular localizations of bacterial proteins: a semantic awareness issue". Trends Microbiol. 17 (4): 139–45. doi:10.1016/j.tim.2009.01.004. PMID 19299134.
8. Sutcliffe IC (October 2010). "A phylum level perspective on bacterial cell envelope architecture". Trends Microbiol. 18 (10): 464–70. doi:10.1016/j.tim.2010.06.005. PMID 20637628.
9. Gupta RS (August 1998). "What are archaebacteria: life's third domain or monoderm prokaryotes related to gram-positive bacteria? A new proposal for the classification of prokaryotic organisms". Mol. Microbiol. 29 (3): 695–707. doi:10.1046/j.1365-2958.1998.00978.x. PMID 9723910.
10. Gupta RS (August 2011). "Origin of diderm (gram-negative) bacteria: antibiotic selection pressure rather than endosymbiosis likely led to the evolution of bacterial cells with two membranes". Antonie Van Leeuwenhoek. 100 (2): 171–82. doi:10.1007/s10482-011-9616-8. PMC 3133647 . PMID 21717204.
11. Marchandin H, Teyssier C, Campos J, Jean-Pierre H, Roger F, Gay B, Carlier JP, Jumas-Bilak E (June 2010). "Negativicoccus succinicivorans gen. nov., sp. nov., --~~~~isolated from human clinical samples, emended description of the family Veillonellaceae any classis nov., Selenomonadales ord. nov. and Acidaminococcaceae fam. nov. in the bacterial phylum Firmicutes". Int. J. Syst. Evol. Microbiol. 60 (Pt 6): 1271–9. doi:10.1099/ijs.0.013102-0. PMID 19667386.
12. Johnston C, Martin B, Fichant G, Polard P, Claverys JP (2014). "Bacterial transformation: distribution, shared mechanisms and divergent control". Nat. Rev. Microbiol. 12 (3): 181–96. doi:10.1038/nrmicro3199. PMID 24509783.
13. Seitz P, Blokesch M (2013). "Cues and regulatory pathways involved in natural competence and transformation in pathogenic and environmental Gram-negative bacteria". FEMS Microbiol. Rev. 37 (3): 336–63. doi:10.1111/j.1574-6976.2012.00353.x. PMID 22928673.
14. Madigan M; Martinko J (editors). (2006). Brock Biology of Microorganisms (11th ed.). Pearson Prentice Hall. ISBN 0131443291.
15. pdf
16. Gibbons, N. E.; Murray, R. G. E. (1978). "Proposals Concerning the Higher Taxa of Bacteria". IJSEM. 28 (1): 1–6. doi:10.1099/00207713-28-1-1.
17. Woese, C. R. (1987). "Bacterial evolution". Microbiological reviews. 51 (2):

221–271. PMC 373105 . PMID 2439888.

18. Gupta, R.S. (1998). "Protein phylogenies and signature sequences: A reappraisal of evolutionary relationships among archaebacteria, eubacteria and eukaryotes". Microbiol. Mol. Biol. Rev. 62: 1435–1491.
19. Gupta, R.S. (2000). "The natural evolutionary relationships among prokaryotes". Crit. Rev. Microbiol. 26: 111–131. doi:10.1080/10408410091154219. PMID 10890353.
20. Desvaux, M; Hébraud, M; Talon, R; Henderson, IR (2009). "Secretion and subcellular localizations of bacterial proteins: a semantic awareness issue". Trends Microbiol. 17: 139–145. doi:10.1016/j.tim.2009.01.004. PMID 19299134.
21. Sutcliffe, IC (2010). "A phylum level perspective on bacterial cell envelope architecture". Trends Microbiol. 18: 464–470. doi:10.1016/j.tim.2010.06.005. PMID 20637628.
22. Gupta, R. S. (1998). "What are archaebacteria: life's third domain or monoderm prokaryotes related to gram-positive bacteria? A new proposal for the classification of prokaryotic organisms". Molecular Microbiology. 29 (3): 695–707. doi:10.1046/j.1365-2958.1998.00978.x. PMID 9723910.
23. Gupta, R. S. (2011). "Origin of diderm (gram-negative) bacteria: antibiotic selection pressure rather than endosymbiosis likely led to the evolution of bacterial cells with two membranes". Antonie van Leeuwenhoek. 100: 171–182. doi:10.1007/s10482-011-9616-8. PMC 3133647 . PMID 21717204.
24. Marchandin, H.; Teyssier, C.; Campos, J.; Jean-Pierre, H.; Roger, F.; Gay, B.; Carlier, J. -P.; Jumas-Bilak, E. (2009). "Negativicoccus succinicivorans gen. Nov., sp. Nov., isolated from human clinical samples, emended description of the family Veillonellaceae and description of Negativicutes classis nov., Selenomonadales ord. Nov. And Acidaminococcaceae fam. Nov. In the bacterial phylum Firmicutes". International Journal of Systematic and Evolutionary Microbiology. 60 (6): 1271–1279. doi:10.1099/ijs.0.013102-0. PMID 19667386.
25. Yabe, S.; Aiba, Y.; Sakai, Y.; Hazaka, M.; Yokota, A. (2010). "Thermogemmatispora onikobensis gen. nov., sp. nov. And Thermogemmatispora foliorum sp. nov., isolated from fallen leaves on geothermal soils, and description of Thermogemmatisporaceae fam. Nov. And Thermogemmatisporales ord. Nov. Within the class Ktedonobacteria". International Journal of Systematic and Evolutionary Microbiology. 61 (4): 903–910. doi:10.1099/ijs.0.024877-0. PMID 20495028.
26. Sutcliffe, I. C. (2011). "Cell envelope architecture in the Chloroflexi: A shifting frontline in a phylogenetic turf war". Environmental Microbiology. 13 (2): 279–282. doi:10.1111/j.1462-2920.2010.02339.x. PMID 20860732.
27. Hugenholtz, P.; Tyson, G. W.; Webb, R. I.; Wagner, A. M.; Blackall, L. L. (2001). "Investigation of Candidate Division TM7, a Recently Recognized Major Lineage of the Domain Bacteria with No Known Pure-Culture Representatives". Applied and Environmental Microbiology. 67 (1): 411–419. doi:10.1128/AEM.67.1.411-419.2001. PMC 92593 . PMID 11133473.

28. Cavaletti, L.; Monciardini, P.; Bamonte, R.; Schumann, P.; Rohde, M.; Sosio, M.; Donadio, S. (2006). "New Lineage of Filamentous, Spore-Forming, Gram-Positive Bacteria from Soil". Applied and Environmental Microbiology. 72 (6): 4360–4369. doi:10.1128/AEM.00132-06. PMC 1489649 . PMID 16751552.
29. Gladwin, Mark; Bill Trattler (2007). Clinical Microbiology made ridiculously simple. Miami, FL: MedMaster, Inc. pp. 4–5. ISBN 978-0-940780-81-1.
30. Sahebnasagh R, Saderi H, Owlia P. Detection of methicillin-resistant Staphylococcus aureus strains from clinical samples in Tehran by detection of the mecA and nuc genes. The First Iranian International Congress of Medical Bacteriology; 4–7 September; Tabriz, Iran. 2011. 195 pp.
31. MacDonald, Mhairi (2015). Avery's neonatology : pathophysiology and management of the newborn. Philadelphia: Wolters Kluwer. ISBN 9781451192681; Access provided by the University of Pittsburgh
32. Johnston C, Martin B, Fichant G, Polard P, Claverys JP (2014). "Bacterial transformation: distribution, shared mechanisms and divergent control". Nat. Rev. Microbiol. 12 (3): 181–96. doi:10.1038/nrmicro3199. PMID 24509783.
33. Michod RE, Bernstein H, Nedelcu AM (2008). "Adaptive value of sex in microbial pathogens". Infect. Genet. Evol. 8 (3): 267–85. doi:10.1016/j.meegid.2008.01.002. PMID 18295550.
34. Centers for Disease Control and Prevention. Emerging Infectious Diseases Journal Style Guide. Preferred Usage
35. Lee, Jin-Sook; Jeremic, Aleksandar; Shin, Leah; Cho, Won Jin; Chen, Xuequn; Jena, Bhanu P. (2012). "Neuronal porosome proteome: Molecular dynamics and architecture". Journal of Proteomics. 75 (13): 3952–62. doi:10.1016/j.jprot.2012.05.017. PMID 22659300.
36. Anderson, L. L. (2006). "Discovery of the 'porosome' The universal secretory machinery in cells". Journal of Cellular and Molecular Medicine. 10 (1): 126–31. doi:10.1111/j.1582-4934.2006.tb00294.x. PMID 16563225.
37. Nickel, Walter; Seedorf, Matthias (2008). "Unconventional Mechanisms of Protein Transport to the Cell Surface of Eukaryotic Cells". Annual Review of Cell and Developmental Biology. 24: 287–308. doi:10.1146/annurev.cellbio.24.110707.175320. PMID 18590485.
38. McNeil, Paul L.; Steinhardt, Richard A. (2003). "Plasma membrane disruption: repair, prevention, adaptation". Annual Review of Cell and Developmental Biology. 19: 697–731. doi:10.1146/annurev.cellbio.19.111301.140101. PMID 14570587.
39. Chirico, William J (2011). "Protein release through nonlethal oncotic pores as an alternative nonclassical secretory pathway". BMC Cell Biology. 12: 46. doi:10.1186/1471-2121-12-46. PMC 3217904 . PMID 22008609.
40. Wooldridge, K, ed. (2009). Bacterial Secreted Proteins: Secretory Mechanisms and Role in Pathogenesis. Caister Academic Press. ISBN 978-1-904455-42-4. [page needed]

41. Boyd, Chelsea D.; Smith, T. Jarrod; El-Kirat-Chatel, Sofiane; Newell, Peter D.; Dufrêne, Yves F.; O'Toole, George A. (2014-08-01). "Structural Features of the Pseudomonas fluorescens Biofilm Adhesin LapA Required for LapG-Dependent Cleavage, Biofilm Formation, and Cell Surface Localization". Journal of Bacteriology. 196 (15): 2775–2788. doi:10.1128/JB.01629-14. ISSN 0021-9193. PMC 4135675 . PMID 24837291.
42. Salyers, A. A. & Whitt, D. D. (2002). Bacterial Pathogenesis: A Molecular Approach, 2nd ed., Washington, D.C.: ASM Press. ISBN 1-55581-171-X[page needed]
43. Hatakeyama, Masanori; Higashi, Hideaki (2005). "Helicobacter pylori CagA: A new paradigm for bacterial carcinogenesis". Cancer Science. 96 (12): 835–43. doi:10.1111/j.1349-7006.2005.00130.x. PMID 16367902.
44. Cascales, Eric; Christie, Peter J. (2003). "The versatile bacterial type IV secretion systems". Nature Reviews Microbiology. 1 (2): 137–49. doi:10.1038/nrmicro753. PMC 3873781 . PMID 15035043.
45. Christie, Peter J.; Atmakuri, Krishnamohan; Krishnamoorthy, Vidhya; Jakubowski, Simon; Cascales, Eric (2005). "Biogenesis, Architecture, and Function of Bacterial Type Iv Secretion Systems". Annual Review of Microbiology. 59: 451–85. doi:10.1146/annurev.micro.58.030603.123630. PMC 3872966 . PMID 16153176.
46. Christie, Peter J. (2004). "Type IV secretion: The Agrobacterium VirB/D4 and related conjugation systems". Biochimica et Biophysica Acta. 1694 (1–3): 219–34. doi:10.1016/j.bbamcr.2004.02.013. PMID 15546668.
47. Yeo, Hye-Jeong; Yuan, Qing; Beck, Moriah R.; Baron, Christian; Waksman, Gabriel (2003). "Structural and functional characterization of the VirB5 protein from the type IV secretion system encoded by the conjugative plasmid pKM101". Proceedings of the National Academy of Sciences. 100 (26): 15947–52. Bibcode:2003PNAS..10015947Y. doi:10.1073/pnas.2535211100. JSTOR 3149111. PMC 307673 . PMID 14673074.
48. Lawley, T.D; Klimke, W.A; Gubbins, M.J; Frost, L.S (2003). "F factor conjugation is a true type IV secretion system". FEMS Microbiology Letters. 224 (1): 1–15. doi:10.1016/S0378-1097(03)00430-0. PMID 12855161.
49. Rikihisa, Yasuko; Lin, Mingqun; Niu, Hua (2010). "Microreview: Type IV secretion in the obligatory intracellular bacterium Anaplasma phagocytophilum". Cellular Microbiology. 12 (9): 1213–21. doi:10.1111/j.1462-5822.2010.01500.x. PMC 3598623 . PMID 20670295.
50. Thanassi, David G.; Stathopoulos, Christos; Karkal, Aarthi; Li, Huilin (2005). "Protein secretion in the absence of ATP: The autotransporter, two-partner secretion and chaperone/usher pathways of Gram-negative bacteria (Review)". Molecular Membrane Biology. 22 (1–2): 63–72. doi:10.1080/09687860500063290. PMID 16092525.
51. Gerlach, R; Hensel, M (2007). "Protein secretion systems and adhesins: The molecular armory of Gram-negative pathogens". International Journal of Medical Microbiology. 297 (6): 401–15. doi:10.1016/j.ijmm.2007.03.017. PMID 17482513.

52. Pukatzki, Stefan; Ma, Amy T.; Sturtevant, Derek; Krastins, Bryan; Sarracino, David; Nelson, William C.; Heidelberg, John F.; Mekalanos, John J. (2006). "Identification of a conserved bacterial protein secretion system in Vibrio cholerae using the Dictyostelium host model system". Proceedings of the National Academy of Sciences. 103 (5): 1528–33. Bibcode:2006PNAS..103.1528P. doi:10.1073/pnas.0510322103. JSTOR 30048406. PMC 1345711 . PMID 16432199.

53. Mougous, Joseph D.; Cuff, Marianne E.; Raunser, Stefan; Shen, Aimee; Zhou, Min; Gifford, Casey A.; Goodman, Andrew L.; Joachimiak, Grazyna; et al. (2006). "A Virulence Locus of Pseudomonas aeruginosa Encodes a Protein Secretion Apparatus". Science. 312 (5779): 1526–30. Bibcode:2006Sci...312.1526M. doi:10.1126/science.1128393. PMC 2800167 . PMID 16763151.

54. Bingle, Lewis EH; Bailey, Christopher M; Pallen, Mark J (2008). "Type VI secretion: A beginner's guide". Current Opinion in Microbiology. 11 (1): 3–8. doi:10.1016/j.mib.2008.01.006. PMID 18289922.

55. Cascales, Eric (2008). "The type VI secretion toolkit". EMBO Reports. 9 (8): 735–41. doi:10.1038/embor.2008.131. PMC 2515208 . PMID 18617888.

56. Schwarz, Sandra; Hood, Rachel D.; Mougous, Joseph D. (2010). "What is type VI secretion doing in all those bugs?". Trends in Microbiology. 18 (12): 531–7. doi:10.1016/j.tim.2010.09.001. PMC 2991376 . PMID 20961764.

57. Coulthurst, S. (2013). "The type VI secretion system - A widespread and versatile cell targeting system". Research in Microbiology. 164 (6): 640–54. doi:10.1016/j.resmic.2013.03.017. PMID 23542428.

58. Silverman, J.; Brunet, Y.; Cascales, E. P.; Mougous, J. (2012). "Structure and Regulation of the Type VI Secretion System". Annual Review of Microbiology. 66: 453–472. doi:10.1146/annurev-micro-121809-151619. PMC 3595004 . PMID 22746332.

59. Kuehn, M. J.; Kesty, NC (2005). "Bacterial outer membrane vesicles and the host-pathogen interaction". Genes & Development. 19 (22): 2645–55. doi:10.1101/gad.1299905. PMID 16291643.

60. McBroom, Amanda J.; Kuehn, Meta J. (2006). "Release of outer membrane vesicles by Gram-negative bacteria is a novel envelope stress response". Molecular Microbiology. 63 (2): 545–58. doi:10.1111/j.1365-2958.2006.05522.x. PMC 1868505 . PMID 17163978.

CHAPTER 9

Bradford Protein Assay

Chapter Contents

- **Introduction**
- **Principle**
- **Advantages**
- **Disadvantages**
- **Sample Bradford Procedure**
- **Using Data Obtained to Find Concentration of Unknown**
- **Alternative Assays**
- **Biuret Test**
- **Lowry Protein Assay**
- **Bicinchoninic Acid Assay**

The Bradford assay is very fast and uses about the same amount of protein as the Lowry assay. It is fairly accurate and samples that are out of range can be retested within minutes. The Bradford is recommended for general use, especially for determining protein content of cell fractions and assesing protein concentrations for gel electrophoresis.

Assay materials including color reagent, protein standard, and instruction booklet are available from Bio-Rad Corporation. The method described below is for a 100 μl sample volume using 5 ml color reagent. It is sensitive to about 5 to 200 micrograms protein, depending on the dye quality. In assays using 5 ml color reagent prepared in lab, the sensitive range is closer to 5 to 100 μg protein. Scale down the volume for the "microassay procedure," which uses 1 ml cuvettes. Protocols, including use of microtiter plates are described in the flyer that comes with the Bio-Rad kit.

INTRODUCTION

The **Bradford protein assay** is a spectroscopic analytical procedure used to measure the concentration of protein in a solution. It is subjective, *i.e.*, dependent on the amino acid composition of the measured protein. The Bradford protein assay was developed by Marion M. Bradford.

PRINCIPLE

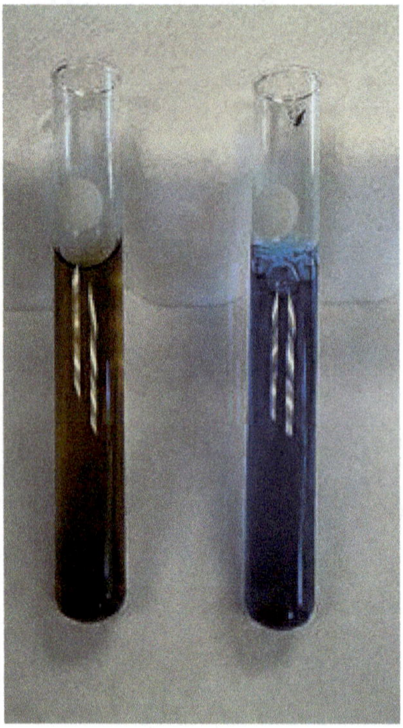

Test tubes containing Bradford reagent alone (left) and with lysozyme added (right).

The Bradford assay, a colorimetric protein assay, is based on an absorbance shift of the dye Coomassie Brilliant Blue G-250. Under acidic conditions the red form of the dye is converted into its bluer form, binding to the protein being assayed. During the formation of this complex, two types of bond interactions take place: van der Waals forces and ionic forces. The red form of Coomassie dye first donates its free electron to the ionizable groups on the protein, which causes a disruption of the protein›s native state, consequently exposing its hydrophobic pockets. These pockets in the protein's tertiary structure bind non-covalently to the non-polar region of the dye via the first bond interaction (van der Waals forces) which position the positive amine groups in proximity with the negative charge of the dye. The bond is further strengthened by the second bond interaction between the two, the ionic interaction. The binding of the protein stabilizes the blue form of the Coomassie dye; thus the amount of the complex present in solution is a measure for the protein concentration, and can be estimated by use of an absorbance reading.

The cationic (unbound) form is green / red and has an absorption spectrum maximum historically held to be at 465 nm. The anionic (bound) form of the dye has an absorption spectrum maximum historically held to be at 595 nm. The increase of absorbance at 595 nm is proportional to the amount of bound dye, and thus to the amount (concentration) of protein present in the sample.

Unlike other protein assays, the Bradford protein assay is less susceptible to interference by various chemicals that may be present in protein samples. An exception of note is elevated concentrations of detergent. Sodium dodecyl sulfate (SDS), a common detergent, may be found in protein extracts because it is used to lyse cells by disrupting the membrane lipid bilayer. While other detergents interfere with the assay at high concentration, the interference caused by SDS is of two different modes, and each occurs at a different concentration. When SDS concentrations are below critical micelle concentration (known as CMC, 0.00333%W/V to 0.0667%) in a Coomassie dye solution, the detergent tends to bind strongly with the protein, inhibiting the protein binding sites for the dye reagent. This can cause underestimations of protein concentration in solution. When SDS concentrations are above CMC, the detergent associates strongly with the green form of the Coomassie dye, causing the equilibrium to shift, thereby producing more of the blue form. This causes an increase in the absorbance at 595 nm independent of protein presence.

Other interference may come from the buffer used when preparing the protein sample. A high concentration of buffer will cause an overestimated protein concentration due to depletion of free protons from the solution by conjugate base from the buffer. This will not be a problem if a low concentration of protein is used.

ADVANTAGES

The procedure for Bradford protein assay is very easy and simple to follow. It is done in one step where the Bradford reagent is added to a test tube along with the sample. After mixing well, the mixture almost immediately changes to a blue color and the absorbance can be read at 595 nm using a spectrophotometer; an easily accessible machine.

This assay is one of the fastest assays performed on proteins. The total time it takes to set up and complete the assay is under 30 minutes. The entire experiment is done at room temperature.

The Bradford protein assay can measure protein quantities as little as 1 to 20 μg. It is an extremely sensitive technique.

The dye reagent is a stable ready to use product prepared in phosphoric acid. It can remain at room temperature for up to 2 weeks before it starts to degrade.

Protein samples usually contains salts, solvents, buffers, preservatives, and metal chelating agents. Using Bradford can be advantageous against these molecules because they are compatible to each other and will not interfere.

The linear graph acquired from the assay (absorbance versus protein concentration in μg/mL) can be easily extrapolated to determine the concentration of proteins by using the slope of the line.

DISADVANTAGES

The Bradford assay is linear over a short range, typically from 0 μg/mL to 2000 μg/mL, often making dilutions of a sample necessary before analysis. In making these dilutions, error in one dilution is compounded in further dilutions resulting in a linear relationship that may not always be accurate.

It is also inhibited by the presence of detergents, although this problem can be alleviated by the addition of cyclodextrins to the assay mixture.

Much of the non-linearity stems from the equilibrium between two different forms of the dye which is perturbed by adding the protein. The Bradford assay linearizes by measuring the ratio of the absorbances, 595 over 450 nm. This modified Bradford assay is approximately 10 times more sensitive than the conventional one.

SAMPLE BRADFORD PROCEDURE

Materials

- Lyophilized bovine plasma gamma globulin
- Coomassie Brilliant Blue 1
- 0.15 M NaCl
- Spectrophotometer and tubes
- Micropipettes

Procedure (Standard Assay, 20-150 µg protein; 200-1500 µg/mL)

- Prepare a series of protein standards diluted with 0.15 M NaCl to final concentrations of 0 (blank = NaCl only), 250, 500, 750 and 1500 µg/mL. Also prepare serial dilutions of the unknown sample to be measured.
- Add 100 µL of each of the above to a separate test tube (or spectrophotometer tube if using a Spec 20).
- Add 5.0 mL of Coomassie Blue to each tube and mix by vortex, or inversion.
- Adjust the spectrophotometer to a wavelength of 595 nm, and blank using the tube which contains no protein.
- Wait 5 minutes and read each of the standards and each of the samples at 595 nm wavelength.
- Plot the absorbance of the standards vs. their concentration. Compute the extinction coefficient and calculate the concentrations of the unknown samples.

Procedure (Micro Assay, 1-10 µg protein/mL)

- Prepare standard concentrations of protein of 1, 5, 7.5 and 10 µg/mL. Prepare a blank of NaCl only. Prepare a series of sample dilutions.
- Add 100 µL of each of the above to separate tubes (use microcentrifuge tubes) and add 1.0 mL of Coomassie Blue to each tube.
- Turn on and adjust a spectrophotometer to a wavelength of 595 nm, and blank the spectrophotometer using 1.5 mL cuvettes.

- Wait 2 minutes and read the absorbance of each standard and sample at 595 nm.
- Plot the absorbance of the standards vs. their concentration. Compute the extinction coefficient and calculate the concentrations of the unknown samples.

USING DATA OBTAINED TO FIND CONCENTRATION OF UNKNOWN

In summary, in order to find a standard curve, one must use varying concentrations of BSA in order to create a standard curve with concentration plotted on the x-axis and absorbance plotted on the y-axis. This standard curve is then used to determine the concentration of the unknown protein. The following elaborates on how one goes from the standard curve to the concentration of the unknown.

First, add a line of best fit, or Linear regression and display the equation on the chart. Ideally, the R^2value will be as close to 1 as possible. R represents the sum of the square values of the fit subtracted from each data point. Therefore, if R^2 is much less than one, consider redoing the experiment to get one with more reliable data.

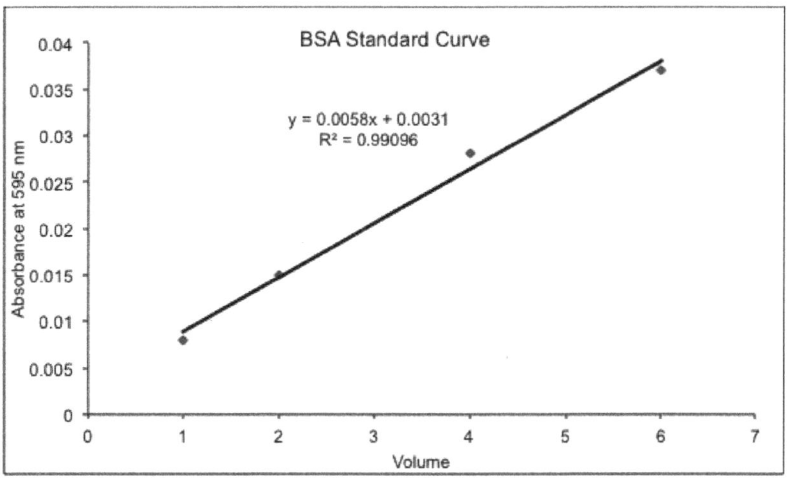

Graph 1: Actual BSA data attained from a micro scale UV-Vis Spectrophotometer.

The equation displayed on the chart gives a means for calculating the absorbance and therefore concentration of the unknown samples. In Graph 1, x is concentration and y is absorbance, so one must rearrange the equation to solve for x and enter the absorbance of the measured unknown. It is likely that the unknown will have absorbance numbers outside the range of the standard. These should not be included calculations, as the equation given cannot apply to numbers outside of its limitations. In a large scale, one must compute the extinction coefficient using the Beer-Lambert Law A=εLC in which A is the measured absorbance, ε is the slope of the standard curve, L is the length of the cuvette, and C is the concentration being determined. In a micro scale, a cuvette may not be used and therefore one only has to rearrange to solve for x.

Table 1: Actual assay data for determine concentration of unknown based on line of best fit of the above standard curve.

Volume BSA (uL)	Absorbance at 595 nm
1	.008
2	.015
4	.028
6	.037

Volume protein in Sample (uL)	Sample Absorbance at 595 nm	Concentration (ug/mL) solving for X	Divide by volume of protein in sample	Corrected for dilution (this was diluted 1:20)	Divide by molecular weight of sample to attain Concentration (M/L)
0	0	Not in standard			
1	.003	Not in standard			
5	.011	1.362	0.272	5.448	8.932E-05
20	.027	4.121	0.206	4.121	6.755E-05
60	.098	16.362	0.273	5.454	8.9412E-05
					Average: 8.209E-05

In order to attain a concentration that makes sense with the data, the dilutions, concentrations, and units of the unknown must be normalized (Table 1). To do this, one must divide concentration by volume of protein in order to normalize concentration and multiply by amount diluted to correct for any dilution made in the protein before performing the assay.

ALTERNATIVE ASSAYS

Alternative protein assays include:

- Ultraviolet–visible spectroscopy
- Biuret protein assay
- Lowry protein assay
- BCA protein assay
- Amido black protein assay

BIURET TEST

The **biuret test** is a chemical test used for detecting the presence of peptide bonds. In the presence of peptides, a copper(II) ion forms violet-colored coordination complexes in an alkaline solution. Several variants on the test have been developed, such as the BCA test and the Modified Lowry test.

The biuret reaction can be used to assess the concentration of proteins because peptide bonds occur with the same frequency per amino acid in the peptide. The intensity of the color, and hence the absorption at 540 nm, is directly proportional to the protein concentration, according to the Beer-Lambert law.

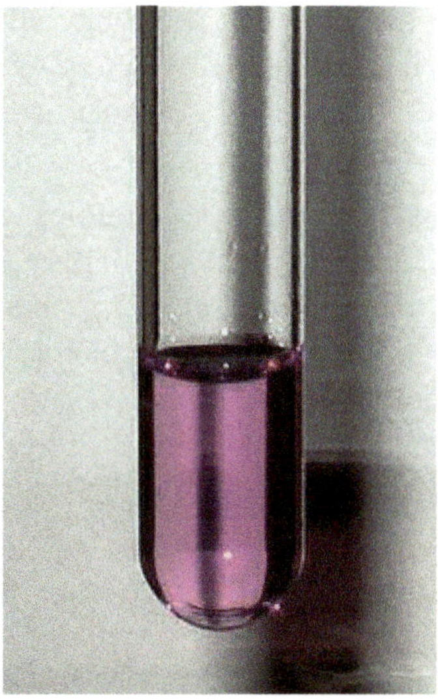

The characteristic color of a positive biuret test.

Despite its name, the reagent does not in fact contain biuret ($(H_2N\text{-}CO\text{-})_2NH$). The test is so named because it also gives a positive reaction to the peptide-like bonds in the biuret molecule.

Procedure

An aqueous sample is treated with an equal volume of 1% strong base (sodium or potassium hydroxide) followed by a few drops of aqueous copper(II) sulfate. If the solution turns purple, protein is present. 5–160 mg/mL can be determined. Peptides with the chain length of at least 3 amino acids are necessary for a significant, measurable colour shift with these reagents.

Biuret Reagent

The **Biuret reagent** is made of sodium hydroxide (NaOH) and hydrated copper(II) sulfate, together with potassium sodium tartrate. Potassium sodium tartrate is added to chelate and this stabilize the cupric ions. The reaction of the cupric ions with the nitrogen atoms involved in peptide bonds leads to the displacement of the peptide hydrogen atoms under the alkaline conditions. A tri or tetra dentate chelation with the peptide nitrogen produces the "biuret" color. This is found with dipeptides (Datta,S.P., Leberman,R., and Rabin,B.R., Trans.Farad.Soc. (1959), 55, 2141.)

The reagent is commonly used in the biuret protein assay, a colorimetric test used to determine protein concentration by UV/VIS spectroscopy at wavelength 550 nm.

High sensitivity variants of the biuret test

Two major modifications of the biuret test are commonly applied in modern colorimetric analysis of peptides: the bicinchoninic acid (BCA) assay and the Lowry assay. In these tests, the Cu^+ formed during the biuret reaction reacts further with other reagents, leading to a deeper color.

In the BCA test, Cu^+ forms a deep purple complex with bicinchoninic acid (BCA), which absorbs around 562 nm, producing the signature violet color. The water-soluble BCA/copper complex absorbs much more strongly than the peptide/copper complex, increasing the sensitivity of the biuret test by a factor of around 100: the BCA assay allows to detect proteins in the range of 0.0005 to 2 mg/mL). Additionally, the BCA protein assay gives the important benefit of compatibility with substances like up to 5% surfactants in protein samples.

In the Lowry protein assay Cu^+ is oxidized back to Cu^{2+} by Mo^{VI} in Folin-Ciocalteu›s reagent, which forms molybdenum blue (Mo^{IV}). Tyrosine residues in the protein also form molybdenum blue under these circumstances. In this way, proteins can be detected in concentrations between 0.005 and 2 mg/mL.Molybdenum blue in turn can bind certain organic dyes such as malachite green and Auramin O, resulting in further amplification of the signal.

LOWRY PROTEIN ASSAY

The **Lowry protein assay** is a biochemical assay for determining the total level of protein in a solution. The total protein concentration is exhibited by a color change of the sample solution in proportion to protein concentration, which can then be measured using colorimetric techniques. It is named for the biochemist Oliver H. Lowry who developed the reagent in the 1940s. His 1951 paper describing the technique is the most-highly cited paper ever in the scientific literature, cited over 300,000 times.

Mechanism

The method combines the reactions of copper ions with the peptide bonds under alkaline conditions (the Biuret test) with the oxidation of aromatic protein residues. The Lowry method is best used with protein concentrations of 0.01–1.0 mg/mL and is based on the reaction of Cu^+, produced by the oxidation of peptide bonds, with Folin–Ciocalteu reagent (a mixture of phosphotungstic acid and phosphomolybdic acid in the Folin–Ciocalteu reaction). The reaction mechanism is not well understood, but involves reduction of the Folin–Ciocalteu reagent and oxidation of aromatic residues (mainly tryptophan, also tyrosine). Experiments have shown that cysteine is also reactive to the reagent. Therefore, cysteine residues in protein probably also contribute to the absorbance seen in the Lowry Assay. The concentration of the reduced Folin reagent is measured by absorbance at 750 nm. As a result, the total concentration of protein in the sample can be deduced from the concentration of Trp and Tyr residues that reduce the Folin–Ciocalteu reagent.

The method was first proposed by Lowry in 1951. The Bicinchoninic acid assay and the Hartree–Lowry assay are subsequent modifications of the original Lowry procedure.

BICINCHONINIC ACID ASSAY

The **bicinchoninic acid assay** (**BCA assay**), also known as the **Smith assay**, after its inventor, Paul K. Smith at the Pierce Chemical Company, is a biochemical assay for determining the total concentration of protein in a solution (0.5 μg/mL to 1.5 mg/mL), similar to Lowry protein assay, Bradford protein assay or biuret reagent. The total protein concentration is exhibited by a color change of the sample solution from green to purple in proportion to protein concentration, which can then be measured using colorimetric techniques.

Mechanism

A stock BCA solution contains the following ingredients in a highly alkaline solution with a pH 11.25:

- Bicinchoninic acid
- Sodium carbonate
- Sodium bicarbonate
- Sodium tartrate
- Copper(II) sulfate pentahydrate

The BCA assay primarily relies on two reactions.

First, the peptide bonds in protein reduce Cu^{2+} ions from the copper(II) sulfate to Cu^{+} (a temperature dependent reaction). The amount of Cu^{2+} reduced is proportional to the amount of protein present in the solution. Next, two molecules of bicinchoninic acid chelate with each Cu^{+} ion, forming a purple-colored complex that strongly absorbs light at a wavelength of 562 nm.

The bicinchoninic acid Cu^{+} complex is influenced in protein samples by the presence of cysteine/cystine, tyrosine, and tryptophan side chains. At higher temperatures (37 to 60 °C), peptide bonds assist in the formation of the reaction complex. Incubating the BCA assay at higher temperatures is recommended as a way to increase assay sensitivity while minimizing the variances caused by unequal amino acid composition.

The amount of protein present in a solution can be quantified by measuring the absorption spectra and comparing with protein solutions of known concentration.

REFERENCES

1. Okutucu, Burcu; Dınçer, Ayşşe; Habib, *Ömer*; Zıhnıoglu, Figen (2007-08-01). Comparison of five methods for determination of total plasma protein concentration “. Journal of Biochemical and Biophysical Methods. **70** *(5): 709–711. doi:10.1016/j.jbbm.2007.05.009.*
2. Protein Assay Technical Handbook “ (PDF).

3. Determination of protein concentration “. elte.prompt.hu. Retrieved 2016-05-19.
4. Ninfa, Alexander J. (2010). Fundamental Laboratory Approaches for Biochemistry and Biotechnology. Wiley. pp. 117–118. ISBN 978-0470087664.
5. Rabilloud, Thierry. A single step protein assay that is both detergent and reducer compatible: The cydex blue assay. “. *Electrophoresis.* **37** *(20): 2595–2601.* arXiv:1610.07373. doi:10.1002/elps.201600270. PMID 27445231.
6. Zor, Tsaffrir; Selinger, Zvi (1996-05-01). Linearization of the Bradford Protein Assay Increases Its Sensitivity: Theoretical and Experimental Studies “. Analytical Biochemistry. **236** *(2): 302–308. doi:10.1006/abio.1996.0171.*
7. Albright, Brian (2009). Mathematical Modeling with Excel. p. 60. ISBN 978-0763765668.
8. Stephenson, Frank Harold (2003). Calculations for molecular biology and biotechnology: a guide to mathematics in the laboratory. p. 252. ISBN 0126657513.
9. Ibanez, Jorge G. (2007). Environmental chemistry: fundamentals. p. 60. ISBN 0387260617.

Index

L

M

N

P

R

S

T

U